First Aid for Mental Health Awareness

CW01095534

First Aid for Mental Health Awareness
is published by: **Nuco Training Ltd**

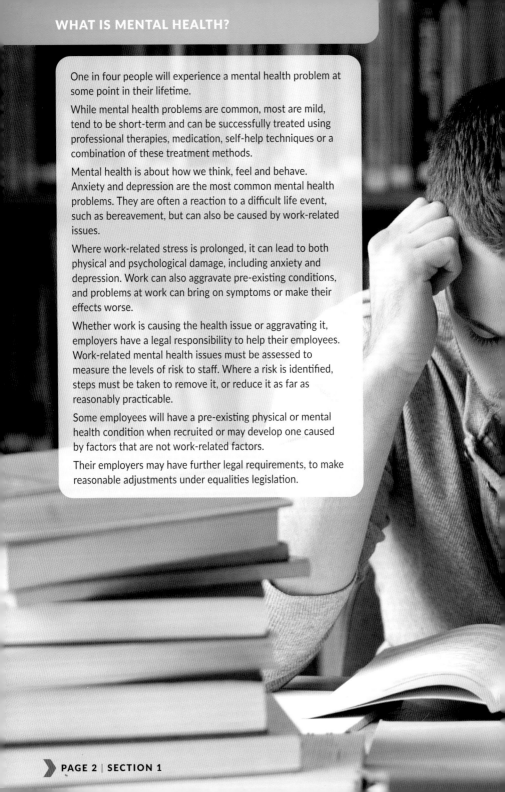

One in four people will experience a mental health problem at some point in their lifetime.

While mental health problems are common, most are mild, tend to be short-term and can be successfully treated using professional therapies, medication, self-help techniques or a combination of these treatment methods.

Mental health is about how we think, feel and behave. Anxiety and depression are the most common mental health problems. They are often a reaction to a difficult life event, such as bereavement, but can also be caused by work-related issues.

Where work-related stress is prolonged, it can lead to both physical and psychological damage, including anxiety and depression. Work can also aggravate pre-existing conditions, and problems at work can bring on symptoms or make their effects worse.

Whether work is causing the health issue or aggravating it, employers have a legal responsibility to help their employees. Work-related mental health issues must be assessed to measure the levels of risk to staff. Where a risk is identified, steps must be taken to remove it, or reduce it as far as reasonably practicable.

Some employees will have a pre-existing physical or mental health condition when recruited or may develop one caused by factors that are not work-related factors.

Their employers may have further legal requirements, to make reasonable adjustments under equalities legislation.

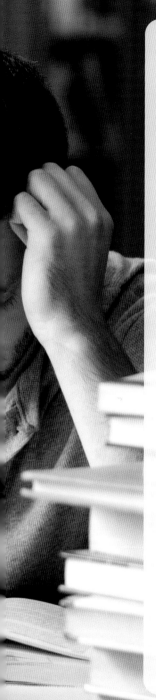

FIRST AID FOR MENTAL HEALTH

First aid for mental health is the initial support provided to a person experiencing a mental health problem until professional help is received or until the crisis is resolved.

In 2017, the government commissioned Lord Stevenson and Paul Farmer *(Chief Executive of Mind)* to independently review the role employers can play to better support individuals with mental health conditions in the workplace.

The 'Thriving at Work' report sets out a framework of actions – called 'Core Standards' – that the reviewers recommend employers of all sizes can and should put in place. The core standards have been designed to help employers improve the mental health of their workplace and enable individuals with mental health conditions to thrive.

The aims of first aid for mental health:

- Preserve life where a person could be a danger to themselves or others
- Alleviate suffering by providing immediate comfort and support
- Prevent the condition from developing into a more serious problem
- Promote recovery of good mental health by signposting and obtaining professional support

Roles and responsibilities of the First Aider for Mental Health:

- The main point of contact for anyone who is going through some form of mental health problem
- Identifying the early signs and symptoms of mental ill health
- Start supportive conversations with people experiencing a mental health problem
- Listen non-judgementally and provide reassurance
- Assess the risk of self-harm and suicide
- To signpost and encourage appropriate professional support
- Reduce the stigma attached to mental health and promote awareness
- Summon for the appropriate emergency services if necessary
- To maintain confidentiality and provide an ongoing supportive working environment

The HSE's stance relating to First Aid Needs Assessment

MENTAL ILL HEALTH AND FIRST AID

Following your employers' first aid needs assessment, you may decide that it will be beneficial to have personnel trained to identify and understand symptoms and be able to support someone who might be experiencing a mental health issue.

You should consider ways to manage mental ill health in your workplace, which are appropriate for your business, such as providing information or training for managers and employees, employing occupational health professionals, appointing mental health trained First Aider's and implementing employee support programmes.

First aid training courses covering mental health, teach delegates how to recognise warning signs of mental ill health and help them to develop the skills and confidence to approach and support someone, while keeping themselves safe.

The impact of mental health issues:

- **Day-to-day:** Mental ill health can make it harder for people to cope with general day-to-day activities
- **Physical health:** Mental illness can impair the ability to protect and develop physical wellbeing
- **Work:** Obtaining or maintaining a job may be more difficult when symptoms of a mental health condition make it harder for someone to function normally
- **Education:** Studying may be more difficult when living with a mental health condition and often students do not reach their true potential
- **Driving:** Mental health conditions themselves do not stop people from driving. However, certain medications that the person may be taking, or if they are a risk to themselves and others, will influence the decision
- **Parenting & children:** Mental illness can affect relationships and family life. Certain medications can also have an affect on pregnancy, but there is now a wide range of medications that are safe to use during pregnancy, such as the antidepressant, sertraline
- **Stigma:** Stigma can create barriers for people to seek help for their mental health condition and can make their situation much worse

MENTAL HEALTH STIGMA

In the context of mental health, there are two main types of stigma:

Social stigma - Includes the negative attitudes and discriminatory behaviours that society or particular individuals hold towards those with mental health problems. A belief that *"all people with mental health problems are violent and dangerous"* could be an example of social stigma.

Self-stigma - This is where people with mental health problems believe what is being said about their condition and agree with their viewpoints. Self-stigma can result in delays or the avoidance of seeking help for their condition due to the fear of being rejected or humiliated.

The effects of stigma

There are a number of adverse effects caused by stigma, including:

- **Feelings of shame and hopelessness**
- **Reluctance to ask anyone for help or to seek professional treatment**
- **Victimisation, harassment and physical violence**
- **Difficulties finding employment and taking part in activities**
- **Lack of understanding from family and friends**
- **Developing a practice of self-stigmatisation caused by the social stigma**

Coping with stigma

No individual should have to tolerate others treating them differently because of a mental health condition.
People can help to combat stigma by:

- **Seeking professional help - not letting the fear of being 'labelled' with a mental illness stop this**
- **Showing family and friends reliable information to improve their understanding**
- **Not equating themselves with their condition**
- **Joining a support group to talk about stigma and relate to others**
- **Organising local campaigns or getting involved with national campaigns about mental health**

MENTAL HEALTH STATISTICS

- 1/2 of all mental health problems are established by the age of 14
- 3/4 of all mental health problems are established by the age of 24
- In Scotland around 101,000 patients received at least one dispensed item for treatment of psychosis and related disorders in 2018/19. This is an increase of 2.5% compared to 2017/18 and an increase of 39.9% since 2009/10
- In England there were 79.4 million antidepressant drug items prescribed to 7.87 million identified patients in 2020/21. The number of antidepressant items issued and the number of patients receiving antidepressant drugs increased for the fifth consecutive year
- In Great Britain there were 822,000 workers suffering from work-related stress, depression or anxiety (new or long-standing) in 2020/21

Source: www.gov.scot, www.nhs.uk, www.scotpho.org.uk and estimates based on self-reports from the Labour Force Survey, people who have worked in the last 12 months.

THE MENTAL HEALTH CONTINUUM MODEL

Mental health does not simply mean the absence of a mental illness – it is possible to have good mental wellbeing whilst living with a diagnosed mental illness. In contrast, someone who has no diagnosable mental illness can still have a low level of mental wellbeing.

EXCELLENT LEVEL OF MENTAL WELLBEING

A PERSON WHO EXPERIENCES AN EXCELLENT LEVEL OF MENTAL WELLBEING, REGARDLESS OF BEING DIAGNOSED WITH A MENTAL ILLNESS

A PERSON WHO EXPERIENCES AN EXCELLENT LEVEL OF MENTAL WELLBEING AND HAS NO MENTAL ILLNESS

CLINICAL DIAGNOSIS

NO DIAGNOSIS

A PERSON WHO HAS BEEN DIAGNOSED WITH A MENTAL ILLNESS AND ALSO EXPERIENCES A LOW LEVEL OF MENTAL WELLBEING

A PERSON WHO HAS NO DIAGNOSABLE MENTAL ILLNESS BUT ALSO HAS A LOW LEVEL OF MENTAL WELLBEING

LOW LEVEL OF MENTAL WELLBEING

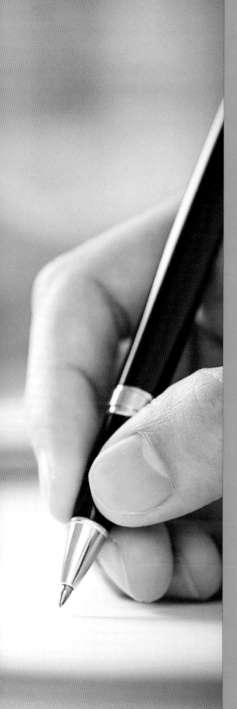

The mental health risk factors:

- Discrimination and stigma
- Social isolation or loneliness
- Abuse, trauma or neglect
- Social disadvantage or financial troubles
- Unemployment or losing a job
- Having a long-term physical health condition or injury
- Severe or long-term stress
- Poverty or homelessness
- Being a long-term carer
- Drug or alcohol abuse
- Domestic violence
- Significant trauma as an adult, such as military combat
- The death of a loved one

THE EARLY WARNING SIGNS OF A MENTAL HEALTH PROBLEM.

Could include:

- Losing interest in activities and hobbies that were previously enjoyed
- Underperforming at work with no apparent explanation
- Increased anxiety levels, feeling exhausted and restless
- Isolating themselves and not wanting to socialise with friends and family
- Changes in appetite such as skipping meals or over-eating/bingeing
- Changes in perception such as hearing or seeing things that others don't
- Self-harming behaviour. Signs of cuts or bruising to uncommon areas of the body
- Reduced, or increased sex drive depending on the mental health problem

HOW TO START A CONVERSATION ABOUT MENTAL HEALTH

Starting a conversation can help tackle the stigma surrounding mental health and make the individual aware that they are not alone – mental health problems are very common and can be treated.

Think carefully about what you want to say before starting the conversation and make sure you are in the right environment without interruptions.

Avoid closed questions which only require a 'yes' or 'no' answer.

Ask open questions such as *"How are you feeling?"* This should provide a basis for a more detailed response.

One of the most important things to do is listen to them carefully without personal judgement. Listening to what the person tells you can sometimes be difficult to hear, so you need to allow time for reflection.

You can provide advice and signpost to professional help but ultimately the individual will need to act for themselves. The exception is when they are in crisis, then you can assist them to seek further help, or call the emergency services if they are a danger to themselves and to others.

WHAT IS NON-JUDGEMENTAL LISTENING?

Non-judgemental listening is when you listen to what someone is telling you with your undivided attention and truly show an interest in what the person is trying to say.

Everybody has different opinions and it is natural to judge what the person is telling you, but you must keep these opinions to yourself and communicate with the person empathetically, without displaying any form of personal judgement.

Non-judgemental listening is not just about listening, the term includes both non-verbal and verbal communication skills.

Here are some points to consider for non-judgemental listening:

- **Give them plenty of time to talk and do not interrupt**
- **Listen carefully to the words spoken**
- **Allow time for reflection**
- **Maintain eye contact but do not stare at the person**
- **Express empathy and do not judge the person**
- **Be aware of your tone of voice and volume level when speaking**
- **Keep an open body position, arms and legs uncrossed**
- **Once they have finished speaking, relay and summarise what they have told you**

Say less. Listen more.

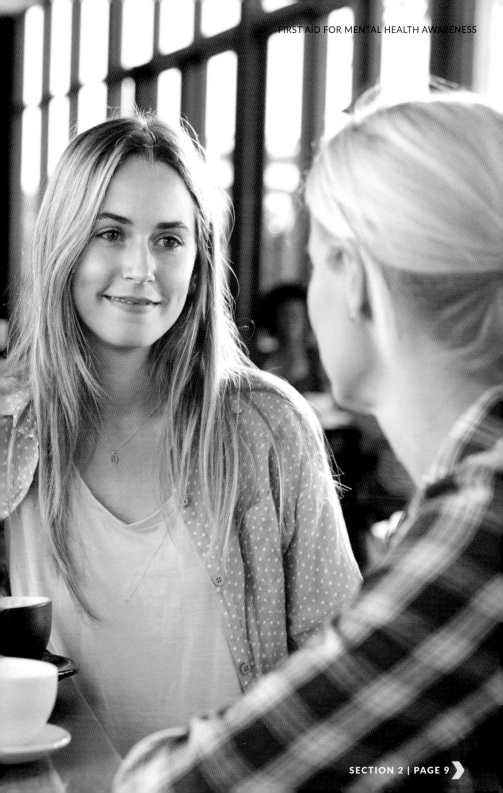

WHEN AND WHO TO CONTACT FOR FURTHER HELP

If a person is in a state of crisis, you may need to seek help for them. This could be from a trusted friend or family member, or a healthcare professional.

The level of help required will depend on their current condition.

Who to contact:

- **Close friend or family member**
  A close friend or family member could be called who knows the person well and can offer them comfort and support

- **Crisis Line** (if they are already assigned to a healthcare professional)

- **The Samaritans** *(116 123)*
  The Samaritans operate a free to call service 24 hours a day, 365 days a year, if they want to talk to someone in confidence

- **NHS**
  You can call NHS 111, or visit www.111.nhs.uk or www.nhs24.scot (Scotland), if you or someone you know requires urgent care, but it is not life-threatening, such as experiencing a mental health problem for the first time. Alternatively, contact your GP practice and ask for an emergency appointment

When you should contact the emergency services.

A mental health emergency should be taken as seriously as a medical emergency.

Call 999 or go directly to A&E if they are:

- **Experiencing serious suicidal thoughts and feelings**
- **Thinking about harming themselves or someone else**
- **Experiencing symptoms of an acute underlying medical condition**
- **They have already hurt themselves**

It is important to note that some people may decline help and they cannot be forced to go to A&E. It is fairly common for people to have suicidal thoughts that come and go and they may never act on them. The situation at the time of crisis should give you an indication of the level of support required.

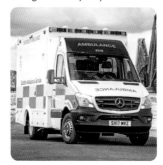

HOW A FIRST AIDER CAN TAKE CARE OF THEIR OWN HEALTH AND EMOTIONS

Supporting others who are experiencing mental health problems can affect your own mental health and wellbeing.

Ideally, employers should factor in first aid for mental health to their policies and procedures to protect you as a First Aider and ensure the role does not affect your main responsibilities in the workplace.

- Speak to your employer or manager about any concerns you may have
- If your own mental health is being affected, seek support from a professional
- Try not to get too involved – your role is to identify the warning signs, provide immediate support and signpost towards professional help
- Make sure you take time out for yourself and look after your own physical and mental wellbeing

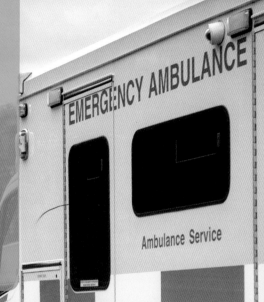

Stress is the *"adverse reaction people have to excessive pressure or other types of demand placed on them". (HSE)*

WHAT HAPPENS TO THE BODY WHEN SOMEONE IS STRESSED?

Adrenal gland produces adrenaline:

This speeds up the heart and increases blood pressure.

Adrenal gland produces cortisol:

This increases glucose in the blood and energy production. Over long periods of stress these reactions can cause illness and reduce life expectancy.

The pituitary gland produces oxytocin:

This can reverse the effects of stress.

Stress affects people differently – what stresses one person may not affect another. Factors like skills and experience, age or disability may all affect whether an employee can cope.

Causes of stress include:

- Work
- Relationships
- Bereavement
- Moving house
- Finances
- Poor physical health
- Divorce
- Bullying
- Family and friends
- Poor behaviour
- Travel
- Personal issues

THE EMOTIONAL, PHYSICAL AND BEHAVIOURAL EFFECTS OF STRESS.

How someone may feel mentally and emotionally:

- Anxious
- Angry
- Lack of concentration
- Difficulty making decisions
- Low self-esteem
- Sad
- Frustrated
- Overwhelmed
- Constant worrying
- Racing thoughts

How someone may feel physically:

- Headaches
- Chest pain
- Tiredness
- Nausea
- Muscle tension
- Dizziness

Behavioural effects:

- Outbursts of anger
- Undereating or overeating
- Changes in sex drive
- Restlessness
- Social withdrawal
- Exercising less often than usual

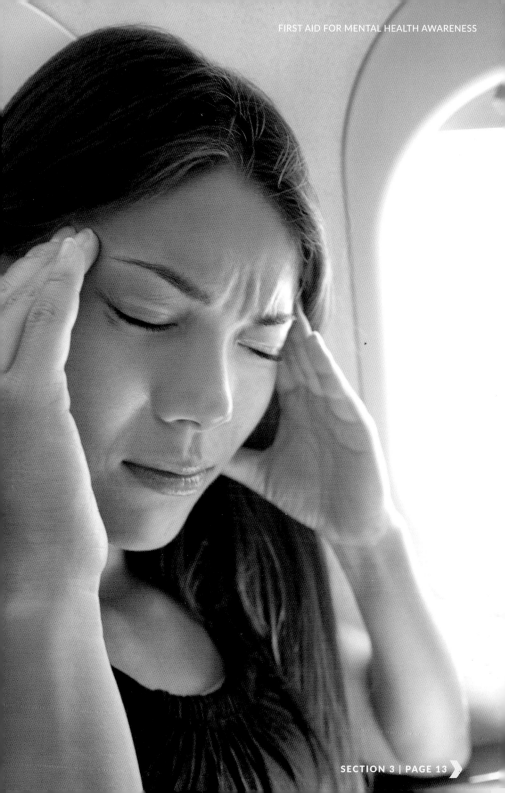

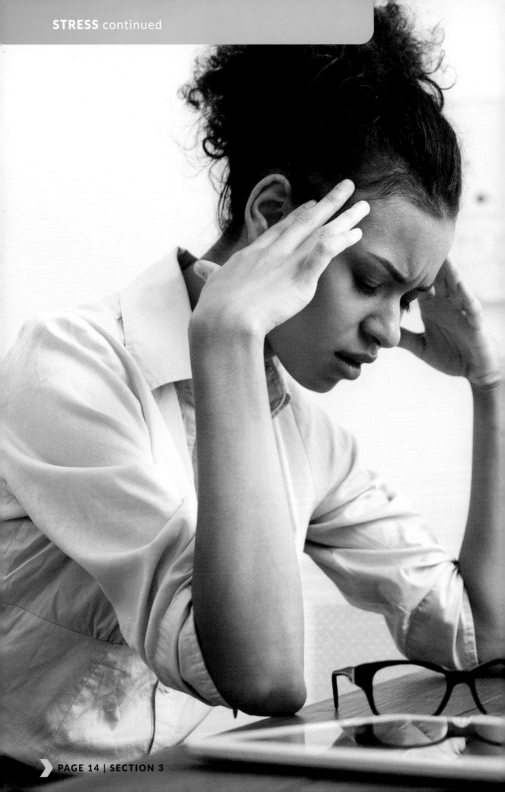

THE LONG-TERM EFFECTS OF STRESS

Lots of things can cause someone to be stressed and generally, this isn't something to be concerned about. However, the effects of long-term stress can put their health at risk.

The long-term effects of stress can include:

- Stress can lead to mental health conditions such as depression, anxiety and personality disorders
- Cardiovascular problems such as high blood pressure, heart disease and stroke
- Problems with the immune system, lower resistance to infection and skin conditions
- Digestive problems such as appetite loss, stomach ulcers, vomiting and diarrhoea
- Excessive changes in behaviour such as alcohol and substance misuse

Coping strategies for stress.

- Realise when stress is becoming a problem and identify the underlying causes
- Build emotional strength and re-organise lifestyle to tackle the causes
- Eat a healthy diet, avoid skipping meals and try to adopt regular eating patterns
- Make time to relax and socialise with friends and family
- Set goals or challenges to help build confidence
- Avoid unhealthy habits such as smoking or excessive alcohol consumption
- Helping other people can relieve stress and help to put problems into perspective
- Look for the positives in life, rather than the causes of stress

THE INTERCHANGEABLE TERMS OFTEN USED IN FIRST AID FOR MENTAL HEALTH

Mental health condition: This could include a minor episode of depression, through to a condition that has, or may develop into a diagnosable mental health illness or disorder.

Mental health illness/disorder: A mental health condition which has been formally diagnosed by a healthcare professional.

The terms 'condition', 'problem', 'issue', 'illness' and 'disorder' are often used interchangeably in relation to first aid for mental health.

It can be very difficult to identify someone who is suffering from a mental health problem, especially in a working environment where there are normal pressures and stresses from the tasks at hand. Knowing the signs and symptoms can play an important part in helping someone obtain professional support and improve their mental health and wellbeing.

This publication covers the signs and symptoms of the following conditions:

- Depression
- Anxiety
- Psychosis
- Eating disorders
- Suicide
- Self-harm

DEPRESSION

Depression is when someone feels persistently sad and unhappy for a long period of time and affects their everyday life. Depression can sometimes be viewed as trivial and not a real health condition - this is not true. Depression is a real illness with real symptoms and is a very common mental health condition.

Signs and symptoms may include:

- Avoiding contact with family and friends
- Avoiding social events and neglecting hobbies
- Not doing as well at work
- Continuous low mood, feeling upset and tearful
- Feeling hopeless and low self-esteem
- Lack of motivation or interest in things
- Feeling irritable and intolerant of other people
- Thoughts of self-harm or suicide
- Changes in appetite or weight loss/gain
- Lack of energy, muscle aches and pains
- Disturbed sleep patterns and low sex drive

ANXIETY

Anxiety is a normal body response and we all experience feelings of anxiety. However, some people find it hard to control their worries. Their feelings of anxiety are more constant and can often affect their daily lives.

In cases such as this, the condition is commonly diagnosed as '**Generalised Anxiety Disorder** *(GAD)'*.

GAD is a common condition affecting approximately 5% of the UK population.

The signs and symptoms of anxiety:

- Feeling tense and unable to relax
- A sense of dread and feeling constantly 'on edge'
- Irritability and difficulties concentrating
- Social withdrawal
- Seeking lots of reassurance from others
- Dizziness and tiredness
- Strong, fast or irregular heartbeat
- Trembling or shaking
- Excessive sweating and shortness of breath
- Lack of energy, muscle aches and pains
- Dry mouth, feeling sick and headaches
- Panic attacks

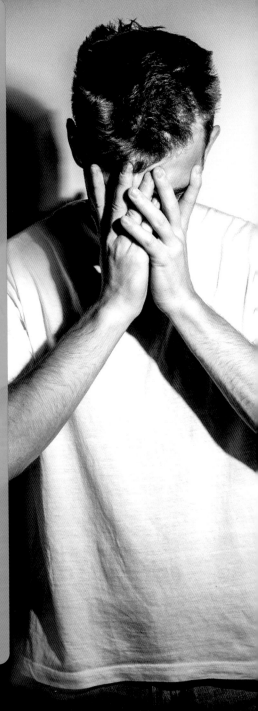

PSYCHOSIS

Psychosis is a mental health problem that causes people to perceive or interpret things differently from those around them. This might involve hallucinations or delusions.

Hallucinations – where a person hears, sees and, in some cases, feels, smells or tastes things that aren't there; a common hallucination is hearing voices.

Delusions – where a person has strong beliefs that aren't shared by others; a common delusion is someone believing there is a conspiracy to harm them

Confused thoughts – confusing speech. Switching from one subject to another mid-sentence. Talking very fast. Sudden loss in their train of thought.

CAUSES OF PSYCHOSIS

People may experience episodes of psychosis if they have:

Bipolar disorder – when someone experiences episodes of mania (elated mood), they may also experience symptoms of psychosis.

Schizophrenia – a mental health condition which causes hallucinations and delusions.

Substance misuse – alcohol or drug misuse can trigger psychotic episodes, particularly if someone stops using substances after a long period of time (withdrawal symptoms).

Postpartum psychosis – a rare but serious mental health illness which can happen to any woman following childbirth. 1:1000 women are affected by postpartum psychosis.

Medical conditions, anxiety, depression or a lack of sleep.

EATING DISORDERS

An eating disorder is when someone has an unhealthy attitude towards food which can take over their everyday life and make them feel very poorly.

Food plays an important part in all of our lives and we often spend time thinking about what we have eaten, or what we are going to eat.

When someone has an eating disorder, they will often eat too much or too little and become obsessed with their body weight and appearance.

Many people believe if someone has an eating problem, they will noticeably appear under or overweight – this is not true! Anyone, regardless of their weight, age or gender can be seriously affected by an eating disorder.

TYPES OF EATING DISORDERS

The most common eating disorders are:

- **Anorexia nervosa – when someone tries to keep their bodyweight as low as possible by not eating enough food, exercising too much, or both**
- **Bulimia – when someone eats a lot of food in a very short amount of time** *(bingeing)* **and are then deliberately sick, use laxatives** *(medication to help with their bowel movements),* **restrict what they eat, or do too much exercise to try to stop themselves gaining weight**
- **Binge eating disorder – when someone regularly loses control of their eating, eats large portions of food all at once until they feel uncomfortably full, and are then often upset or guilty**
- **Other specified feeding or eating disorder** *(OSFED)* **– when the symptoms don't exactly match those of anorexia, bulimia or binge eating disorder, but it doesn't mean it is a less serious illness**

WARNING SIGNS OF AN EATING DISORDER

It can often be very difficult to identify that a loved one or friend, has developed an eating disorder.

Warning signs to look out for include:

- **Dramatic weight loss**
- **Lying about how much and when they have eaten, or how much they weigh**
- **Eating a lot of food very fast**
- **Going to the bathroom a lot after eating, often returning looking flushed**
- **Feelings of anxiety about eating or digesting food**
- **Obsessively exercising and sticking to a rigid diet**
- **Cutting food into small pieces or eating very slowly**
- **Avoiding eating with others or eating in secret**
- **Checking body weight and comparing to others**
- **Developing physical health problems**

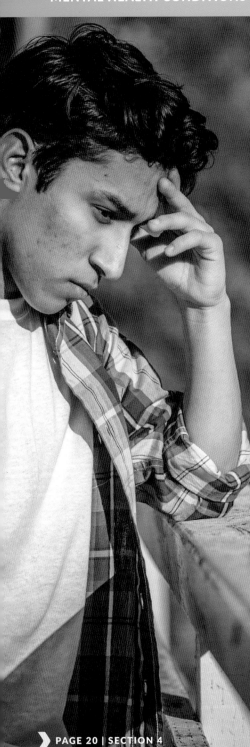

SUICIDE

Suicide is when someone deliberately ends their own life.

In 2020, 4,912 people in England, 805 people in Scotland, 285 people in Wales and 209 people in Northern Ireland took their own life.

Reference: Samaritans, Suicide Statistics, 2020

The possible risk factors for suicide:

- Previous suicide attempts
- Mental health problems
- Physical, sexual or emotional abuse
- Drug and alcohol misuse/addiction
- Imprisonment
- Bullying and discrimination
- Bereavement or the end of a relationship
- Losing a loved one to suicide
- Adjusting to a significant change
- Being diagnosed with a serious medical condition
- Social isolation and loneliness
- Financial problems or homelessness

THE POTENTIAL WARNING SIGNS FOR SUICIDE

Potential warning signs that someone is experiencing suicidal thoughts may include:

- Threatening to hurt or kill themselves
- Talking or writing about dying, death or suicide
- Making financial preparations such as writing or updating a will
- Recent trauma or life crisis such as the death of a loved one
- Talking about feeling hopeless or having no purpose
- Talking about being a burden or nuisance to others
- Anxious, agitated or acting reckless
- Increasing the use of alcohol and drugs
- Withdrawing from activities and feeling isolated

SELF-HARM

Self-harm is when somebody intentionally damages or injures their body. It's usually a way of coping with or expressing overwhelming emotional distress.

Why people self-harm?

Self-harm is more common than many people realise, especially among younger people.

It's estimated around 10% of young people self-harm at some point, but people of all ages do.

This figure is also likely to be an underestimate, as not everyone seeks help.

In most cases, people who self-harm do it to help them cope with overwhelming emotional issues, which may be caused by:

- Social problems – such as being bullied, having difficulties at work or school, having difficult relationships with friends or family, coming to terms with their sexuality or coping with cultural expectations, such as an arranged marriage
- Trauma – such as physical or sexual abuse, the death of a close family member or friend, or having a miscarriage
- Psychological causes – such as having repeated thoughts or voices telling them to self-harm, disassociating *(losing touch with who they are and with their surroundings)*, or borderline personality disorder

SIGNS OF SELF-HARM

If you think a friend or relative is self-harming, look out for any of the following signs:

- Unexplained cuts, bruises or cigarette burns, usually on their wrists, arms, thighs and chest
- Keeping themselves fully covered at all times, even in hot weather
- Signs of depression, such as low mood, tearfulness or a lack of motivation or interest in anything
- Self-loathing and expressing a wish to punish themselves
- Not wanting to go on and wishing to end it all
- Becoming very withdrawn and not speaking to others
- Changes in eating habits or being secretive about eating, and any unusual weight loss or weight gain
- Signs of low self-esteem, such as blaming themselves for any problems or thinking they're not good enough for something
- Signs they have been pulling out their hair
- Signs of alcohol or drug misuse

People who self-harm can seriously hurt themselves, so it's important that they speak to a GP about the underlying issue and request treatment or therapy that could help them.

MENTAL HEALTH HELPLINES

Whether you're concerned about yourself, a friend or a loved one, these helplines and support groups can offer expert advice.

Anxiety UK
Charity providing support for people affected by anxiety disorders.
Phone: 03444 775 774 *(Mon to Fri, 9.30am to 5.30pm)*
Website: www.anxietyuk.org.uk

Bipolar UK
A charity helping people living with manic depression or bipolar disorder.
Website: www.bipolaruk.org.uk

Breathing Space
A free, confidential phone and web based service for people in Scotland experiencing low mood, depression or anxiety.
Phone: 0800 83 85 87 *(Mon to Thurs, 6pm to 2am. Fri to Mon, 6pm to 6am)*
Website: www.breathingspace.scot

CALM
CALM is the Campaign Against Living Miserably, for men aged 15 to 35.
Phone: 0800 58 58 58 *(daily, 5pm to midnight)*
Website: www.thecalmzone.net

Childline
Online, on the phone, anytime.
Phone: 0800 1111 *(24-hour service)*
Website: www.childline.org.uk

Men's Health Forum
24/7 stress support for men by text, chat and email.
Website: www.menshealthforum.org.uk

Mental Health Foundation
Provides information and support for anyone with mental health problems or learning disabilities.
Website: www.mentalhealth.org.uk

Mind
Promotes the views and needs of people with mental health problems.
Phone: 0300 123 3393 *(Mon to Fri, 9am to 6pm)*
Website: www.mind.org.uk

No Panic
Voluntary charity offering support for sufferers of panic attacks and obsessive compulsive disorder *(OCD)*. Offers a course to help overcome phobias and OCD.
Phone: 0844 967 4848 *(daily, 10am to 10pm)*
Website: www.nopanic.org.uk

OCD Action
Support for people with OCD. Includes information on treatment and online resources.
Phone: 0845 390 6232 *(Mon to Fri, 9.30am to 5pm)*
Website: www.ocdaction.org.uk

OCD UK
A charity run by people with OCD, for people with OCD. Includes facts, news and treatments.
Phone: 0845 120 3778 *(Mon to Fri, 9am to 5pm)*
Website: www.ocduk.org

PAPYRUS
Young suicide prevention society.
Phone: HOPElineUK 0800 068 4141 *(Mon to Fri, 10am to 5pm & 7 to 10pm. Weekends 2 to 5pm)*
Website: www.papyrus-uk.org

Rethink Mental Illness
Support and advice for people living with mental illness.
Phone: 0300 5000 927 *(Mon to Fri, 9.30am to 4pm)*
Website: www.rethink.org

Samaritans
Confidential support for people experiencing feelings of distress or despair.
Phone: 116 123 *(free 24-hour helpline)*
Website: www.samaritans.org.uk

SAMH - Scottish Association for Mental Health
Provides a range of mental health support and services
Phone: 0141 530 1000 *(Mon to Fri, 9am to 5pm)*
Website: www.samh.org.uk

SANE
Emotional support, information and guidance for people affected by mental illness, their families and carers.
SANEline: 0300 304 7000 *(daily, 4.30 to 10.30pm)*
Textcare: comfort and care via text message, sent when the person needs it most:
              http://www.sane.org.uk/textcare
Peer support forum: www.sane.org.uk/supportforum
Website: www.sane.org.uk/support

YoungMinds
Information on child and adolescent mental health. Services for parents and professionals.
Phone: Parents' helpline 0808 802 5544 *(Mon to Fri, 9.30am to 4pm)*
Website: www.youngminds.org.uk

ABUSE (CHILD, SEXUAL, DOMESTIC VIOLENCE)

NSPCC
Children's charity dedicated to ending child abuse and child cruelty.
Phone: 0800 1111 for Childline for children *(24-hour helpline)*
              0808 800 5000 for adults concerned about a child *(24-hour helpline)*
Website: www.nspcc.org.uk

Refuge
Advice on dealing with domestic violence.
Phone: 0808 2000 247 *(24-hour helpline)*
Website: www.refuge.org.uk

ADDICTION (DRUGS, ALCOHOL, GAMBLING)

Alcoholics Anonymous
Phone: 0845 769 7555 *(24-hour helpline)*
Website: www.alcoholics-anonymous.org.uk

Gamblers Anonymous
Website: www.gamblersanonymous.org.uk

Narcotics Anonymous
Phone: 0300 999 1212 *(daily 10am to midnight)*
Website: www.ukna.org

ALZHEIMER'S

Alzheimer's Society

Provides information on dementia, including factsheets and helplines.

Phone: 0300 222 1122 *(Mon to Fri, 9am to 5pm. Weekends, 10am to 4pm)*
Website: www.alzheimers.org.uk

BEREAVEMENT

Cruse Bereavement Care

Phone: 0844 477 9400 *(Mon to Fri, 9am to 5pm)*
Website: www.crusebereavementcare.org.uk

CRIME VICTIMS

Rape Crisis

To find your local services phone: 0808 802 9999 *(daily, 12 to 2.30pm, 7 to 9.30pm)*
Website: www.rapecrisis.org.uk

Victim Support

Phone: 0808 168 9111 *(24-hour helpline)*
Website: www.victimsupport.org

EATING DISORDERS

Beat

Phone: 0808 801 0677 *(adults)* or 0808 801 0711 *(for under-18s)*
Website: www.b-eat.co.uk

LEARNING DISABILITIES

Mencap

Charity working with people with a learning disability, their families and carers.
Phone: 0808 808 1111 *(Mon to Fri, 9am to 5pm)*
Website: www.mencap.org.uk

PARENTING

Family Lives

Advice on all aspects of parenting including dealing with bullying.
Phone: 0808 800 2222 *(Mon to Fri, 9am to 9pm. Sat to Sun, 10am to 3pm)*
Website: www.familylives.org.uk

RELATIONSHIPS

Relate

The UK's largest provider of relationship support.
Website: www.relate.org.uk

MANAGING WORKPLACE STRESS AND MENTAL HEALTH ISSUES

HSE

Website: www.hse.gov.uk/stress/mental-health

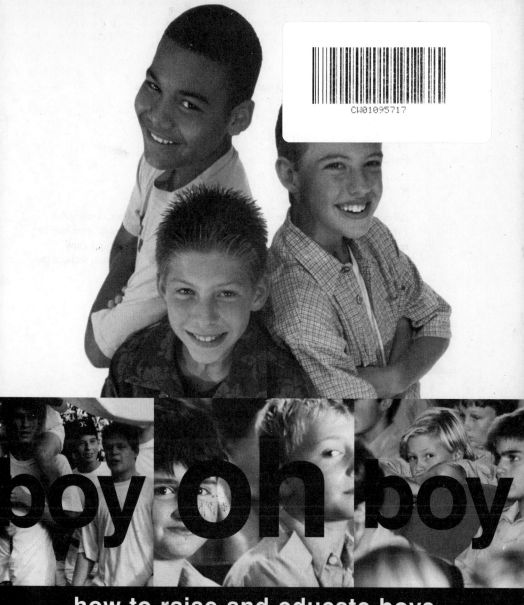

boy oh boy

how to raise and educate boys

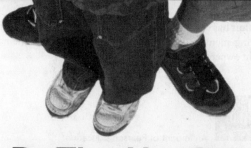

Dr Tim Hawkes

Pearson Education Australia
Unit 4, Level 2
14 Aquatic Drive
Frenchs Forest NSW 2086

www.pearsoned.com.au

Acquisitions Editor: Diane Gee-Clough
Managing Editor: Susan Lewis
Copy Editor: Loretta Barnard
Cover and text designed by Ingo Voss
Typeset by Midland Typesetters

Printed in Australia

4 5 05 04 03 02

National Library of Australia
Cataloguing-in-Publication data

Hawkes, Tim
   Boy oh boy: how to raise and educate boys.

   Bibliography.
   Includes index.
   ISBN 1 74009 554 5.

   1. Boys – Psychology. 2. Child rearing. 3. Boys – Education. I. Title.

649.132

Prentice
Hall

An imprint of Pearson Education

Contents

About the author

DR TIM HAWKES
B Ed (Hons) (Durham), Grad Dip
Ed Studies (UNE),
PhD (Macquarie), FACE,
MACEA

Dr Tim Hawkes is a leading authority on educating boys. His highly entertaining, yet very scholarly contribution to debate in this area has made him enormously popular as a speaker and writer on gender issues in education.

Dr Hawkes is headmaster of one of Australia's most well-known and respected boys' schools, The King's School, Parramatta. Prior to his appointment to Australia's oldest independent school, Dr Hawkes was principal of St Leonard's College in Melbourne. Being a large co-educational school, St Leonard's enabled Dr Hawkes to compare and contrast the needs of boys with the needs of girls.

Dr Hawkes has served on the governing board of the International Baccalaureate Organisation; his other educational experiences have included the roles of senior boarding master at Knox Grammar School in Sydney and of teacher at Loughborough Grammar School in England. There are many other interests in Dr Hawkes's life—he has participated in the British Undergraduates' Jotenheimen Expedition to the mountains of Norway, been involved with drug rehabilitation work and Christian outreach with the Society of St Stephen in Hong Kong and has accepted an Officer's Reserve Commission in the British Army.

Dr Hawkes studied for his first degree at Durham University in England and completed his doctoral studies at Macquarie University, Sydney.

Acknowledgments

I would like to thank the following people for their assistance with the writing of this book:

Lise Berkeley
Rob Chandler
Mark Dwyer
Diane Gee-Clough
Margaret Higgerson
Di Letham
Megan Perry
Lorna Wales
Cecilia Wilson
Peter Wordsworth

Perhaps my greatest expression of appreciation is reserved for all my students, both past and present, for they have inspired me to write the book and supplied me with much of the wisdom within it.

This book is dedicated to my family.

Jane, Peter, Alicia and Philippa have given me
the love and support necessary to write *Boy oh Boy*.

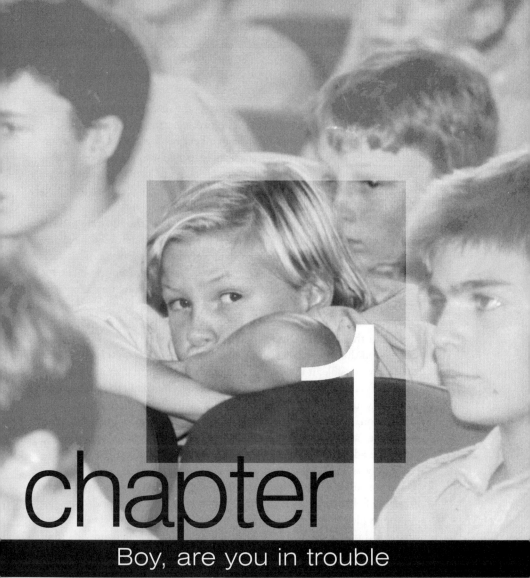

chapter 1

Boy, are you in trouble

Boy (boi)   1.   Male child, usually toxic.
               2.   One who burps in public.
               3.   Person who misses toilet bowl.

Male (mâl)   1.   Of the sex that begets offspring.
               2.   See above (few grow up).
               3.   Person who leaves toilet seat up.

BOYS IN TROUBLE

Boys appear to suffer from two problems — the first is that they are male, the second is that they are young. The two together have been judged by some to be particularly bad news. If one believes some social commentators, being male makes a person susceptible to predatory sexual dominance, power play and aggression. Being young makes a person susceptible to immaturity, high risk behaviours, and boundless energy. Together, this 'high risk' cocktail of characteristics describes a boy.

Somewhere between the hype and the denial lies the accurate picture of how boys are travelling. There are some who deny that boys have any problems, and even if they do, so what, everyone has problems. This view is irresponsible, but so too is the sensationalisation of the boy problem, for the hype is not difficult to find. More and more headlines are trumpeting the news of academic failure and social inadequacy in boys.

Some are suggesting that all the principal evils of the world can be linked to the so-called toxic touch of testosterone. There is a growing conviction that the state of boyhood is a disease which must be healed as quickly as possible: it is a very inconvenient ailment that should be eliminated. Even the law is in some way hobbled in its ability to control boys, for their youth makes them immune from many forms of prosecution. For this reason, some are advocating a lowering of the age whereby boys can be tried as adults,[1] namely if you commit an adult crime then you should serve the adult time.

Are boys so frightening as to cause society to want to lock them up? Have the cultural rules changed to the extent that boys must now be sent from the field of play? Is it true that girls are made of sugar and spice and all things nice, whereas boys are constituted less generously of worms and snails and puppy dogs' tails? Is it true boys are from Mars and girls from Venus? Is it true that males are now the weaker sex and an endangered species? Can any evidence be given to refute the jibes and rhymes of today such as:

> Girls have their faults,
> Boys have only two:
> Everything they say
> And everything they do.

Why is it that 'girl power' brings to mind the self-assertive, confident scholar, whereas 'boy power' brings to mind the thug who delights in occasioning physical hurt?

FEMINIST SUPPORT FOR BOYS

Boys have been so pilloried and punished for their inadequacies that some must wonder whether it has all gone too far. Such is the bruised state of boyhood that some feminists have even declared a cessation of hostilities. Their victim, battered and beaten, is now no longer giving satisfaction as a target. Pity makes it hard to land the killer blow. Best to smooth the dying pillow. Boys in particular and males in general are dying out anyway, with young men committing suicide at five times the rate of girls and having a 300% higher death rate from motor vehicle accidents.[2] Even in their first year of life about 12 boys out of every 1000 die, compared with nine girls out of every 1000.[3] This is not an auspicious start, and the future brings no respite in worrying news.

Boys are far more susceptible than girls to end up on a slab in the morgue or a bed in the hospital. Boys will top the class in accidents and assaults and they will be bottom of the class in literacy and learning.[4]

The capacity of boys to harm themselves is alarming. The capacity of boys to harm others is even more alarming. In their search for maturity and meaning, boys are leaving in their wake an unacceptable carnage. Car smash, assault and suicide figures make dismal reading not just from the male perspective, but from any perspective, for there are no winners with figures like these.

The figures relating to the suicide of boys are particularly disturbing. In 1998 in Australia, 364 boys killed themselves compared with 82 girls. In the USA, of those aged between five and 24 who committed suicide, 701 were female, 3792 were male.[5] These statistics are obscene, and to ignore these findings or to trivialise them by deliberately deflecting concern on to other societal problems is as irresponsible as it is inappropriate.

Also inappropriate and also irresponsible has been the over-reaction of some within society to the behaviour of boys. The American social commentator Christina H. Sommers tells a variety of shocking accounts of boys being accused of crimes by a society that appears to be in danger of becoming boy phobic. One of the stories is of a nine-year-old Virginian boy who had been on a trip to the National Gallery of Art. Presumably inspired by what he saw there, he drew a picture of a nude woman in art class. This was considered offensive. His second alleged infraction was that he had rubbed up against a girl while in a queue in the cafeteria. The school notified the police who handcuffed the boy, fingerprinted him and charged him with aggravated sexual battery.[6]

Motivated by compassion and an innate desire to help, some women are coming to the rescue. Mary Pipher, in her foreword to William Pollack's book *Real Boys*, suggests that contemporary society is doing a very ordinary job in raising its sons.[7] The evidence is in the quality of man that many of these boys grow into. They are unattractive. It is difficult to argue against such claims when men continue to furnish evidence in such quantity that all is not well in the male domain. Check out the prisons, the domestic violence shelters, the adult bookstores, the pubs. The evidence is compelling, and all too often, the verdict must be 'guilty'.

Babette Smith, author of *Mothers and Sons*, has called for a rethinking of what it means to be male. She has been joined by high profile Australian women such as Ita Buttrose. All are career women who have sons of their own. They can see that their sons are in danger of growing up imprisoned by both a social convention and a gender convention, which limits not only the display of emotion by boys, but also many other attributes such as compassion, despair, joy, wonderment, and intellectual curiosity. Mothers value these qualities and want their sons to be allowed to possess these characteristics, free from the ridicule and risk of rejection which forces a boy to be hard, dull and unfeeling.

Things must be bad when some of the opposite gender need to give males some support to make a game of it. But to these voices must be added the concerns of many male commentators. Steve Biddulph has done some magnificent pioneering work in causing parents to reflect on how to help their sons. Richard Fletcher has been dynamic in organizing seminars on improving boys' education at Newcastle University, and Peter West at the University of Western Sydney has become one of the most respected authorities in *maleness* and other related topics. State governments have also begun to tackle the problem through such initiatives as the *Enquiry into Boys' Education: Challenges and Opportunities: A Discussion Paper produced by the New South Wales Government Advisory Committee on Education, Training and Tourism, 1994*. More recently, the federal government of Australia has announced an enquiry into boys' education chaired by Dr Brendan Nelson, MP.

EXPECTATIONS OF BOYS

Boys are feeling somewhat alarmed at what is expected of them. Not many wish to deny their maleness or their heterosexual proclivities. Most have little wish to dress in an ambiguous manner, read Mills and Boon, or remain passive and unmoved when their team is playing in the grand final of the Soccer World Cup. Not only do many boys not want this, interestingly, neither do many girls. What usually attracts girls to boys in their teen years and beyond is evidence of a boy's maleness. True, a girl's perception of maleness is not necessarily linked to a boy's capacity to flatulate proudly, drink prodigiously and drive like a maniac. However, her primeval chemistry is likely to be excited by evidence that the boy could be a great carer (thoughtful, considerate) and a great provider (athletic, healthy, intelligent) as well as by evidence that the boy could well be good at reproduction and the maintenance of a strong and successful species.

CHANGING MODELS OF MASCULINITY

Boys are caught up in a redefinition of what it means to be male. This rewriting of the male characteristics is not a new phenomenon, for maleness, and indeed femaleness, is constantly being redefined as humankind continues to evolve.

Steve Zolezzi, a counsellor at St Aloysius College, a large non-government boys' school in Sydney, believes boys are caught up and confused by changing societal values and changing attitudes about masculinity.[8] It is difficult for a boy to find his feet when the world is spinning so fast.

Zolezzi describes the 1950s as a decade devoted to acquiring wealth and possessions. Then the Woodstock era of the 1960s moved the energy to protest marches, social reform and a drive towards greater gender equity. The 1970s found people in thermal baths holding hands. Encounter groups flourished and humanism was the creed of the day. The 1980s saw a hard edged pragmatism creep in and a move back to cruel reality. The 1990s was an era of political correctness and deconstruction. Truths were validated not against past wisdom, but on present interpretation. The current decade has yet to be defined although it does seem to be ushering in a new sensitivity and a new spirituality. Quite what the new God is, has yet to be fully revealed.

The impact of all these cultural and value shifts is likely to impact on many boys. A 1960s flower power baby becomes the transcendental teenager who then gets married in the very practical climate of the 1980s. This adult then produces a child in the redefinition period of the 1990s, who becomes a teenage boy in the new millennium crying out for a values system and some moral absolutes in a time when an 'e-year' will shortly be measured in just a few weeks.

To understand the confused morality of boys and their questioning of authority is to understand that the children of today are gypsies, blessed and cursed by travel. Their world is not constant. The only things that are constant are the scholastic caravan and their families. Sometimes even these will change.

Those who would suggest there is a moral hardening in contemporary children, and a hesitancy to commit, those who see today's youth as belonging to the 'options generation' must understand that the youth of today are on a journey. They are travellers, staying light, staying mobile, hanging loose. The children of today are footloose. Commitment and the establishing of roots are not big on their agendas. But there is some motion sickness, and a certain world-weariness. There is also a quiet desperation to enjoy the present, for the future is so uncertain.

Of course change is not new. Biologically, humans have emerged from a reptilian sensory brain to an emotional brain. Socially, humans have evolved from hunter-gatherers to those involved in agri-industrial activities. Now, society is moving beyond the agri-industrial age to the information age. Part of this change involves the redefinition of what it means to be male. The territorial male has now become the pilgrim, no longer sitting still but travelling, even into the wilderness, for it is in nature that the new spirituality is beginning to emerge. There is a growing search for the sacred and even a return to the value of courage and the virtue of wonder.[9]

Some have pilloried the new male as the 'sensitive new-age guy, the SNAG'. Some have been repulsed by the growing femininity of the male, for a few are not able to define male as anything other than 'not female'. Some have, in an age rampant with nostalgia, tried to return to the definition of a male who will 'shoot if it moves and ring-bark it if it doesn't'; the 'ocker' male with his parties on a Friday night, football on a Saturday and barbecues on Sunday.

Into all of this comes the boy caught up in a maelstrom of change, a boy disorientated by what it means to be a citizen of this planet, what it means to be a male in this world. If he is confused, it is only because society is confused. Boys find it difficult enough to learn and abide by the current gender expectations made of them, but when those expectations are themselves changing, one can begin to understand the confusion that some boys feel. This confusion can be exacerbated by their adult male role models celebrating one model of masculinity as they and their peers are celebrating a new model.

THE MEN'S MOVEMENT

The men's response in the 1990s to the women's movements of the 1970s and 1980s can generally be described as disappointing but, as some of the more uncharitable have noted, men have often had difficulty in organising anything. The only two things men can do at the same time is die in their sleep. It seems that all men have managed to do is to form into groups and cry a bit. Nora Ephron, in her 1983 book *Heartburn*, warns that it is as well to beware of crying men. Although it suggests they are in touch with their feelings, Ephron suggests the only feelings they tend to be in touch with are their own.

Social commentator Garrison Keillor laments the lack of leading men and asks where is the contemporary Van Gogh, the Plato, the St Francis, the Leonardo da Vinci?[10] Is it that the calibre of men has dropped? Have the mutations been such that the male chromosomes have lost their quality? Have generations of beer swilling, crotch scratching, sports mad, comic reading males evolved to a stage where they can no longer sire someone who can paint a *Mona Lisa* or compose a *Don Giovanni*?

A number of men have tried to stop this evolution and have sought to discover their 'feminine side' only to find that women are shrinking in horror from this ghastly transformation. Women are grieving over the loss of authority in their men and complain that the support given by the contemporary male has less strength than a sundowner without the gin.[11]

Hugh Mackay, in his book *Generations,* suggests that many of today's males feel victims, for they bear the accusations from feminists, and then from within their own ranks comes the guilty prose of authors like Steve Biddulph. Being sandwiched between testosterone and oestrogen is no fun. Trying to adapt to the new definition of male is not easy. Garrison Keillor writes of the brooding presence of critics in the lives of boys who are grading them and monitoring their behaviour for signs of poor attitude and macho tendencies.[12] Keillor suggests that this type of criticism is pointless for the biochemistry is such that boys can never exhibit the vestal virtues some would expect of them.

BEING MACHO

One of the dangers of the increased interest in redefining maleness is that a reaction can occur in the form of extreme chauvinism and grotesquely insensitive behaviour. An example, albeit humorous, is found in Bruce Feirstein's book *Real Men Don't Eat Quiche*.

American men are all mixed up today . . . there was a time when this was a nation of Ernest Hemingway's REAL MEN. The kind of men who could defoliate an entire forest to make a breakfast fire — and then wipe out an endangered species while hunting for lunch. But not any more. We have become a nation of wimps. Pansies. Alan Alda types who cook and clean and 'relate' to their wives, Phil Donahue clones who are 'sensitive' and 'vulnerable' and 'understanding' of their children. And where's it gotten us? I'll tell you where. The Japanese make better cars, the Israelis better soldiers . . . and the rest of the world is using our embassies for target practice.

Source: Feirstein, B. (1982) *Real Men Don't Eat Quiche*, Pocket Books, New York.

Being 'macho does not prove mucho' says Zsa Zsa Gabor. The much married Gabor might be interested in an observation made by a number of researchers, that the more traditionally masculine a husband, the less a marriage works.[13] There is the painful realisation by many men that Zsa Zsa Gabor is not alone in her views. Women are the chief initiators of divorce in Australia, walking out on their husbands with a frequency that is beginning to send clear messages that men might need to lift their game. Even a few males are beginning to wake up to the fact that a beer gut is not sexy, maintenance payments are expensive and the prospect of prostate cancer is not a bag of laughs. A few too many fathers have seen delinquency in their own children and unhappiness in their own marriage to feel comfortable that they are living an exemplary lifestyle. The macho thing is not working so well. There is increasing evidence that physical toughness, stoicism and the suppression of emotions is being correlated with educational problems, behavioural problems, and health problems.[14] The time may now be appropriate for a new model of maleness, where a slightly less macho level of maleness is passed from father to son.

Boys will learn how to be macho from their peers and from men, particularly their fathers. Herein might lie the cause of macho attraction: the desire to identify with, the desire to relate to, the desire to belong. The desire to belong can drive boys to adopt the code of the nearest gang and to melt chameleon-like within the group by adopting the group colours, the group language, the group attitudes. Given that these groups exist outside the control of the establishment, they often attract leaders and members who have failed to gain kudos within the establishment. An anti-intellectual sentiment can develop and the pressure is on all members to limit smartness to the street and not to the school. The societal pressures on boys to be dumb can be great. To be bright is to be a fool. Better to be moronic. The rewards in terms of social acceptance are greater. Better to be more interested in what's in your pants than what's in your head. The rewards in terms of social acceptance are greater. Better to kick, punch and tease than to be kicked, punched and teased. The rewards in terms of social acceptance are greater.

Macho is still alive and well in society. Despite the winds of change that are beginning to cause a redefinition of what it means to be male, the reforming breezes are too light and too fitful to tempt many to sail a new course. Until the forces are stronger, the macho thing will still be in.

THE PROBLEMS OF PASSING ON 'MANHOOD'

Faced with the current image of maleness — tough, steely-eyed, unflinching — there is little wonder that many boys find themselves bewildered and confused by those who wish boys to be sensitive renaissance beings, immune from the siren call of sport, sheds and sheilas. Finding answers as to how to best influence boys so that they grow up realising their potential, contributing in a positive and responsible manner to society, is like trying to pick the truths out of a party political broadcast. Even the 'Biddulphian' solution of fathers modelling more appropriate examples of manhood is challenged by writers such as Elizabeth Ryan who says that it is all very well to highlight the need for fathers to rumble with their sons and transfer the mysteries of manhood to them, but the question not asked by Steve Biddulph is just whose manhood is passed on?[15] The manhood displayed by some men can be described, even by the most generous, as having a few flaws. For this reason some care is needed to not just pass on any manhood.

To be fair to Steve Biddulph, his best selling book *Manhood* does indicate some characteristics of manhood that should be passed on to sons. This does not satisfy Ryan who complains that Biddulph appears to suggest that all boys have the same needs, hopes and preferred styles of learning. It is argued that they do not, so that the 'one size fits all' approach to fathering is not appropriate. Then again, are the base level needs of boys really different? Do not all boys need love, security, direction and encouragement? Is not Ryan being a little harsh? And so the debate rages on.

What is not in dispute is that boys need help, and can benefit enormously from having a positive role model in their lives. This can be particularly important in early adolescence when the boy begins to venture further from his mother, in particular, and from his parents, in general, in search of what it means to be masculine.

THE SOCIETAL BACKDROP

The litany of problems facing boys today is written on a parchment already decorated by a description of many societal problems, including:

- a growing secularisation with the resultant loss of a common frame of moral reference
- no absolutes and a reduced acceptance of ultimate truth
- the challenging of normative values resulting in confusion and moral ambiguity
- changes in the constitution of families with a significant increase in single parent and reconstituted families
- a growing tendency to celebrate individual rights at the expense of recognising individual responsibilities
- the great power wielded by peers resulting in a form of tribalism which requires members to conform or be expelled
- a growing social tension caused by an increased polarisation of wealth and a shrinking middle class
- the heavy influence of the media so that traditional values such as fidelity, forgiveness, chastity, service and love are being deconstructed, and even dismissed as no longer having relevance

■ the growth in materialism
■ increasing pluralism
■ a growing sense of boredom and pointlessness among some young people
■ evidence of a growing narcissism as expressed by feelings of entitlement, an inflated sense of self-importance, and an insensitivity to others

. . . to name but a few.

Quite apart from the insecurity of knowing who they should be as males, there is the attendant insecurity of not quite knowing who they should be as people. Boys are growing up in a world in turmoil, in transition. Trying to find a few firm islands within this world's swamp, from which a boy might take his bearings with any degree of confidence, is not easily found. Even the great meta narratives are going. God is shrinking and with it goes the concept of ultimate truth. There are now no generic answers, they are all case specific. No wonder boys are finding it tough.

LACK OF RESEARCH

Something must be done. Statistics both educationally and socially would suggest that the current initiatives to meet the needs of boys are inadequate. Some commentators are beginning to suggest that political and educational inaction on the matter of helping boys is now both embarrassing and irresponsible. Writing in the *Sydney Morning Herald*, Frank Devine suggests there is little excuse for this lack of action, for the steady decline in learning performance by males has been tracked for 15 years.[16] Despite this evidence being there for so long, all it seems to have elicited is a celebration of how well girls appear to be doing, and some mild tut-tutting about the performance of boys.

The awful truth might be that Devine may be stating only the half of it. Australian research undertaken by Georgia Kamperos indicates that the problem of the relatively poor academic performance of boys has not just been observed for 15 years, but ever since girls were allowed to matriculate from the University of Sydney in 1884. The only reason there is some limit to the dismal news of the relatively poor academic performance by males is that there are very few comparable records before this date. If girls had been enrolled at the University of Sydney earlier, the evidence of poor academic performance by males could well span many more years. This does not bring much comfort to the male camp. Kamperos found that even in the early days of public examination in Australia, girls outperformed boys in most subjects. The twentieth century brought no respite, with girls still outperforming boys in most subjects.

POLITICAL INACTION

Much of the interest in the past few decades has centred on the feminist cause and on meeting the needs of girls. In the early 1990s the Australian federal government published a report entitled *The Gender Equity in Secondary School Assessment, Project 'ESSA'*. It is now generally recognised that the report confined most of its comments on bias in school exam assessments to the handful of subjects where girls were still perceived to be disadvantaged, while totally ignoring the underperformance of boys in many subjects.[17] It is significant that the underperformance of boys in English received only a one-sentence comment whereas the ESSA made major recommendations to the government for strategies to increase girls' participation in mathematics.

In writing on this inequity, Bettina Arndt found out that the Gender Equity project seemed little more than a feminist controlled initiative to search out those few subjects that girls were not doing relatively well in. This led the ESSA team to make a number of indignant remarks about there being gender bias against girls, and getting stuck into those subjects to ensure that girls could presumably make a clean sweep of all subjects.

Feminist extremism, just like chauvinism, does little to add intellectual integrity to the gender debate. Both extremes must be avoided, for sanity and sense are invariably the victims of extremist views. An example was the concern reported by some feminists that boys were being advantaged in schools. The evidence presented to support this interesting claim was that a large amount of money was being spent on remedial classes in schools. Given that very few girls were in these remedial classes, it was unfair. Girls were not getting the benefit of the money.[18] The astonishing blind spot was that no one appeared to be concerned with the 'fairness' of the remedial classes being filled up with boys in the first place.

The gains made by the feminists need to be acknowledged and applauded. If there is now a growing interest in the problems faced by men and boys, feminists should not feel threatened, for there is mutualism in this new cause. There is a need to move out of the gender trenches and to find peace through a mutual recognition of the needs of both boys and girls. The histrionics of those who react violently against any initiative to advance the solving of problems for girls or solving problems for boys, must be viewed with suspicion. Some feminists have warned of the 'backlash', seeking to dismiss any initiative that might meet the needs of boys as an inappropriate over-correction. What is correct about some of the dismal academic results and suicide rates of boys today?

The feminist angst is quite understandably fuelled by the fact that despite significant gains made in education, there is still too much evidence of gender inequity in society. They have every right to feel angered. However, if this results in an unwillingness to acknowledge the needs of boys in schools, because it is thought that boys will end up with privileged positions in society, it would be unfortunate. The needs of boys in schools should not be sacrificed on the altar of a gender equity push in society. It is necessary to remove all forms of inequity and unfairness.

Some researchers, including female researchers, are alarmed at the relatively poor performance of boys in schools. Jennifer Buckingham was so shocked at the lack of empirical research on the topic that she produced a monograph entitled *The Puzzle of Boys' Educational Decline* which was written as part of the Taking Children Seriously program run by the Centre for Independent Studies in Australia. Within this paper Buckingham makes the startling suggestion that the great reluctance to release the figures showing the very ordinary educational performance of boys was to protect poorly performing teachers and schools.[19] These are serious claims, so it is as well not to accept these statements at face value. However, the fact that enough evidence is amassing to even cause a suspicion of a 'cover up' is deeply disturbing.

Further doubts as to whether Australian educators have really been serious in their desire to meet the academic needs of boys are raised by Richard Porter, the teacher in charge of 'boys' strategy' at Manly High School in Sydney. What Porter observed was that in girls' high schools and in government-run co-educational schools of over 1000 pupils, schools are allowed to appoint a senior teacher whose job it is to look after the welfare of girls. This is an executive position attracting an emolument and period allowance of a head teacher. The inequity which so perplexed Porter was that no similar position exists for boys in government co-educational schools, nor is an equivalent position even found in large government-run boys' schools.[20] Why? Is it that boys do not have needs? What has been allowed to happen in Australian schools that has allowed this inequity to exist? Is there not anyone looking after the academic and pastoral needs of boys in government schools? The answer is, there probably is, but why has this task not been acknowledged as being important?

In Australia

It has been slow, and it has been limited, but Australian governments are gradually waking up to the fact that they have been sleeping through a national scandal, and that scandal has been the poor performance of boys relative to girls in academic tests and exams. This inaction is hard to explain. The evidence has been clear and compelling for some time that all is not well in the academic and social world of boys.

In June 2000 an inquiry into boys' education chaired by Dr Brendan Nelson was launched by the federal Education Minister, Dr David Kemp. The inquiry was commendable and followed a New South Wales initiative a few years earlier led by state Liberal back-bencher Stephen O'Doherty. However, the curse of many such initiatives is that they can all too easily be snuffed out by the changing political winds. As Bettina Arndt recounts, Stephen O'Doherty was unable to follow through on the implications and suggestions arising from his inquiry.[21] O'Doherty was expelled to the nether world of Shadow Education Minister, and the winning Labor Party appointed as its consultant on the matter of boys' education an academic called Victoria Foster. If one is to believe Arndt, Victoria Foster had been critical of the growing level of concern being shown to boys by the previous state government. It was of no real surprise that the gender equity policies, which then emanated from Labor's time in office, seemed only to address the boys' issues which, if solved, would greatly advantage girls.

Arndt suggested that some feminists may be displaying a partisan support for the girls' cause, and, in an age of political correctness and affirmative action, they may have been successful in neutralising an initiative to address the needs of boys. An example cited by Arndt was a report examining girls' educational progress, prepared by a Professor of Education at the University of Sydney, Peter Cuttance. Professor Cuttance saw his report largely buried because it showed just how well girls were doing relative to boys and the feminists feared that releasing this report might lead to a moving of the focus from girls to boys.[22]

Overseas

The issue appears to be no different overseas. When asking why it had taken so long for politicians to take up the matter of boys' education in the USA, an answer was suggested by Christina Sommers in her book *The War Against Boys*. Sommers attributes the ever increasing gender gap in American schools to an educational bureaucracy, which is controlled by gender experts who have discouraged initiatives to help boys. Sommers is both confrontational and unapologetic in her claim that even research findings are being distorted in the USA to promote the belief that it is really only girls who are being disadvantaged in schools.[23]

Sommers talks of there being a covert animus against American boys, with the agenda being grabbed by gender police who only seem interested in meeting the needs of girls. Some of these people appear to have a natural antipathy towards boys, and even an anger against males, which fuels their enthusiasm in writing anti-harassment policies and such other rules to try and curb, perhaps even punish, maleness.

OPPOSITION TO HELPING BOYS

Initiatives to help boys have attracted opposition. For some extraordinary reason there are some who remain committed to the advancement of one gender by denying the needs of the other gender. Opposition can sometimes be avoided. A way of sidestepping the gender ideologies was shown by the Victorian government when in 1999–2000 it committed $102 million to a literacy scheme for young children. The results have been encouraging. Peter Hill, Professor of Education at the University of Melbourne, suggests that it is good to try and avoid tackling the ideologues on the matter of gender equity in schools, for it only results in a bloody battle with very few winners. It is far better, says Professor Hill, to get on with it and tackle low achievers in school. In doing so, many boys will be assisted. In other words, Hill argues for a distribution of resources on the basis of need, not gender.[24]

While recognising the political expediency of such an approach, it remains a tragedy that strategies to help boys need to be disguised in any way. Surely society has come of an age that it can recognise that academic and social impoverishment of any gender is something it can ill afford. Such is the growing evidence of the problem in relation to boys' education, that it is unlikely that those not supporting initiatives to help boys will triumph. Commonsense is likely to prevail and governments and educational authorities will be allowed to tackle the important question of how to meet the needs of boys rather more effectively. The fact that it has taken the authorities this long to act is alarming enough without compounding culpability by demurring on this issue much longer.

BOYS HURTING THEMSELVES

One of the leading Australian authorities on the needs of boys, Richard Fletcher, argues that there is little that is natural about 29% of 14–24-year-old males drinking on at least two days a week, as compared with 16% of females. There is nothing natural in boys having 700% more convictions for assault than girls. There is nothing natural with boys excelling in drownings, drug related crime, suicides, assaults both physical and sexual, alcohol abuse, work injuries and spinal cord damage.[25] Added to this is the aberration of the educational problems including school expulsions, poor literacy skills and attention deficit disorder often found with boys.

The problem seems to be exacerbated by some boys remaining silent in their pain and not admitting to their difficulties. Not only does the current boy culture require the pain to be borne without a whimper, there is also the complicity of adults and even parents who do not encourage boys to show their emotions . . . 'There, there, big boys don't cry . . . now come on . . . take it like a man'. This last statement is often rather ludicrous because not all men cope with their pain or discomfort well. Stories are legion of men classifying their cold as flu, their headache as meningitis and their indigestion as a regional catastrophe of some significance. Despite these observations, the general picture is that most are usually very stoic. Many boys have been humiliated and conditioned by their peers to the extent that they dare not show their true feelings, their individuality, their hurt.

This conditioning of males starts at birth with mothers pacifying their infant sons in a manner different from their infant daughters. Crying seems to be tolerated more in baby girls and the display of emotions is tolerated more in baby girls. Peter West suggests that boys learn to mask emotions by the age of four to six years.[26] In studies described by West, mothers found it relatively easy to read the emotions of their daughters but not nearly so easy to read the emotions of their sons. The research described by West involved pictures being shown to young boys and girls, and mothers trying to read the emotional response to these pictures by the children. The evidence was clear that boys even as young as four had already learned to hide their feelings. They had learned to keep their emotional expression to a minimum.

Society may need to question the subtle messages that it is giving to its boys. The inability to readily express emotions has undoubtedly contributed to shocking statistics such as suicide being the leading cause of death among young Australian males in the 15–24 age range.

CAN BOYS CHANGE?

There is some debate as to whether boys can be changed. William Pollack, author of *Real Boys*, believes boys can be changed and thinks it is a myth that boys' behaviour is predetermined, or that nature must necessarily win out over nurture. Furthermore, Pollack suggests there is great danger in accepting biological determination. It assumes an impotency in being able to nurture a boy's emotional development.[27]

Moir and Jessel, in their book *Brainsex*, argue differently and state that changing boys is problematic. Boys are not psychosexually neutral, they are wired differently from girls within their mother's womb. It is pointless getting apoplectic about maleness. It is as useless as raging against the existence of mountains or the inclement nature of the weather. Far better to abandon the bulldozer, acquire a brolly and get on with life. Attempts to de-male males through the genetic manipulation of selected sperm or fiddling with the foetal child in a petrie dish of feminising chemical hormones is not, in the opinion of Moir and Jessel, likely to achieve much. Sex differences will continue to emerge like hostile Indians in western movies.[28]

In the blue corner there are those who do not believe nurture can impinge much on the biology of a child. In the red corner there are those who disagree, and will fight to have it recognised that something can be done to help boys escape their biological predisposition. Parents and educators can let both parties slog it out, for the likely result is a draw. However, recent attempts to completely 'map' the basic helix of human creation are looking encouraging for those who feel humankind can alter its own make-up and character. This opens a Pandora's box on the ethics associated with such ventures.

It is worth pointing out that fatalism is seldom a constructive response to a problem. Undoubtedly initiatives can be taken to meet the needs of boys so that they become more effective as learners and have more of their pastoral needs met. However, society must be careful to avoid the implication that changing boys means to make them more feminine. It may be entirely possible to encourage appropriate behaviours, values and attitudes in young men without attacking their quintessential maleness.

NATURE VERSUS NURTURE

Authors of the Australian Temperament Project (ATP) believe that the nature versus nurture debate should now cease. The reality is that temperament and behaviour is 100% the product of an interaction between nature and nurture.

The ATP studied children from 2000 families from 1982–2000 and found that problems such as anxiety, hyperactivity and aggression could be predicted in children just a few years old. Thus early intervention is important.

The ATP found boys had more development problems than girls, with girls being more socially mature, responsible and empathetic. Girls were also better adjusted to school for they were less hyperactive and more task-oriented.

Source: Gunn, M (2000), 'Growing up in public', Australian, 29 November 2000, p 13.

In an effort to encourage greater sensitivity among boys in school, an Australian researcher, Jeff Borg, invited students to draw pictures which revealed their values and beliefs. Examples of the themes used by Borg for the pictures included 'What does masculinity mean? What does femininity mean? What is academic achievement?' By encouraging students to reflect on these issues and by staging dramatic skits on related themes, students were able to explore their values through discussion and were able to reflect on, reform and refine their definitions of 'male' and 'female'.[29]

Any school program designed to 'change' boys, needs not only to be reactive but also to be proactive. John Fleming, a teacher at Camden

High School, Sydney, suggests that the most effective programs for boys in schools have been programs that have involved:

- training in leadership
- peer mentoring initiatives
- mentoring through role modelling
- showing leadership by motivating others
- reinforcing daily responsibilities
- running workshops on specific boy-related issues
- organising adventure activities and expeditions
- adjusting the welfare policy to meet the needs of boys more effectively.

Whatever stratagems are used in schools, they must involve initiatives to meet not only the learning needs of boys, but also their social and emotional needs. Fleming advises that the following initiatives can help meet the needs of boys in school:

- integrated strategies which are long term
- development of a 'whole school' approach to the boy problem
- proactive rather than reactive intervention
- individual mentoring of boys
- deliberate attention to social learning
- developing a sense of achievement in boys
- use of peers
- early intervention and remediation.[30]

THE 'BOY' CODE

Pollack's book *Real Boys* claims that societal pressures are such that they require boys to hide behind masks of masculinity. These masks portray maleness, strength, toughness and stoicism, whereas their real feelings may well be those of loneliness, insecurity and fear. These masks are presented to boys in infancy as part of their gender uniform. Vulnerability and fear are unacceptable emotions that must be trapped behind a mask of bravado and feigned self-confidence. Should the mask be dropped, shame and ridicule will force the boy to put it back on. A chorus of 'big boys don't cry' and 'take it like a man' will cause the boy to hide his face, hide his feelings, hide himself. Pollack argues that boys will do just about anything to avoid shame, for boys are phobic about not being accepted by their peers. A boy's sensitivities are such that he will do whatever it takes to be liked by his peers. If the price to be paid is to adopt standards that are contrary to family standards, then so be it. If the price paid is to act dumb, then so be it. If the price paid is to engage in high risk behaviours, then so be it.[31]

To avoid shame, a variety of masks is presented to boys to be worn for life. Pollack suggests that one such mask is the 'sturdy oak' mask designed to mute any whimper or complaint. This mask portrays a face that is stoic, stable and strong. Another mask is the 'give 'em hell' mask which can be quite frightening as it signals an attraction to daring and violence. Then there is the 'big wheel' mask which gives the impression of dominance, status and power, encouraging man and boy to drive themselves mercilessly in the pursuit of status. Finally, there is the 'no sissy stuff' mask which is an anti-feminine creation designed as such because Pollack defines becoming masculine as quite simply avoiding the feminine. For this reason, the feminine traits of compassion and empathy are unlikely to be the sort of descriptors a boy would be happy with. The anti-'wuss' brigade would tease him back into line, back behind the mask.[32]

Unfortunately the list of qualities deemed by boys as feminine is rather long, and so being a boy requires some concentration as well as the wit and wisdom to:

- avoid showing emotions
- not talk about feelings
- not apply yourself to reading and writing tasks
- not be a compliant student in class
- not be sensible in terms of behaviour
- engage in attention seeking activities
- not control anger
- not be compassionate and empathetic
- not care for others

. . . to name but a few.

Masks are worn by boys to protect themselves from shame and to gain acceptance among peers. However, masks can hide not only a face but also individuality and ability. Society does not like the masks to be very different from each other. So there is a colourless conformity. Behaviours are adopted which encourage compliance and which avoid matters intellectual or creative. Pollack quotes one boy as saying there would be no way he would sit at the front of the class and become the teacher's pet. If he did, the 'peer police' would move in and he would have his backside kicked and his head decorated with spit balls. Liking neither spit balls nor bruised backsides, boys will align themselves with the dominant culture which all too often is anti-intellectual and disruptive of the learning process.[33]

For many boys, one of the great sins of the age is to be different. If boys are not prepared to run with the pack, they can find themselves rounded upon with some savagery and driven away from scented boundaries with resentful animosity. Tall poppies are harvested with alacrity, lest it be proved that others are growing better. Derision for the disadvantaged; destruction for the distinguished. The goal is a grey conformity and a comfortable mediocrity.

Loneliness is profound if the family rejects, and it is profound if the peer group rejects. Thus, the pressure to conform with the group and to be accepted is enormous. Boys learn the language of the group; boys watch the appropriate TV programs; boys listen to the relevant music and wear the group's uniform. Individualism and personal standards are sacrificed for popularity.

This conformity will not always occur. There is still the occasional individualist. It must also be said that conformity is not always damaging, providing that the peer group chooses standards which respect both people and property. However, standards chosen by many peer groups may not always be worthy of the individuals who form the group.

CONCLUSION

In conclusion, it may be said that there are very real problems faced by boys both academically and socially. To understate these problems is as irresponsible as to overstate them. The number of 'gloom and doom' books on boys is growing, and many do little more than alarm. Their major trap is to suggest that all boys are the same. They are not, and neither are the definitions of acceptable maleness.

Not everyone defines the only permissible male as having the physical frame of Crocodile Dundee and the wit of a brick. Other legitimate expressions of maleness are beginning to emerge. Leonardo di Caprio seems popular enough, and still manages to get the girl even though he cries a bit and does not appear to have body hair.

Feminism has been terrific for boys. The mother's voice is now stronger; the girl's point of view is rather more acknowledged. There is growing evidence that many girls are not only quite tolerant of a boy who can't play football, they even prefer it. If they were to be honest, standing on the duck-boards watching the boys on a wet Saturday afternoon is not quite so compelling as they pretend.

The female voice is being heard. Not everyone is hearing it, not everyone is listening to it. Not everyone is persuaded by it even if it is heard, but the voice is getting louder and ever more compelling. The post-industrial age of the microchip is also expanding the options of what it means to be acceptably male. The 'chip head' is now finding a very real place in contemporary society, and the badge of 'nerd' is worn by some boys with pride. Boys thinking and boys reading is beginning to be tolerated. For those in doubt, try following a game of Pokémon, and try counting the number of pages in the latest *Harry Potter* book. In other words, it is not all bad news. There are boys who bring nothing but pride to their parents, and pleasure to their teachers. There are boys who are sensitive and intelligent and yet remain very male.

Assisting to increase the list of acceptable attributes for males is the growing multiculturalism of many western countries. The phlegmatic white Anglo-Saxon protestant is beginning to be enlivened by a touch of Asian work ethic, a dash of Latin flair and a smidgen of Middle Eastern passion. Yes, there is also evidence of increased tribalism and intolerance in the land, but this should not obscure the fact that some coalescing of cultures is occurring. Perhaps the tolerance is still only at the 'restaurant stage' where some will only eat foreign food but not accept foreign culture. But remember, there was a stage when not even the food was eaten.

There are very real problems facing boys today, but the picture should not be one of complete despair. Some boys are in trouble, just as some girls are in trouble. Both need help. This book is a contribution to helping the former. No apology is offered for this. Boys appear to need more help at the moment, and the following chapters suggest various ways that this help might be given.

ADDITIONAL INFORMATION

For those wishing to have further details on some of the points raised in this chapter, the following references may be helpful. Each number in the text of the chapter relates to a reference number below which will give further information related to the topic.

1	Loane, S (1995)	'The trouble with boys'	*Sydney Morning Herald*, Spectrum, 7A, 19/8/95.
2	Legge, K (1995)	'Some mothers do have 'em'	*Australian Magazine*, 11/3/95, p 21.
3	Maslen, G (1995)	'Boy, you're in big trouble'	*The Bulletin*, 25/4/95, p 28.
4	Loane, S	(op cit)	
5	Sommers, C H (2000)	*The War Against Boys*	Simon and Schuster, New York, p 10.
6	Sommers, C H	(op cit)	p 8.
7	Pollack, W (1998)	*Real Boys*	Owl Books, Henry Holt and Co., New York, p xvii.
8	Zolezzi, S (2000)	'What It Means To Be a Man — Role Model of Masculinity'	IES Conference, The Gazebo Hotel, Sydney,. 22–23 June 2000.
9	Zolezzi, S	(op cit)	

10	Keillor, G quoted in West, P (1996)	*Fathers, Sons and Lovers*	Finch Publishing, Sydney, p 180.
11	Mackay, H (1997)	*Generations*	Macmillan, Sydney.
12	Keillor, G quoted in West, P	(op cit)	p 180.
13	Callaghan, G (2000)	'A family by any other name'	*Australian Magazine*, 1/1/00, p 16.
14	Hall, S (1993)	'Bully in the mirror'	*New York Times Magazine*, section 6, 22/8/99, p 31.
15	Ryan, E (1999)	'Boys' education: handle with care'	*The Practising Administrator*, Vol 21, No 4, p 23.
16	Devine, F (2000)	'Disconcerting lack of interest in male lag'	*Australian*, 7/2/00, p 13.
17	Arndt, B (1994)	'Gender war in class'	*Weekend Australian Review*, 19/2/94, p 1
18	MacLean, S (1994)	'Beware the backlash'	*Age*, 3/5/94, p 14.
19	Buckingham, J quoted in Devine, F	(op cit)	
20	Porter, R (2000)	'Making boys' education work — Inculcating a success attitude'	IES Conference, The Gazebo Hotel, Sydney, 22–23 June 2000.
21	Arndt, B (2000)	'The trouble with boys'	*Sydney Morning Herald*, 17/6/00, p 34.
22	Arndt, B (2000)	(op cit)	
23	Sommers, C H	(op cit)	
24	Hill, P quoted in Arndt, B (2000)	(op cit)	
25	Fletcher, R (1997)	*Improving Boys' Education, A Manual for Schools*	Family Action Centre, University of Newcastle, Publication No 973.
26	West, P	(op cit)	p 31.
27	Pollack, W	(op cit)	
28	Moir, A and Jessel, D (1989)	*Brainsex*	Mandarin, London.
29	Borg, J (2000)	'Bringing sensitivity into the schooling process'	IES Conference, The Gazebo Hotel, Sydney, 22–23 June 2000.
30	Fleming, J (2000)	'Boys who fall behind In school — Working with difficult boys'	IES Conference, The Gazebo Hotel, Sydney, 22–23 June 2000.
31	Pollack, W	(op cit)	p 33.
32	Pollack, W	(op cit)	p 24.
33	Pollack, W	(op cit)	p 16.

chapter 2

Schoolboys

A PSALM

1. Why art thou so vexed, oh my soul; and why art thou so disquieted within me?
2. Thou must be joking when thou sayest that Edward has broken another window.
3. Oh, what sins have I committed that I am chastened with teaching heavily testosteroned boys last period on a Friday afternoon?
4. After interminable years of scuffed shoes and scraped knees, wormwood and gall will be as nectar and ambrosia.
5. Whither shall I go for peace and quiet or where shall I hide at the sound of boys' voices?
6. If I climb the stairs I will hear them, and if I go down, even to the Common Room, they are heard there also.
7. My days are gone like a shadow and I am withered like grass.
8. Iniquities are more in number than sand, particularly those of Wayne and Shane and their sullen little friends with querulous temperaments, piercing voices, allergy to work and incessant nasal whines.
9. Remove them from my sight lest I smite them upon the hip.
10. They who maketh the windows to break and their jackets to smell of Benson & Hedges.
11. They that pulleth hair and chewing gummeth the carpets.
12. Under whom I then swore in my wrath; and snappeth my pencils asunder.
13. Boys lay waste my study like a whirlwind; storm and tempest fulfilling their words.
14. Oh, how amiable is the weekend.
15. By the notice boards I sat down and wept; by the pigeonholes I uttered my reprove.
16. One day with boys feels something like a thousand. *Amen*

(Adapted by the author from the psalms and a poem of unknown origin.)

SCHOOLS NOT BOY-FRIENDLY

William Pollack, in his book *Real Boys*, suggests that schools are often not boy-friendly.[1] Schools can fail to be stimulating places of learning for boys, as many teachers do not really understand how boys learn. This is hardly surprising, for in most primary and middle schools there is a dearth of male teachers. Eighty per cent of teachers in New South Wales primary schools are females.[2] This lack of male teachers can send messages to boys in their formative years that serious learning is really for girls only, and that it is not really acceptable for boys to learn as they must follow a code of bovine indifference to things academic.

Social commentator Ian Lees found that in his local school, 100% of those in the school's discipline program were boys.[3] Lees suggests that if the reverse were so and there were 100% of girls in the discipline program, there would be a royal commission of enquiry.

Parents in particular and society in general may need to be more discerning about the schools they send their sons to, and more politically active in ensuring that schools really understand the emotional needs of boys. Determining the emotional needs of boys is not always easy. There is an enforced social conditioning which forces boys to conceal their true feelings and to mask their insecurities and fears. It is disturbing that one can still find within schools a fear of boys' toxicity with some educators being quite hostile towards boys. This can be particularly prevalent when boys become teenagers and begin to take on the characteristics of men. The tragedy is that this disengagement from teachers comes just at a time when boys need even more understanding and reassurance from adults.

It is important to recognise not only the learning challenges that boys face but also their emotional challenges. Pollack talks of this and of the cycle of shame and hardening that many boys have to endure in school. What educators may need to be reminded of is that behind a boy's bravado can be found a vulnerable and insecure child struggling with his own body chemistry and a bewildering world of threats and opportunity.

BOYS' RELATIVELY POOR ACADEMIC PERFORMANCE

The Australian evidence

Perhaps the clearest evidence that schools are not boy-friendly are the academic performances by boys which make fairly unimpressive reading when compared with the performances of girls. An editorial in the *Sydney Morning Herald* on 23 December 1999 joined a plethora of other articles indicating that boys were not travelling well academically. The editorial stated that girls in New South Wales outperformed boys in the 1999 Higher School Certificate (HSC) honours list. The top student in over two-thirds of all HSC courses was female. The editorial went on to suggest there was nothing new in these statistics, that the domination by girls had been going on for nearly 10 years. In the 1998 HSC results the girls average mark in 64 of the 70 subjects exceeded that of boys by up to 11%, and in the New South Wales Board of Studies list of the top 9% all-round achievers, only one-third were boys.[4]

The situation was no different interstate with the top performance bands in 36 of the 45 subjects in Queensland being dominated by girls in their final school grades in 1998. In South Australia, in the same year, girls outperformed boys in 27 of the 34 subjects taken by students at the end of Year 12.

FIGURES FROM THE CHAIRMAN OF THE NATIONAL INQUIRY INTO BOYS' EDUCATION, AUSTRALIA

- In Australia in every area of the assessed cognitive curriculum, boys are achieving lower standards than girls.
- In the 1999 Year 12 HSC results, in 36 of the 40 subjects with the largest candidatures, girls outperformed boys by up to 11%.
- Fourteen-year-old boys were failing basic literacy in New South Wales at an increased rate with 30% failing in 1975 and 35% failing in 1995.
- Boys outnumber girls two to one in the bottom 10% of HSC scores.

Source: Dr Brendan Nelson (2000) 'Why boys achieve B-grade results', *North Shore Times*, 22 November 2000. p 15.

Professor George Cooney at a meeting of the Headmasters' Conference of New South Wales in March 1998 stated that the percentage of girls in the top 5000 had increased from 52% to 57%. Tertiary entrance rankings were also examined from the period 1981 to 1994. Throughout the 1980s girls typically had an average tertiary entrance rank two percentage points better than boys. In 1992 the difference increased to 12%, in 1993 to 18% and in 1994 to 20%.

Professor Cooney conceded that boys continued to dominate the score in the top 5%. It was also pointed out that the differences in academic standard seemed to vary according to age. Up to Year 6 there was no significant difference between the verbal and mathematical skills of girls and boys. By School Certificate age, that is about 15–16 years of age, there was no difference in maths and science ability between boys and girls, but a significant difference existed in English ability in favour of the girls. The situation remained for the HSC exams when students were aged 17 and 18.

An Australian federal report suggests that, on average, boys are five percentage points behind in academic performance in schools. Other educational researchers such as Dr Ken Rowe are indicating that the gap is even larger with girls some 15–22% ahead of boys.[5] Research undertaken at the Australian Centre for Independent Studies by Jennifer Buckingham led to the paper entitled 'The puzzle of boys' educational decline'.[6] The paper confirmed that throughout the 1990s at least, there had been a very real deterioration in academic performance by boys. At the very start of 1990 boys tended to dominate the bottom and the top achievement bands. By the late 1990s boys at the top were thinning out and the number of boys at the bottom was nearly twice that of girls. In addition, for every three boys in reading support schemes and language support initiatives in New South Wales there was only one girl. Some 60% of referrals to the student counsellor were boys and three-quarters of all school suspensions were boys.

In a paper produced by the Victorian Association of State Secondary Principals in 1996 entitled 'Improving the school performance of boys', it was pointed out that the retention rates for boys in schools were significantly less than that for girls and that boys were underrepresented in studying the humanities. It was also stated that boys were over-represented in courses that were likely to experience the greatest decline in terms of vocational relevance over the next few years and were under-exposed to competencies which had the best employment prospects. For example, boys were under-enrolled in courses which required skills in:

■ working cooperatively in a group situation
■ parenting and domestic tasks
■ communication of a relational and interpersonal nature
■ learning based on literacy
■ conflict resolution
■ personal well-being and health.[7]

Employment in the twenty-first century is putting a premium on skill rather than muscle, yet this reality has not quite penetrated a number of male craniums. In the USA, the five industrial sections which are declining the fastest are shipbuilding, ammunition, footwear, leatherwork and photographic supplies.[8] Men account for at least two-thirds of the workforce in these industries. Not only are boys choosing subjects that appear not to develop skills most prized in contemporary society, more boys than girls are not even completing their schooling to Year 12. In 1967 about 26% of boys completed their schooling in Australia as compared with 18% of girls. By 1993 the situation had changed significantly with 81% of girls completing their education and only 72% of boys completing secondary school.[9]

Small wonder boys are bailing out of schools. Even the subjects they once used to dominate such as mathematics and science are being taken over by girls. Whatever indicator is chosen, the news on the scholastic front for boys is reasonably gloomy. Boys do not complete school as much as girls, and they tend not to be choosing subjects which will lead to careers that are experiencing good employment potential. Girls are entering university in greater numbers and boys are far more likely to develop behavioural problems while at school.

The overseas evidence
There is similar news from places such as the USA and Great Britain. In a study reported in 1999 in Great Britain, researchers examined the

gender gap at General Certificate of Secondary Education (GCSE) level in eight different English secondary schools and found that boys tended to attract most of the teachers' time relative to girls and tended to dominate student-teacher interaction.[10] This was not generally seen as a positive quality by teachers who increasingly seemed to be defining the 'ideal student' as being female.

Some of the reasons for this rather jaundiced view of a boy as a learner was the conviction by many of the teachers that:

- girls were far better organised, with boys often failing to bring equipment to class;
- boys took far longer to settle down and were prone to poor behaviour, limited attention span and disruptive behaviour;
- girls had more sophisticated communication skills and were more articulate;
- boys were less skilled in being independent learners and were less confident in the classroom.

General feedback from the British study also supported the view that girls were better as independent learners. This was reflected in superior planning, greater diligence in completing work and spending more time on homework. In short, girls conformed more to the demands made of them by the school and were able to anticipate what was required of them. Boys, on the other hand, were seen as demotivated, disordered and disruptive as well as being less academically advanced. Boys seemed far more concerned with pleasing their peer groups than their teachers. Indeed, there was the clear impression that boys were often in opposition to the school, challenging its educational offering, its relevance and its ethos.

> Man is a clever animal who behaves like an imbecile.
> Albert Schweitzer

As a consequence, a number of teachers confessed that they were somewhat tougher on boys. There was an expectation that boys would misbehave and thus teachers would seek to head off misbehaviour by aggressive posturing.[11]

Among the implications of the British study was the need to support teachers more and to help them devise strategies to raise boys' achievement levels. It was suggested that first-year out teachers needed more assistance. Collaborative teaching with experienced educators was identified as a possible way forward.

Some possible reasons for a relative decline in boys' academic performance

The fact that boys are under-performing relative to girls in schools is one matter, but what has happened to exacerbate this situation in the last decade or so? Has there been an outbreak of male 'moronicness'? Has some significant progression been made on the evolutionary journey in this last decade whereby males are being readied for extinction? Even the proud function of perpetuating the species is something which technology is replacing. Is the ultimate destiny of males to be a buttress to a cathedral or to be corralled into stadia throughout the land to engage in Romanesque sporting spectaculars?

It is unlikely that cranial inertia has suddenly afflicted boys in a manner hitherto unknown, so what are the other possibilities? Far more research is needed on this topic, but the major suspects may well be:

■ An escalation of the culture among boys that it is 'cool to be a fool' fuelled by incessant images in the media of the studious boy being a 'geek'.

> If this belief from heaven be sent
> If such be Nature's holy ploy
> Have I not reason to lament
> What boy has made of boy?
> Adapted from William Wordsworth's poem Early Spring

■ A feminisation of the curriculum with literacy skills, a traditional area of weakness for many boys, being given a greater influence on marks. For example, subjects like physics and mathematics are having their material rewritten to make them more 'girl-friendly'. No one appears to have noticed that in so doing they may be making this material 'boy-unfriendly'. When a physics test loses its distinctive content and merely requires students to write an essay on the life and times of Sir Isaac Newton, one can be forgiven for wondering whether all subjects are slowly evolving into an English exam.

■ The growing dominance of the teaching profession by females. With new child protection laws and the frequent reminders about child abuse in schools, it is a very special and very courageous man who becomes a primary teacher. The pedophile suspicion is such that not many men wish to risk possible societal condemnation by becoming a primary teacher. Added to this is the growing conviction that teaching is really only a 'secondary income' profession. The wages are such that the major bread winner must do something other than teach. The secondary bread winner is permitted to teach, but only as an adjunct to the main income, and only until the baby is born.

DO NOT TOUCH

The rest of the world is allowed to use five senses, male teachers can only use four. They are not allowed to touch.

The shadow of suspicion has led to some schools not even trying to discern the difference between 'good touching' and 'bad touching'. There is now the blanket rule of 'no touching', particularly by male teachers in primary schools.

Little wonder that many males are too frightened to become primary school teachers.

- The success of the feminists in demanding that the needs of girls be met. Girl-conscious teaching, equal opportunity, affirmative action, harassment laws, stalking laws, enquiries into girls' education have all combined with the female vote to ensure there is a societal sensitivity to meeting the needs of girls.
- The professions available to girls are no longer limited to nursing, secretarial work or teaching. The confident, power dressed girl with executive skills is now a common sight. This opening up of increased alternatives for future employment has motivated girls far more in their studies. Conversely, boys have found employment prospects declining given that many boys lack the attributes necessary to be considered an asset to an organisation.
- Some scrutiny is needed of changes in assessment techniques over the last decade. Tests need to ensure that they do something more than examine literacy skills and memory recall. If these two elements, important though they are, were to be removed from all school tests, teachers would probably have to think of other ways to distribute well over half of their marks. Are these two skills being over-tested? Are there other skills such as problem solving and creativity which might need to be rewarded more in schools? If other skills were to be rewarded more and literacy and memory rewarded less, would boys experience a renaissance in learning as measured by tests? Are schools keeping boys in the Dark Ages by not allowing the testing of all intelligences, restricting most exams to literacy-based answers and putting a premium on inert, quiet behaviours?

AN HERETICAL THOUGHT

An heretical thought is who really cares if the current academic test results of boys are really bad? The tests are no good anyway and do not prove anything except that boys do not do well at badly designed assessment tasks. Are the current methods used to test students really showing anything other than a boy's incapacity to remember scraps of information and to regurgitate this information under exam conditions? The information is largely irrelevant and will probably be dated within a few years. In the end boys finally get there, so why worry? Success in life is governed, if one believes Daniel Goleman, rather more by emotional quotient (EQ) than by intelligence quotient (IQ) anyway, so why the concern?[12]

Alfie Kohn argues that an emphasis on achievement can actually undermine a student's interest in learning and can prevent a student from challenging himself and being creative.[13] Kohn suggests that achievement-oriented students can become preoccupied with what they shouldn't be preoccupied with, such as their performance rather than their effort.

Reviewing the last few paragraphs, one can begin to realise that the argument is getting rather desperate. It does not matter what 'spin' is put on it, it **does** matter that some boys are underperforming in schools. There is no adequate excuse and something must be done about it.

SCHOOLS TOO BOY-FRIENDLY

Having spent a good proportion of this chapter detailing how schools are not boy-friendly, another point of view needs to be explored. This different point of view is likely to cause conniptions among the more liberal minded educators devoted to child-centred learning, for it supports the view that many schools are quite simply too soft, too friendly, too 'you don't have to if you don't want to'. Schools that see teachers and students negotiating on equal terms, that rely heavily on rewards even for normal behaviour let alone good behaviour, may be providing an educational environment which is not only unhelpful for boys, but is also dangerous. It is also dangerous if teachers fail to tell a boy that he considers himself well ahead of his actual accomplishments.

It must be recognised that what is being suggested is not educational brutalism or a 'thrash them on the hour and beat them in between' approach to teaching. What is being suggested is the right to expect appropriate standards of effort, attitude and behaviour from boys to the extent that their academic potential is realised and that they are well equipped to make a positive contribution to society.

The argument as to whether schools should be more or less child-centred boils down to the ageless philosophy of original sin and the basic nature of humankind. Are children born good, or are children born bad? Does the state of humankind need to be redeemed by a loving God and by some no-nonsense instruction in schools, or should one celebrate the innate goodness in all creation including the belligerent over-testosteroned Year 9 boy who has a penchant for relieving fellow students of their lunch money? The ideological battle lines have stood for centuries, the romantic Rousseauian 'aren't we beautiful' view on the one side and the dark St Augustine view of the fallen and imperfect nature of man on the other. Do boys need deliverance from hell, deliverance from themselves and deliverance from trendy child-centred approaches to teaching boys?

Opinions will be divided on this issue, but there is evidence to suggest that some boys are not as able to cope with a child-centred approach to learning as some girls. One reason for this is that many girls are intuitively aware of what their teachers want and thus there is a happy accord between girl and teacher. This results in a child-centred approach becoming a teacher-centred approach, because the girl has learnt to want what the teacher wants. Meanwhile, the boy hasn't noticed anything — his 'receptors' are not nearly so well attuned to what his teachers want and even if they are, he does not want to please his teachers anyway.

- Girls want to please their teachers.
- Boys want to please their friends.

> A boy's will is the wind's will,
> And the thoughts of youth are long, long thoughts.
> Henry W Longfellow, My Lost Youth

Longfellow might have been a trifle generous, for all too often a boy's will is not the wind's will, it is the will of his mates to whom he has pledged allegiance. This hardly fosters any thoughtfulness as a mindless conformity is called for, and frequently given.

This is a generalisation, but it is imbued with enough truth to begin to understand that a child-centred style of education for boys may well be fraught with difficulty.

Boys need the security of rules, they need the confidence that comes with the establishing of firm boundaries. Yes, it is better if boys understand why these boundaries are in place, but understanding or not, clear non-negotiable standards of academic and social behaviour need to be set. It is not always possible to wait until a boy understands why a stricture is in place. Some boys may need to be reminded that thousands of years of accumulated wisdom can be more realiable than the knowledge accumulated by a boy who has celebrated only 14 birthdays. Society can, and indeed must, be unapologetic in the demands it makes on its children. If this is done with warmth, compassion and understanding, greater security, direction and purpose can be given to boys.

Evidence is beginning to emerge that four decades of child-centred learning have helped girls rather more than boys. Many boys tend to respond well to more traditional methods of teaching. This does not mean a return to slates, quill pens and regular beatings. It does mean a return to:

- more teacher-directed education
- regular checking of work done in class and at home and the regular checking of learning through tests and exams
- a more structured environment with clear rules and procedures and sanctions in place to support them
- single sex classes
- uncompromisingly high standards and competition
- formal periods of silent work with minimal distractions.[14]

A recommendation from Britain

Many schools are too 'soft' on boys. This was the conclusion of a council of British Headmasters who met in 1988 to tackle the issue of the under-performance of boys in education. Some might want to suggest that these conclusions are not surprising given the conservative disposition of some headmasters. However, it would be both unwise and inappropriately judgmental to dismiss the views of the headmasters. Not only are these colleagues vastly experienced, there is clear evidence emerging that the schools that have been guided by the recommendations of these headmasters do seem to be producing better academic results for boys.[15]

The British initiative has been supported by the publication of literature such as *Can boys do better?* written by Robert Bray et al of the Secondary Heads' Association in Bristol and by a 'back to basics' push by the British government. Arising from these initiatives has been the establishment of the Literacy Hour in many English schools. This is a quiet, supervised reading time which is timetabled into the school day. It is not unlike the Drop Everything and Read (DEAR) program found in many schools today.

THE NEED FOR FENCES

Boys need some boundaries within which they should operate. If the fences are weak and undefended, the young bulls will break through. Asking them not to lean on the fence is about as useless as playing the flute and expecting rats to follow. It only happens in fairy tales. Unless some behavioural endocrinology is engaged in, such as lopping off a few testicles, bulls will always test fences. If a fence is weak, as behavioural and academic fences can be in some child-centred learning environments, then boys will cross the boundaries of acceptable behaviour. A weak fence tells a boy that 'this particular restriction is not thought very important by adults . . . I wonder why it's not worth defending . . . I'll give it a gentle nudge . . .' The natural streak of inquisitiveness, when combined with a propensity for aggression and independence, will ensure that a bull will soon run wild and a wild bull can do a great deal of damage in places other than a china shop.

If someone has taken the trouble to run a little persuasive electricity through the fence or to build a strong fence that will withstand the odd bump from a bull, the boundaries become both known and respected. Boys generally admire strength, and teachers who are strong are the ones who they remember with genuine fondness at alumni gatherings for decades to come. The compliant teacher who is weak in discipline, if remembered at all, will only be remembered as an object of pity or as a target of scorn.

Care needs to be taken not to confuse oppressive bullying behaviours with being strong. The strong teacher need not be a stranger to compassion and sensitivity. One can see this in the strong men in history. Mandela, Ghandi, Jesus: each had a moral and ethical strength which was extraordinary. They were resolute men who remained constant to their calling. This did not stop any of them showing love, shedding tears or dealing with those they met with kindness.

Something of this moral and ethical strength may have been missing from the lives of Eric Harris and Dylan Klebold who in April 1999 perpetrated the Columbine High School massacre, where a number of students and a teacher were killed. Such was the callousness of the slaughter in Littleton, Colorado, that the event gave birth to 'The Columbine Syndrome'. This syndrome was a deep disquiet that something was going horribly wrong with many teenage boys, something which society could not control. A string of 'dear oh dear' books appeared and a country went into mourning, not only for the death of children but for the death of societal innocence. A collective pathology was attributed to boys and the question was asked 'How can boys be controlled?'

Christina H. Sommers in her book *The War Against Boys* suggests that where the parents and the school went wrong in Littleton was to fail to put boundaries in the lives of Harris and Klebold. Such boundaries might have stopped them wearing 'serial killer' T-shirts and producing extremely violent videos.[16] While celebrating the virtues of self-expression, the adults in the lives of these two boys had failed to put constraints on their lives. Everyone is wise after the event and there is nothing like a tragedy to unleash sermons, but the question must still be asked. 'Are boys being best served by homes and schools that are so child-centred as to prevent boys from being required to accept the wisdom of adult experience?' Many boys serve as excellent illustrations of 'the principle of least effort'. Unless compelled into the experience, some boys will not extend themselves or expand the boundaries of their ability.

Not all boys underachieve in schools. In fact, there is a worrying polarity occurring in school boys. On the one hand there are the valium-fuelled and irrepressible workaholics; these are blurred images between two points, ricocheting from one job to another. Work is consumed with a voracious appetite as task after task is fed through their hands en route to the teacher's desk. On the other hand there are the sloths, the chronic work avoiders, prompting schools to put notices on boards such as:

PLEA FOR WORK

Some time between morning roll call and the afternoon dash for the bus, without infringing on recess, lunch break, class change-over time, toilet breaks, chatting with your mates, retelling the magic moments of the first XI win and going to matron for an aspirin, we ask that you find time for some academic work. This might seem radical to some but it may lead to success, employment and the enjoyment of future life.

Hard work is not always congenial to boys whose hedonistic tendencies combine with a deep suspicion that work is seriously 'un-cool', to ensure that scholastic tasks are given a priority towards the bottom of the 'must do' list.

For this reason, parents and educators may need to be given a new freedom to insist on certain standards both academic and social. The right of parents and educators to do this is bestowed by history which has dutifully handed down bountiful lessons in what is good for the human condition and what is not. To fail to pass on these lessons in preference to a student working out the lessons for himself, can sometimes be as stupid as it is impractical. There is just far too much to learn. For this reason society should feel free to tell boys things from time to time, rather than requiring them to discover everything for themselves.

It must also be said, and this might come as a shock to some, that the trail of wreckage left by some boys as they blunder through life's learning experiences is unacceptable. A boy drives his mates to a party; beer and booze makes him speed. He crashes and kills his friends. At their funeral the boy says he is sorry. There are times when boys need to know that sorry is not good enough. Sorry is good, but not good enough to assuage the hurt, the grief, the anger. Sorry cannot always be slapped on a wound in the hope that the wound will now heal. 'But I said I was sorry!' will not always be taken as acceptable rhetoric to escape sanctions, or to escape putting in place some limitations to personal freedom.

There is nothing wrong with a child-centred education providing that the education is also society-centred. The individualising and customising of education can be beneficial, but not if it is going to produce boys who have never fully extended themselves, or who have never had to take within the orbit of their concerns, the contrary views of others.

Just as society should cherish its children, children must cherish society. This should not translate into a slavish acceptance without question, for this would snuff out the creativity and individualism that society needs. What it means is that base level behaviours should be established without apology by parents and teachers, and within the boundaries of these behaviours boys should be free to roam.

Quite what these principles should be will need to be decided by teachers and parents. There are several good starting points. Jesus suggested that all the laws hinged on one basic requirement which was to love God and one's neighbour as oneself. To this can be added honouring oneself and not being content until the boundaries of one's own ability have been fully realised.

This might mean that some schools may need to think through what it is they want the school to stand for. This will be dealt with in the following chapter. A community that stands for nothing will fall for anything. Schools may need to be reminded that they have the mandate to expect their boys to work with diligence and to the best of their ability. Boys must be taught to value themselves, their peers and their teachers enough to take their learning seriously. To assist boys in this regard, schools should ensure that what is taught to boys is important and is not just work designed to keep boys busy. School is not a boy-sitting exercise, it is a learning exercise designed to prepare a boy for life and, possibly, even death.

Some boys go to schools that require them to wear a tie. The tie is often associated with private boys' schools rather than government schools. It is strange that the neck-tie should be accorded such prominence in post-school society. It adorns the neck and constricts the throat of most contemporary executives and those whose professions, wealth or fashion incline them to wear a suit. Despite performing no obvious function, the tie steadfastly refuses to go the way of gaiters and bloomer straps, but merely contents itself to expand and contract in width according to the fashion of the time. Schools should be TIE schools. It is not suggested that there be a shift in dress code but rather that schools should be known as places that are:

- Thinking
- Individualised
- Energetic.

By thinking, it is advocated that schools consciously encourage students to develop their cognitive skills. Individualised schools are schools that find out how each child learns and adopts customised teaching strategies to optimise that learning. Energetic schools means energetic schools.

> I do not know what I may appear to the world, but to myself I seem to have been only a boy playing on the seashore, and diverting myself in now and then finding a smoother pebble or a prettier shell than ordinary, whilst the great ocean of truth lay all undiscovered before me.
> Isaac Newton

BOYS ARE DIFFERENT

Society has a habit of making generalisations and most of these generalisations are as unhelpful as they are inappropriate. 'Boys are bad at reading.' No they are not; some of the most able literary students in schools are boys. 'Boys love sport.' No they do not; some boys are not at all interested in sport and prefer other activities such as playing with the computer or making music. 'The Columbine High School massacre in April 1999 confirms that boys are toxic and out of control.' This is errant nonsense. Sommers reminds her readers that one boy, Seth Houy, used his body to protect a terrified girl from the bullets, and that Daniel Rohrbough died as he heroically held the door open to allow many children to escape.[17] There were boys on that tragic day who acted heroically and selflessly.

It is very tempting to treat all boys as the same. This simplifies the treatment. Give all boys the same dose of medicine. The reality is that no single formula can work in meeting the academic and pastoral needs of boys. The wonder of creation is in its diversity and complexity and evidence of this is to be found in boys.

Given the vast number of permutations of preferred learning styles in boys that can be influenced by variables such as personality, area of competence and hemisphericity of the brain, one can begin to understand that there is no simple answer as to how best to educate boys. Having noted this, the weight of research does seem to suggest that a fair proportion of boys prefer:

- structure
- closed tasks
- kinesthetic learning
- multi-sensory approaches to learning
- analytical tasks
- practical hands-on types of activities
- shorter tasks.

> Clever boys believe only half of what they hear.
> Wise boys know which half to believe.

ADD AND ADHD

It is sad that any treatise on school boys would be considered incomplete unless it were to tackle the issue of Attention Deficit Disorder (ADD) and Attention Deficit and Hyperactivity Disorder (ADHD). Both these terms have entered the educational lexicon with an impact which has been quite frightening. Large numbers of boys are being diagnosed with ADD or ADHD to the extent that psycho-stimulants and tricyclic anti-depressants are pouring millions of dollars into the pharmacology industry.

In the United States alone, the psycho-stimulant Ritalin is being used by between two and three million American boys. This represents a huge industry which seems to give no indication of contracting. There are many who doubt the wisdom or the appropriateness of using such drugs. The American therapist and educator, Michael Gurian, estimates that nearly two-thirds of those diagnosed with ADD or ADHD brain disorders have probably been misdiagnosed.[18] Gurian is not alone in his view that many children diagnosed with ADHD are perfectly fine from a neurological point of view.[19] It is sentiment such as this that has led to ADD being dubbed 'Another Dubious Diagnosis'.

Just when one is settling down to the task of the total denigration of the ADD and ADHD industry, one is tapped on the shoulder and shown the obvious presence of these types of neurological problems and the undeniable efficacy of many contemporary drugs in their treatment. ADD and ADHD do exist and can be treated well through the use of medication. To be able to advance the debate in a responsible manner some understanding is needed of ADD and ADHD.

Both ADD and ADHD seem to be a male problem, with by far the greatest proportion of those being diagnosed being adolescent and pre-adolescent boys. As the names suggest, ADD and ADHD both involve attention disorders, the inability to pay attention, and the ability to be easily distracted. There are chemicals in the brain, such as serotonin, that appear to have a calming effect, and which allow the brain to concentrate. A boy's brain often produces less serotonin and so some doctors seek to provide substitute chemicals to make up the deficit.

There are several dimensions to ADD including, but not limited to:

- **A cognitive dimension** — difficulty in understanding; inattention; finding it hard to remember data and difficulty in following routines. In other words the functions of being able to absorb, process and apply information are impaired.
- **A behavioural dimension** — inattention, fidgeting, squirming, restlessness, impulsiveness, interruptiveness and a tendency to distract others are features of this dimension.
- **An academic dimension** — problems with reading and spelling, difficulty remembering facts and things such as multiplication tables. Those affected in this dimension sometimes do the work in an incorrect manner due to failure to follow directions.
- **A social and emotional dimension** — frustration, depression, low self-esteem, moodiness, belligerence.

There are other dimensions, and not all the symptoms described above necessarily indicate an ADD or ADHD child. It should also be noted that some of these symptoms can be indicative of problems other than ADD or ADHD.

One of the key questions is where lies the boundary between normal exuberant boy behaviour and behaviour which is neurologically abnormal? Just when does a child need to be labelled as ADD or ADHD and given drugs, and just when does a child need to be reprimanded and given some firm discipline?[20] The problem is that this boundary is not always easy to see and an even greater problem is that there are some who do not want to be told where the boundary is lest they be told their child falls on the less desirable side.

Quite what the 'less desirable side' is can be debated. Some parents cannot wait to have their child diagnosed with ADD or ADHD for this will then win the child compensation in school — extra reading time in exams, extra help and extra pity. Other parents cannot wait to have their child diagnosed with ADD or ADHD as it then absolves them from any accusation that a child's poor behaviour is due to mediocre parenting and inadequate discipline within the home. Fortunately, most parents cannot wait to have their child diagnosed because they love the child and are keen to discover the cause of the child's problems so that an appropriate cure can be sought.

For other parents, the less desirable side is to have their child labelled ADD or ADHD. These parents are worried by ADD and ADHD labels and are concerned by the treatment offered when it comes in the form of powerful psycho-stimulants like Ritalin. These concerns are understandable but it is important that the legitimacy of ADD and ADHD be recognised, particularly for boys, as nearly 10 times as many boys are likely to be diagnosed with ADD as girls.

Why is it that so many boys are put on drugs to treat ADD and ADHD? The answer is complex and probably centres on some excellent marketing by the pharmacology industry. There is also the love of many parents that can cause a near neurosis to try to 'normalise' their son. To this must be added the joyous simplicity of treatment. Gone is the confrontation, the need for hours of corrective behaviour, the drudgery of discipline — just swallow this. Then there is the difference in knowledge about ADD and ADHD by those within the medical profession who range from the irresponsible and opportunistic to the hugely professional and well informed. Perhaps the main reason why so many boys are put on drugs like Ritalin is because the drug often works.

The bad name that is sometimes associated with treating ADD or ADHD with drugs comes from:

■ concerns over the possible creation of a drug-dependent child. These concerns are all the more understandable given the strength of some of the drugs;

■ concerns over the tragic effect of labels on a child resulting in them having to wear the ADD or ADHD label as a leper would carry his bell;

■ concerns over the giving of drugs to treat a condition which might be better treated another way;

■ concerns over there being no valid diagnosis, no definitive symptom for ADD or ADHD;

■ concerns that what is being labelled as pathological in fact falls well within the range of acceptable behaviours for a boy;

■ concerns that the root cause of the problem stems not so much from a neurological disorder but from a nurturing disorder.

Is ADD or ADHD a valid diagnosis? The answer to this question will vary depending on who is asked. Disorders of self-control are recognised by most doctors but whether they should be classified as ADD or ADHD is another matter.

Care must be taken not to expect Ritalin and other drugs associated with the treatment of ADD and ADHD to do things for which they were never designed. The drugs are not designed to help a boy who is intellectually challenged to become an Einstein. Nothing short of a cranial lobotomy is likely to achieve that and even that is doubtful. The drugs

AN ADD STORY

A wonderful story is told by Steve Biddulph in his book *Raising Boys*. Paraphrasing the tale somewhat, it begins with a dad being told his son had ADD. The father had not even heard of the term. In his business, which was truck driving, one did not come across such phrases. However, being intuitive, the father deduced that his son had a learning disorder caused by him not receiving enough attention. So he decided he could solve this problem by giving his son some extra attention.

Day after day, the dad would bring his son to school in the truck and pick him up in it. They would chat merrily away in the cab as the dad, driven by a love for his son and a desire to have this ADD thing beaten, gave his son a great deal of one-on-one attention. During the holidays they would ride off together in a great big pantechnicon and spend happy days travelling the roads together. Several months passed before the father was informed by a delighted school teacher that the ADD problem in his son had completely disappeared.

The question Biddulph leaves is obvious. Had the father, in his ignorance of the real meaning of ADD, stumbled upon the real cure for ADD?

Source: Biddulph, S, (1997), *Raising Boys*, Finch Publishing, Sydney, p 18.

---

are not designed to make the sociopath a serious contender for the citizenship award. The drugs are not designed to turn very ordinary progeny into dream children.

Having noted the above, it is quite defensible to diagnose ADD and ADHD and to treat this condition with drugs, but the following checks may be useful in ensuring that both diagnosis and treatment are appropriate.

Advice to parents on ADD and ADHD

■ Be careful to compare boys with boys rather than with girls. Many boys are naturally more easily distracted and given to forgetting books and wanting to play touch footy all the time.

■ Ensure the diagnosis is done properly. The doctor must see the child several times and obtain feedback from both his home and the school about the nature of the problem. In the USA the guidelines for diagnosis include:

- the symptoms being present before the child's seventh birthday
- the symptoms being present for over six months
- the symptoms being observed independently in the home and the school or in two other separate environments
- the symptoms causing serious social problems
- the symptoms not being traceable to other primary factors such as poor parenting, abuse, bullying, insecurity and so on.

- Drugs and their dosages should be 'customised' for each child to minimise unwanted side effects.
- Drugs should not necessarily be the first option in the treatment of ADD or ADHD.
- Drugs should only be used in combination with other therapies such as counselling and behaviour modification schemes.
- If drugs are administered, they should be very carefully monitored and administered by responsible adults. The black market in ADD and ADHD drugs is significant.

Quite apart from the above, other practical steps can be taken to help boys who may have ADD or ADHD including:

- minimise their distractions — study walls decorated with scantily clad young women is probably tempting fate in terms of keeping a boy focused on his homework. Desks in front of windows or mirrors are also high risk in this regard;
- improve consistency through routines;
- encourage meditation and calming activities;
- learn behaviour modification tricks. Even counting to 10 before saying or doing something can help;
- use practical methods to help, such as lists of things that must be in the school bag each day;
- encourage and give what is probably one of the most precious gifts an adult can give a child besides love, and that is time.[21]

ADDITIONAL BIBLIOGRAPHY

At the end of each chapter, there is a recording of the major references used in the chapter. However, there are a number of other worthwhile resources that deal with the issue of educating boys including some very useful Australian research. A list of these follows.

Alloway, N and Gilbert P (1997)	'Boys and literacy: Lessons from Australia'	*Gender and Education*, 9(1):49–58.
Arnold, R (1997)	*Raising levels of achievement in boys*	National Foundation for Educational Research, Slough, UK.
Arnot, M et al (1998)	'Recent research on gender and educational performance'	The Stationery Office, Office for Standards in Education:110, London.
Arnot, M et al (1999)	*Closing the Gender Gap: Post War Education and Social Change*	Polity Press, Oxford.
Blair, M, Holland, J et al (eds) (1995)	*Identity and Diversity: Gender and the Experience of Education*	Open University Press, Multilingual Matters Ltd, Clevedon, UK.

Bleach, K (ed) (1998)	*Raising Boys' Achievement in Schools*	Trentham Books, Stoke-on-Trent
Buckingham, J (2000)	Boy Troubles: Understanding Rising Suicide, Rising Crime and Rising Educational Failure	Policy Document, Sydney, Centre for Independent Studies, NSW.
Collins, C, Kenway, J and McLeod, J (2000)	Factors Influencing the Educational Performance of Males and Females in School and Their Initial Destinations After Leaving School	A project funded by the Commonwealth Department of Education, Training and Youth Affairs, Commonwealth of Australia.
Connell, R (1997)	'Teaching the boys: New research on masculinity, and gender strategies for schools'	*Teachers College Record*, 98(2):206–235.
Davies, B (1997)	'Critical literacy in practice: Language lesson for and about boys'	*Interpretations*, 30(2):36–57.
Epstein, D, Elwood, J et al, (eds) (1998)	*Failing Boys? Issues in Gender and Achievement*	Open University Press, Buckingham, Philadelphia
Fletcher, R, Hartman, D and Brown, R (eds) (1999)	*Leadership in boys' education: 16 case studies from public and private, rural and urban, primary and secondary schools*	The University of Newcastle, NSW.
Fletcher, R (1997)	*Improving boys' education: A manual for schools*	Family Action Centre, University of Newcastle, NSW.
Foster, V (1995)	*What about the boys!: Presumptive equality as the basis of policy in the education of girls and boys*	Social policy and the challenges of social change: proceedings of the National Social Policy Conference, Sydney, 5–7 July 1995, Volume 1. P Saunders and S Shaver, Sydney, University of New South Wales, Social Policy Research Centre (SPRC) (SPRC reports and proceedings n.122) Oct:81–87.
Frater, G (1997)	*Improving boys' literacy: A survey of effective practice in secondary schools*	The Basic Skills Agency, London.
Gilbert, P (1997)	'Gender and schooling in new times: The challenge of boys and literacy: The 1997 Radford Lecture'	*Australian Educational Research*, 25(1):15–36.
Gilbert, R and Gilbert, P (1998)	*Masculinity Goes to School*	Allen & Unwin, Sydney.
Kenway, J et al (1997)	*Answering Back: Girls, Boys and Feminism in Schools*	Allen & Unwin, Sydney.
Lillico, I (2000)	*Boys' Education*	Churchill Fellowship Report. City Beach High School, Kalinda Drive, City Beach, WA 6015.

MacDonald, A, Saunders, L and Benfield, P (1999)	*Boys' achievement, progress, motivation and participation: Issues raised by the recent literature*	National Foundation for Educational Research, Slough, UK (ISBN 0 7005 1543 7).
Martino, W (1994)	'Masculinity and learning: exploring boys' under-achievement and under-representation in subject English'	*Interpretations*, 27(2).
Martino, W (1999)	'"Cool boys", "party animals", "squids" and "poofters": Interrogating the dynamics and poiltics of adolescent masculinities in school'	*British Journal of the Sociology of Education*, 20(2).
Millard, E (1997)	*Differently Literate: Boys, Girls and the Schooling of Literacy*	The Falmer Press, London.
Mitchell, P (2000)	'Building capacity for working with boys at risk of depression and suicide'	*Conference Handbook: Teaching Boys*, Developing Fine Men Conference, Callaghan, NSW, Men and Boys Program, Family Action Centre, University of Newcastle, NSW pp 124–127.
O'Doherty, S (1994)	*Challenges and Opportunities: A Discussion Paper: Inquiry into Boys' Education*	A report to the Minister for Education, Training and Youth Affairs by the New South Wales Government Advisory Committee on Education, Training and Tourism, Sydney.
Power, S and Whitty, G et al (1998)	'Schoolboys and schoolwork: Gender identification and academic achievement'	*Journal of Inclusive Education*, Vol 2 (No 2) pp 134–153.
Robinson, P and Smithers, A (1999)	'Should the sexes be separated for secondary education? Comparisons of single-sex and co-educational schools'	*Research Papers in Education*, 14(1):23–49.
Rowe, K (1995)	'Factors affecting students' progress in reading: Key findings from a longitudinal study'	*Literacy, Teaching and Learning*, 1(2):57–110.
Rowe, K (2000a)	*'I hate school!' Addressing the emergent research evidence about the education and schooling of boys*	Invited keynote workshop presented at the National Student Welfare Conference 2000, Melbourne Exhibition and Convention Centre, 1–2 June 2000.
Rowe, K and Rowe, K (2000b)	*Inquiry Into the Education of Boys: Submission to the House of Representatives Standing Committee on Employment, Education and Workplace Relations*, Melbourne, MIMEO	This paper is available on the House of Representatives web site at: http://www.aph.gov.au/house/committee/eewr/Eofb/subs/sub111.pdf
Rowe, K and Rowe, K (2000c)	'Useful findings from research in literacy and numeracy teaching and learning for boys and girls'	*Conference Handbook: Teaching Boys*, Developing Fine Men Conference, Callaghan, NSW, Men and Boys Program, Family Action Centre, University of Newcastle, NSW, pp 82–92.

▶

Rowe, K (2000d)	Schooling Performances and Experiences of Males and Females: Exploring 'Real' Effects from Evidence-Based Research in Teacher and School Effectiveness	Background paper of invited discussant presentation for AIPS and DETYA Education Symposium, Eden on the Park Hotel, Melbourne, 22 November 2000.
Sukhnandan, L, Lee, B and Kelleher, S (2000)	An investigation into gender differences in achievement, Phase 2: School and classroom strategies	Berkshire, National Foundation for Educational Research (ISBN 0 7005 1551 8).
West, P (1998)	'Boys, sport and schooling: the popular debate and some recent research'	*Improving Outcomes in Boys' Education: Where to Now?*, The National Conference, Sydney.
West, P (1999)	'Boys' underachievement in school: Some persistent problems and some current research'	*Issues in Educational Research*, 9(1):33–54.

ADDITIONAL INFORMATION

For those wishing to have further details on some of the points raised in this chapter, the following references may be helpful. Each number in the text of the chapter relates to a reference number below which will give further information related to the topic.

1	Pollack, W (1998)	*Real Boys*	Owl Books, Henry Holt and Co., New York.
2	Kearney, S (2000)	'Teacher sexism a blow to boys'	*Sunday Telegraph*, 27/8/00, p 5.
3	Lees, I (2000)	'Killing our boys'	*Alive Magazine*, May 2000, p 57.
4	Editorial	'Girl power in the classroom'	*Sydney Morning Herald*, 23/12/99.
5	Rowe, K quoted in Kearney, S	(op cit)	
6	Buckingham, J quoted in Arndt, B (2000)	'The trouble with boys'	*Sydney Morning Herald*, 17/6/00, p 34.
7	VASSP (1996)	'Improving the school performance of boys'	An occasional paper produced by the Victorian Association of State Secondary Principals. State Education Office, Victoria.
8	West, P (1997)	'Class struggle epitomises the male identity crisis'	*Education Review*, 11/4/97.
9	Teese, R, Davies, M Charlton, M and Polesel, J (1995)	*Who Wins at School? Boys and Girls in Australian Secondary Education*	Department of Education, Policy and Management, University of Melbourne JS McMillan Printing Group.

10	Younger, M et al (1999)	'The gender gap and classroom interactions: Reality and rhetoric'	*British Journal of Sociology of Education*, Vol 20, Issue 3, September 1999, p 325.
11	Younger, M et al	(op cit)	p 327.
12	Goleman, D (1995)	*Emotional Intelligence*	Bloomsbury Publishing, London.
13	Kohn, A (1999)	*The Schools Our Children Deserve*	Houghton Mifflin Co., Boston.
14	Sommers, C H (2000)	*The War Against Boys*	Simon and Schuster, New York, p 161.
15	Sommers, C H	(op cit)	p 163.
16	Sommers, C H	(op cit)	p 199.
17	Sommers, C H	(op cit)	p 13.
18	Gurian, M (1999)	*A Fine Young Man*	Jeremy P Tarcher/Putnam, New York.
19	Gurian, M quoted in Newberger, E (1999)	*The Men They Will Become*	Bloomsbury Publishing, London, p 174.
20	Pollack, W (1992)	(op cit)	p 255.
21	Irvine, J (1992)	*Coping with School*	Simon and Schuster, Sydney.

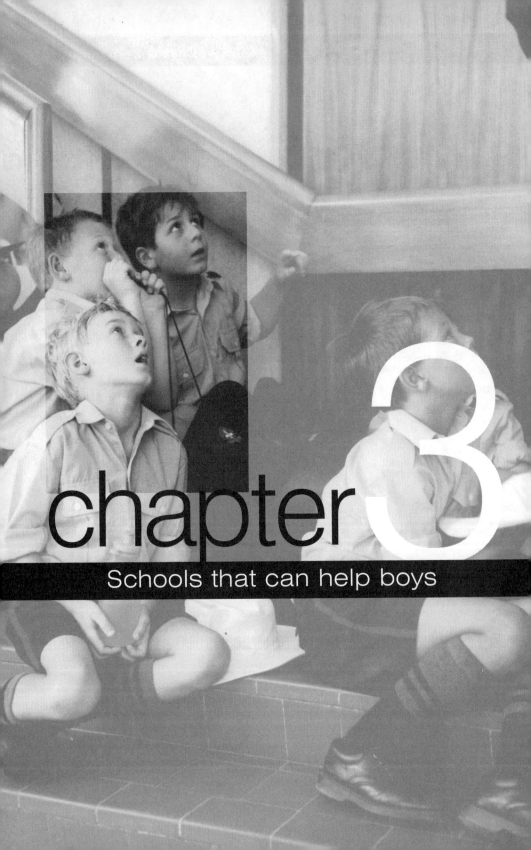

chapter 3

Schools that can help boys

INTRODUCTION

This chapter looks at how schools can fashion themselves to help meet the learning needs of boys. Issues relating to educational objectives, the curriculum, school policy and practice and learning climate are explored.

THE SCHOOL'S CULTURE

There is a 'Kulturkampf' on. A cultural war is being waged in schools. The warring factions are a tired and increasingly dispirited army of teachers who are taking on the audacious energy of an even greater number of young males. The war is over the value of current curriculum, the value of school and the value of learning. It is not quite clear who is winning the war. Every now and again some inspirational teachers take significant ground, but on the other flank teachers are bruised and in retreat to the common room bunker to anesthetise their pain with coffee and to plan their career conversion to bank teller.

Laborare orare (work is worship) may be chiselled into the school's gateway but there are not many worshippers. The secular culture has taken hold, but it is a culture devoid of any great narratives, resulting in a generation of boys who see learning as pointless. Too many boys do not know why they are learning or where learning will take them. These questions need to be answered before any other in the quest to get boys to learn in school.

An added problem is that of a culture of under-achievement by boys. Much has been written on the tendency of some adolescent girls to deliberately underperform in order not to shame their 'brain-dead' boy friends. It also needs to be recognised that many boys choose to underperform in order that they are not labelled a 'spock'. The frightening spectre of being a social pariah is such that some boys will do anything to be accepted by the herd and most herds amble at a speed that enables even the slowest to keep up.

Compounding the above is the thought in some boys that achievement in school and appreciation of school is a feminine characteristic and not a sentiment worthy of any self-respecting male. The boy culture of anti-intellectualism must be fought on many fronts. This chapter details a number of ways by which some ground might be taken in this battle.

THE SCHOOL'S LEARNING CLIMATE

If one wishes to stimulate learning within a school, conscious attention might need to be given to school design and architecture. There is a magic about many of the world's more famous schools, for their very architecture seems to elicit a predisposition to study. So schools should be designed to have a high degree of visual amenity which encourages students to want to learn. Synonymous with many schools, however, are characterless buildings that are high on utility and low on aesthetics. Some schools have bitumen playgrounds that grow battered litterbins and bent basketball hoops. They also grow resentment and a lack of respect for property, and ultimately people, and certainly for learning. Such vistas can encourage a mindless anonymity and a grey mediocrity where creativity is limited to the back of toilet doors. Schools should be designed to avoid signalling a lack of respect for learning.

Care might be needed to ensure that the academic focus of the school is not marginalised by the school's co-curricular program. A quick check in the school magazine can give a useful indication as to whether a school is celebrating curricular activities as much as co-curricular activities. Are as many academic colours awarded as sporting colours? There may well be merit in undertaking an audit of the 'learning climate' of one's school, and to consider such strategies as peer support and cross-age tutoring as well as peer mentoring programs. Boys are strongly influenced by peer pressure and the presence in the school of senior students who are reflective thinkers can be enormously useful in encouraging younger boys to be scholarly.

One of the most pernicious forces preventing higher academic performance in males is that of low expectations from parents, from teachers and from the boys themselves. The educational offering has been cut to the same height so all may graze on its pasture. The mantra of 'mean, median, mode' is heard all too frequently in schools. There is evidence of a growing lack of rigour in some schools, of a 'dumbing down' with expectations of boys that are minimal. Giving equal esteem to all states of the mind, the dull as well as the informed, is yielding very poor fruit. It would seem important that teachers be empowered to suggest that some academic standards are better than others and not be coerced into rewarding ordinary performance with extraordinary marks.

A quite astonishing blind spot with many child developmental theorists and educators is their preoccupation with the normal rather than the possible. Why shouldn't boys enjoy reading? Why shouldn't teachers expect the expression of feelings in boys? Why shouldn't it be fine for a boy to be gifted in an area? It is vital that there be no compromise in what teachers expect of boys while remembering that at all times there must also be compassion and an understanding that excellence can be expressed in many ways.

An example of a questionnaire that might be useful in finding out about the learning climate of a school is shown in Figure 3.1 on pages 49–50. The questionnaire is designed to be filled in by the student.

Figure 3.1 Learning climate review

NAME: **CLASS:**   **DATE:**

It is useful for a school to look at its learning climate from time to time in order to check whether there is a positive and supportive environment for study and academic achievement.

You are asked to record your responses to the questions below using the scale of responses provided.

Thank you for your input into this review. It is only when we have honest and mature feedback of this nature that we can continue to upgrade the quality of our educational offering.

| 6 Very effective | 5 Effective | 4 Slightly effective | 3 Slightly ineffective | 2 Ineffective | 1 Very ineffective |

To what extent do you believe your school has been effective in providing an environment in which:

1. Academically high achieving students are respected by their peers

2. Academically average students are respected by their peers

3. Academically low achieving students are respected by their peers

4. You feel comfortable asking a teacher for extra help with your work

5. You feel comfortable asking classmates for extra help with your work

6. You feel comfortable answering the teacher's questions in class

7. You feel comfortable sharing your ideas in class

8. You feel comfortable working on your own

9. You feel comfortable working in a group

10. You feel comfortable getting high grades for work

11. Good academic performance is recognised by the school and valued

12. Academic improvement is recognised by the school and valued

13. Academic effort is recognised by the school and valued

14. Classrooms are good learning environments

15. Common rooms/prep rooms are good learning environments

16. The library/study centre/computer room are good learning environments

17. Critical and reflective thinking is encouraged

18. Creative thinking and problem solving are encouraged

19. You find class work interesting

▶

20. You find class work is set at the right level of difficulty ☐

21. You find homework rewarding ☐

22. You find homework is set at the right level of difficulty ☐

23. You are given regular feedback on academic performance ☐

24. Students are proud of their school's academic reputation ☐

25. If there was one piece of advice you would like to give on how your school might improve its learning climate, what would it be?

Back to basics movement

Demands for greater academic discipline in boys has come from the 'back to basics' movement. However, the simple retreat to the past is not the answer. If one went to see the Moscow Circus in the late 1990s, one would have seen a 100 kilogram Russian bear driving a motorbike and Yuri Malinkovich doing back flips from a spring board wearing two and a half metre stilts. Neither of these acts had been seen in previous years and so the audience was enthralled and wondered what exciting acts would be presented when the circus visited next.

Just as the Moscow Circus needs new acts for its survival as an entertainment venture, society needs new thinking to survive the problems that threaten to destroy it. It is critical that schools encourage this new thinking and allow students to experiment with new acts above a safety net of love and acceptance. The 'back to basics' movement is worrying. Schools cannot just put on the old acts again. Patrons will be slumped on their benches and muttering 'been there, seen that', stifling yawns and dozing quietly on a cushion of corn chips and fairy floss. Literacy and numeracy must be encouraged in schools, just as a circus must encourage daring and skill in its program. But schools must not be seduced into merely turning the clock back. Society has moved from an industrial society with its accent on factory productivity, to a post-industrial age which is characterised by information storage and retrieval. Students need knowledge but they do not need to have their minds stuffed with anachronistic, encyclopedic knowledge. Society needs students who can use knowledge to create new acts through critical and creative thinking.

Some educational commentators like Alfie Kohn question whether the traditional style of teaching has served children well.[1] This is a brave line of questioning when nostalgia is so popular and a 'back to basics' push is in full swing. Nonetheless these claims are worth investigating, particularly from the point of view of trying to find out how best to educate boys. It could well be that the student docility that characterises the 'chalk and talk' approach to learning may be particularly ineffective with boys. The push for tougher standards in schools often sees a return to traditional teaching methods with its accent on filling students up to an acceptable level of factual knowledge. All too often learning options are limited to one source — the teacher — and a premium is placed on memory, literacy and passivity.

Boys are not good at being inert. What some teachers prize most is docility and obedience. Control is the name of the teaching game and the child who obliges through good behaviour is the child who is thought to have good character. In truth, the compliance in all things by some children can hint at a marked lack of creativity and self-confidence. Chaos can be creative, and significant learning can come via peers rather than the teacher. Schools might encourage individualism but society encourages teamwork and cooperative work skills. Brittle teaching styles need to become bygone teaching styles and tolerance given in the classroom to some creative noise and movement.

A well governed people are generally a people who do not think much.
André Siegfried, 1920

Tasks given to boys by teachers can be made more effective in terms of their educational value if they involve the solving of a problem which is seen by boys as deserving to be solved. Kohn gives an example of how the physics related to heat conduction might be taught with a little more meaning by getting boys to design a food container that will keep food hot when being delivered.[2] This is practical, hands on, interesting and impossible to complete without gaining some appreciation for the physics associated with heat transfer. These are the sorts of learning experiences which appeal to most boys.

Docility and inactivity are not generally recognised as strengths in boys, and thus initiatives to turn the clock back in the classroom may need to be viewed with caution if that classroom is full of boys. Although all children need firm boundaries, these boundaries should not enforce passivity. For learning to be effective, the student must engage with what is being taught and effective engagement often reveals itself in noise, excitement and movement — traits that are often associated with boys.

Making learning fun

Is the answer to make lessons more interesting for boys, to introduce action and a great deal of kinesthetic learning? Many educators would suggest so. An innovative program at Donvale Christian School in Victoria has boys getting involved in physical activities which are not just limited to sport, but which are extended to looking after the 'chooks' and tending the gardens. Boys enjoy these activities and learning becomes fun.

Yet the question should be asked, should learning always be fun? There are boys who can cope with academic rigour without the need for fun and frolics. It could be argued that the 'it must be made fun for boys' approach is demeaning and fails to realise that most learning is not necessarily fun. The fun element is only realised when certain levels of proficiency are attained and this attainment is usually only possible by dint of hard work and sober hours spent in the close company of teachers and books. Humour is to be recommended when teaching and even some fun, but the sense should never be engendered that the only learning one can reasonably expect from a boy is learning which comes from puppet choirs, two metre chickens and musical jingles.

The answer lies somewhere between the two extremes. There needs to be enough fun within the total learning experience to encourage an attraction to school but not so much commitment to entertainment that the integrity of the learning experience is lost. Instead of making schools places that pander to the incessant demand for making learning fun, boys need to be paid the compliment that they have the capacity to cope with the learning situation without having to rely on 'infotainment'. There is also a need to ensure that boys do not lose the value of working towards a deferred reward. In this age of instant gratification there may be merit in upholding the truth that the great and worthy things of life are seldom achieved without significant sacrifice.[3]

Some laughter is good and happy children should be a feature of schools. What makes for happiness is not always a romp with the chooks, it can be the quiet glow of satisfaction which comes from mastering a skill and in doing well in an arduous academic task.

Care needs to be taken to ensure that the whiff of authoritarianism in the educational breezes does not become overpowering. Allan Bloom's book *The Closing of the American Mind* (1988, Pocket Books, UK) has sold well and combines with a number of other books that dare to run counter to the climate of political correctness and suggest it is necessary to introduce rather more accountability in our schools.

American universities are offering courses in 'The pleasure horse: Appreciation and use'. One should not necessarily have anything against the pleasure horse, or indeed the informal and enjoyable learning opportunities available to students provided that there is some serious study and academic rigour to be found somewhere in the educational experience. One can empathise with educators who condemn contemporary curriculum in many schools as saccharine and shallow.

Not every learning exercise can be made fun — and nor should it — for then a student would never learn to cope with rigour, to build self-discipline or to realise that all that is good in this world is not necessarily decorated in seven minutes of song and dance between generous commercial breaks.

THE SCHOOL'S MISSION AND PURPOSE

Knowing where you are going and why

Alice, while wandering in Wonderland, didn't quite know where to go, so she asked the Cheshire Cat. The cat thought a little and then suggested that it all rather depended on where Alice wanted to go. Alice confessed she didn't much care where she was going which prompted the Cheshire Cat to conclude that it, therefore, didn't matter which way Alice went. Alice was protected from the realities of not knowing where she was going by the benevolent pen of Lewis Carroll. Boys, on the other hand, are classified under biographies rather than fiction and are not afforded the security of not knowing where they are going.

If teachers and parents want to help boys to learn, then they had better brace themselves for the inevitable response 'Why?' Why should a boy go to school? Why should a boy learn? It seems such an obvious question yet it is alarming that many adults do not actually have a coherent, let alone persuasive, answer. Boys are rather pragmatic and need to be persuaded of the worth of a thing before they will commit themselves to it. For this reason, parents and teachers might need to think through a response as to why it is they want boys to learn.

The most common answers given to the 'Why should I learn?' question tend to fall into one of the following categories:

■ 'it's an investment' response
■ 'it's good fun' response
■ 'because I told you' response.

All of these answers have their place and their effectiveness will depend on the oratory and reasoning skills of the apologist. The investment response works well with those boys who have the emotional quotient necessary to be able to work for a deferred reward. They will accept that learning is necessary if they wish to prepare themselves for future employment, for the acquisition of great wealth and the capacity to float around Sydney Harbour in a well appointed ship lighting cigars with smouldering $20 notes.

The 'building block' argument is often advanced as part of the investment response, with adults suggesting to boys that learning increases the capacity to learn. However, this response is usually only a stalling tactic, for the question 'Why?' will almost certainly reappear when the next building block is put in place.

Another variation to the investment response is 'because it is good for you'. This response is all well and good but it probably will require the adult to know what is good about knowing the name of the highest mountain in Africa and the physics of the light refracting qualities of a prism. If teachers are not able to answer these questions beyond the ultimate defence 'because it's in the exam' then they themselves need to question the value of what they are doing. The investment response is a valid response but it needs some thought and a raison d'être needs to be worked out for each subject area.

The 'it's good fun' response to 'Why should I learn?' may take some selling if a boy is patently not finding the learning experience much fun. Teachers can talk about the sense of achievement, the satisfaction there is in developing one's skills and knowledge base. However, not every boy staggers from the stage on speech night under the weight of prizes embossed with the school crest. For many boys, school has been little else than an affirmation of their inadequacies. For this reason, the 'it's good fun' response is only likely to work with the successful student and that is the very student who is least likely to be troubling his teachers with the question 'Why should I learn?'

The last resort for many adults is the 'because I told you to, that's why, so get on with it and stop your whinging' response. It's not subtle, but it can work. The response, quite understandably, has its critics. Blind obedience is not a popular virtue these days and proponents of this approach are very likely to be lectured on the effectiveness of intrinsic (internal) motivation over the limitations of extrinsic (external) motivation.

While the 'I told you so' response is one which should not be relied upon exclusively, there may be virtue, on the odd occasion, in telling a boy 'I know you may not like learning at the moment. I am going to ask you to continue with it because I am confident there are rewards that will come. Let's get on with it and find out what these rewards might be.'

If pressed to articulate what these rewards might be, the following provides some indication of the sort of responses that might be considered:

■ Most of us have a natural curiosity that makes us want to find out about things. Learning at school can help us to find answers to questions we might have, or should have, about life.

■ Learning is the fulfilment of our ultimate design. We are made by God and given gifts which we should develop to honour God and to serve humankind.

■ Learning is socially responsible. If we are ignorant, we can harm ourselves and others and not be in a good position to pass on to our children the lessons which will keep them happy and healthy.

■ Learning gives us skills that are needed by society. Each member of society has an obligation to contribute to the well-being of that society by offering skills and services which are useful.

Knowing where a boy should be going with his learning is probably only slightly easier to answer than why a boy should learn. Opinions will vary greatly, but the following represents the sort of educational goals which might be considered appropriate for boys.

An example of educational goals that could be set for boys

We have academic goals to encourage boys to:

■ realise their academic potential

■ develop a sense of wonder, a love of learning, and a respect for ability

■ be lifelong learners who can work productively both individually and collaboratively

■ be able to solve problems and be critical and creative thinkers

■ cope with the lifelong challenge of managing change

■ use modern technology effectively and wisely

■ communicate well in spoken, written, non-verbal and electronic form

■ plan responsibly and be able to collect, evaluate and organise information

■ take responsibility for their own learning

■ develop an international perspective.

We have spiritual goals to encourage boys to:

■ develop knowledge of their own faith and their own God

■ reflect on the spiritual dimension of life and on how this dimension might enrich their lives

■ grow in their understanding of other religions

■ engage in reflection and meditation on spiritual truths

- develop an informed conscience and purpose
- explore ethical issues and adopt worthy values.

We have social and emotional goals to encourage boys to:

- grow in character within a community that seeks to promote faith, hope, compassion and service to others
- promote and enact values which edify and enrich both the individual and the community
- develop leadership skills so that students are empowered and encouraged to contribute to society as responsible servants
- respect personal differences in others irrespective of sex, age, ability, appearance, culture or socio-economic situation
- develop pro-social skills and social maturity
- know, desire and do good
- respond appropriately to verbal and non-verbal communication
- operate effectively as a member of a team
- respect both their own and other people's property
- respect the law and the rights of others
- be empathetic, kind, courteous and well mannered
- be prepared to accept the accountability which comes from taking on responsibility
- form friendships and have the capacity to develop meaningful relationships
- have an appropriate sense of self-esteem
- develop acceptable mechanisms for dealing with anger and anxiety
- appreciate beauty in its many manifestations
- abhor bullying and seek to eradicate it when found.

We have physical well-being goals to encourage boys to:

- understand the links between the physical, social, emotional, academic and spiritual elements of their life
- know and desire the habits of a health promoting lifestyle
- seek that which promotes physical well-being
- exercise and work appropriately
- eat, be involved in recreation and rest in a responsible manner
- enjoy and develop skills in sport
- enhance personal fitness
- obtain an appropriate balance in life
- avoid addictions.

WHAT STUDENTS AND TEACHERS SHOULD KNOW AND DO

In 1999, the Center for Development in New Orleans held a number of public forums and set up a 31-member think tank to consider:

- what students should know and do
- what teachers should know and do.

Their conclusions were as follows.

What students should know and do:

- communicate effectively
- solve problems creatively
- master a defined body of knowledge
- commit to lifelong learning
- understand how they learn
- plan their lives skillfully
- achieve interpersonal and intrapersonal success
- exhibit global citizenship.

What teachers should know and do:

- provide a moral compass
- communicate effectively
- love teaching
- understand how students learn
- foster creative problem solving
- master a body of knowledge
- make the classroom a learning community
- commit to lifelong learning
- achieve interpersonal success and strong collegial ties
- create an effective community presence
- exhibit global citizenship.[4]

A NEW CURRICULUM

Some years ago, I started developing a vague sense of unease about the current curriculum being offered in schools. This sprung from watching the light of enthusiasm in the eyes of children slowly dimming as they progressed into secondary school. I also saw too much evidence of work being given to keep students busy, rather than to keep them learning. Added to this was a growing tiredness of dancing to a tune played by tertiary institutions. These institutions seemed to be orchestrating the agenda in schools in a way which was discordant with my own views on education, for the tertiary sector seemed less interested in preparing students for life and more interested in preparing students for university.

▶

Perhaps my strongest concerns came from the mounting evidence that too many students, in too many schools, seemed bored.

Now we need to be a little careful here for I do not see my charter as one to entertain, but rather to educate. I would also want to remind the 'add water and mix' age, that some of the more worthy achievements in life must be paid for by hours of uninspiring toil, with just our dreams to urge us on. But there is the trick you see, they must be **our** dreams — not our teachers' dreams, or our parents' dreams — but **ours**. Schools must seek to be full of the stuff our students' dreams are made of.

The Greeks had only one faculty and it was the Faculty of Wonder. I found this to be an inspirational thought which led me to the dangerous idea of scrapping the existing curriculum and replacing what we teach with at least six new faculties of which one would be the Faculty of Wonder.

It seems to me that a Faculty of Wonder has the learning sequence right, that is, create the wonder to effect the learning. All too often we try to effect the learning to create the wonder and I don't know if this is so effective. There is little in this world more dispiriting than spending all our time in schools painstakingly answering questions our students are not asking. Thus it was that I began suggesting a total rethink of the curriculum — one which would radically restructure learning in schools. As George Bernard Shaw stated, 'What we want to see is the child in pursuit of knowledge and not knowledge in pursuit of the child'.

My second faculty would be the Faculty of Communication. Yes, it would accommodate the hardy annals of literature and language that bloom both in foreign and native fields but I would seek more. I would seek the study of body language, of voice tone, gesture, symbol and the language of behaviour. Why is it that when body language can be a stronger form of communication than written or verbal communication, we ignore the learning of it in our schools? Interpreting mood, sensing another's meaning and intent — these contribute greatly to emotional and social maturity. Even the language of prayer can be taught. The Old Testament saints talked to God and they read God's reply in nature, circumstance, scripture and sound. We don't, we have lost the art. Then, of course, there is the new language of technology. Are we in control, or does this technology control us?

Another faculty would be the Faculty of Relationships — not just between people — but between us and the natural world. Do we own the world, or does the world own us? We are only dimly aware of the vital relationship that exists in human health and environmental health, between human beauty and natural beauty. Much of the breakdown in the civilised world is due to a lack of connectedness, of failing to see ourselves belonging in relationship with others, with nature and with God. Perhaps one of our most neglected relationships is with ourselves, the result of which has seen Australia having one of the highest teenage suicide rates in the world.

Other faculties that I would consider include the Faculties of Creativity and Problem Solving. Knowing things is becoming less important than knowing what to do with the things we know. Filling minds with knowledge has its merits, but there is greater merit in being able to use that knowledge to solve a problem or create a means of allowing us to acquire more knowledge. Given that information is expanding so rapidly, learning information is now less important than learning how to learn and training ourselves for a lifelong adventure in learning.

Ethics too, is a faculty I would introduce, for I believe that we are in an age of real moral ambivalence, for the absolutes of spiritual decree have gone and been replaced, at best, by situational ethics and, at worst, by nothing. There is a need to consider what should be valued and what should not. Valuing too little leads to black despair and nihilism. Valuing too much is naive. Valuing values is essential for any society that wishes to consider itself civilised.

I am sure that there are other faculties we should consider just as I must acknowledge that lurking within our existing curriculum are many of the sentiments described above. However, I would certainly list Wonder, Creativity, Problem Solving, Communication, Ethics and Relationships as among my Key Learning Areas.

What would you include in your curriculum for schools?

Source: Hawkes, T F, *Newslink*, St Leonard's College, Melbourne, 25 July 1997.

The middle school option

It is entirely possible that some success in meeting the needs of boys can be found through the establishment of middle school programs. Some countries have middle schools but many do not. A middle school involves the setting up of a discrete school for students aged somewhere between Years 5 and 10. There are many different permutations. Some schools have established middle schools to cater for students in Years 7 to 10. Others have sought to blur the transition from primary to secondary school and established middle schools ranging from Year 5 through to Year 9.

The establishment of a middle school can set up an environment which is oriented to meeting the needs of students at this age. The requirements of students of middle school age are unique, particularly in Years 7 and 9. These are the two years where referrals to those specialising in the treatment of learning difficulties appear to be at its greatest. Year 7 is a transition year from primary to secondary school. Quite apart from the insecurity related to changing school, there is the need to adjust to subject-based teaching after having been used to class-based teaching. Often the move is associated with the comparison of the student with a larger body of students and this can help diagnose learning difficulties. Year 9 marks a peak in students testing the boundaries and seeking independence. There can also be an expression of adolescent insecurity which can drive both teacher and parent to distraction.[5]

The establishing of a middle school can benefit children in at least two ways. First, a middle school can foster the knowledge necessary to meet the unique needs of children of middle school age. This ability to specialise may well mean that a middle school can put in place policies and practices which are particularly focused on the pre-adolescent and adolescent child. Typically it is in the middle school years where a boy begins to take on the characteristics of a man. It is a time of growing independence, a time of rebellion against authority figures and the testing of boundaries. It is a time of growing sexual awareness and self-consciousness about body shape and size. There are insecurities at this age and significant changes in body chemistry. The potential for emotional hurt is great. An effective middle school with staff training in how best to nurture specific needs of boys this age may be effective in reducing the potential for emotional and social hurt as well as increasing academic effectiveness.

The second way a middle school can help students is by smoothing the transition from primary to secondary school by putting in place an intermediate school structure with something of the character of both a primary and secondary school. The increased use of specialist teachers in the middle school can prepare students for a complete move to subject-based teaching when they move to senior school. Leadership opportunities can also be provided for the senior students in the middle school. A smaller learning environment can be created which can lead to more effective pastoral care and a stronger sense of identity within the school. For these reasons, a middle school structure can be effective in meeting the needs of boys from about 10 to 15 years of age.

A later starting age in schools

It is suggested by Steve Biddulph that because young boys are less well developed in the area of their fine motor and cognitive skills when they start school that consideration should be given to starting boys later at school. This delay might allow for greater maturation and could make the schooling experience a more positive one.[6]

This advice may well be sound, particularly as it is made clear by Biddulph that this should not be a blanket ruling for all boys. However, some clear and honest thinking is required as to what to do with boys when they are awaiting the cognitive 'readiness' to start school. The ticking of the clock is not the only variable influencing school readiness. The preschool boy, if not given a daily regime of love, nurturing and stimulating learning, may never be ready for school. If a boy is not going to school, alternative activities will need to be provided to cause the boy to become ready for school.

Single sex schools

The debate as to which form of schooling — co-educational or single sex — is best for boys is a debate that is probably unwinnable, and thankfully so. That is because some boys will do better in a single sex environment and others in a co-educational environment. It should also be pointed out that there is no magic or guarantee given to students because of the absence or presence of children from the other sex in their school. There are other more significant variables such as teacher quality and climate of a school which impacts on the quality of the learning experience. There are good co-educational schools and bad ones. There are good single sex schools and bad ones. It is the job of the discerning parent to find the good school as their first priority and then consider other factors such as its gender make up as one of a series of secondary priorities.

Having noted the above, there are some persuasive studies that would suggest that many boys fare better in a boys' school. The Cotswold Experiment in Leicestershire, England is reported by Biddulph. This involved a co-educational school moving to single sex classes in English with the result that the number of boys in the high scoring range of English increased by 400%.[7] It is suggested that the boys-only class allowed the teacher to focus on boys' weaknesses in literacy such as language acquisition and to encourage boys not to play the fool in front of girls to cover up their inadequacies.

It does seem a pity that in the public as well as the private sector of education the declining number of single sex schools may be resulting in a society that has closed a very important option for some children. The American educational commentator Ruhlman questions whether the lack of schooling choice in America is really serving its country well.[8] The fact that few, if any, all-boys government schools are allowed is something that Ruhlman finds regrettable. This regret is fuelled by the conclusions reached by Cornelius Riordan who, in his book *Girls and Boys in School: Together or Separate*, suggests that the scales tip in favour of single sex schools. On the other hand, there are those who argue that 'it is important not to over-interpret the "importance" of these gender and gender/class/school-grouping effects since they pale into insignificance compared with class/teacher effects — regardless of student gender' (Rowe, K J [2000], see reference in Figure 3.2).

There is a need to be careful of tipping scales for it all depends on what is being weighed and by whom. It should also be pointed out that gifted teachers who have the knack of meeting the individual needs of

Figure 3.2 Plot of mean 'ability-adjusted' VCE scores for four gender/school/class groupings of students (1994–1999)

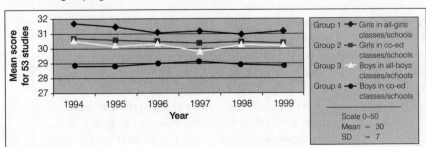

Source: This research, involving about 270 000 students, was based on the VCE scores in 53 subjects with the largest candidature drawn from 600 VCE providers. The study is reported in Rowe, K J (2000), 'Schooling performances and experiences of males and females: Exploring "real" effects from evidence-based research in teacher and school effectiveness', a background paper to invited discussant presentation for the Australian Institute of Political Science and the Department of Education, Training and Youth Affairs Education Symposium, Eden on the Park Hotel, Melbourne, 22–23 November 2000.

their students, will have the capacity to meet the needs of boys as well as girls in their class. This can, therefore, make the gender debate irrelevant . . . except, of course, not all teachers are gifted.

If boys tend to be more disruptive in class, to act the class clown, to soak up huge amounts of the teacher's time and to divert the teacher's energy to discipline issues rather than learning, then there might be merit in addressing teacher training before considering wholesale school changes such as converting to single sex education. Teachers need to recognise the truth in Biddulph's observation that boys ask for help in a different way from girls. Boys will act for help whereas girls will ask for help.[9]

Parents should be given the choice between single sex education for their sons or a co-educational environment. The question is not so much whether single sex or co-education is better, but whether parents are being given adequate choices in the matter.

Exercise

There are indications that obesity is on the increase among boys and this can be attributed to inappropriate diet and a lessening in the amount of exercise. Being a 'couch potato' can have an adverse affect on learning. There is some truth in the sayings 'the fitter the legs, the clearer the brain' and 'the prerequisite of a healthy mind is an active, healthy body'. Regular exercise in non-excessive amounts has been shown to stimulate the mind and to assist learning. Physical exercise can improve mental performance in three ways. Five to 10 minutes of exercise can give an immediate short-term improvement to mental performance which may last up to one hour. A slightly longer period of help with learning lasting about a day can occur when a student has an active lunch hour rather than a sedentary one.[10] The third is a long-term effect when mental performance is improved through a daily regime of physical activity. Physical activity should be a part of a boy's educational program but care should be taken that it does not become obsessive.

Use of music to enhance learning

When Congreve wrote 'music has charms to soothe a savage breast' he may have only been stating the half of it, for there is some evidence to suggest that listening to music while one works can actually assist the cognitive process. This has become known as 'The Mozart Effect' with the original researchers, Shaw and Rauscher, showing that there was a slight improvement in spatial-temporal reasoning after students listened to a few minutes of Mozart. Alex Messine writing in the *Age* on page 7, 29 September 1995, reported on the research being undertaken by Rauscher who found that young children regularly playing a keyboard instrument could boost their intelligence by an average of 47%. Rauscher also found that listening to a Mozart sonata for 10 minutes would cause a similar increase in IQ but the effect was more short term.

The National Commission on Music Education in the USA in its publication *Growing Up Complete* suggests that children need sentiments and sensibilities to enable them to be fully human, and that appropriate music can help in this regard. It is also suggested that music can help children understand and use symbols and assist in developing their problem-solving skills and their ability to understand a number of mathematical concepts.

It is important not to sensationalise these findings, for listening to a few minutes of Mozart is unlikely to rescue a boy who has not revised for an exam. However studies have shown that music training can enhance memory, and that long-term music instruction can have a very positive impact on learning and intelligence. What is also being noted is that Mozart is not the only music to enhance learning but that many kinds of music can serve this purpose.

Parents might be well advised to encourage their sons to take up a musical instrument, but this should only happen if the child has a predisposition towards wanting to play a musical instrument, otherwise the experience could become counter productive.

At a small Roman Catholic school in Kingston, Jamaica, a rich and innovate music program has been introduced which has had a very positive impact on boys. Alpha Boys School regularly invited local musicians, most of them male, to perform to the boys and to conduct music workshops with them. The boys in the program did not just experience music, but also friendship and some positive role modelling. Boys who would otherwise be on the street and into crime were making music instead. It took the example of a small island nation to remind the larger developed continents that music plus a little kindness can work wonders.[11]

Information technology, literacy and learning

Some schools are investing heavily in information technology (IT) equipment, with computers in some form or another becoming a standard fixture in many classrooms. Does the computer represent the death knell of literacy and the marginalisation of handwriting skills? With voice recognition now a feature on some computers, is there even a need to learn to write at all? What are the implications of the advent of this new technology for teaching boys?

Writing is a life skill which is likely to remain important in the foreseeable future. Reading is even more of a basic life skill for it impinges directly on matters such as safety and survival, quite apart from the ability to absorb the recorded knowledge stored in printed form for thousands of years.

Having noted the importance of retaining writing skills, the increased use of IT in schools represents a significant learning opportunity for boys, for many boys are captivated by modern technology and enjoy using computers.

Contemporary software allows boys to present written work in a legible form and gives them immediate 'conferencing' of their written work by informing them if a word is not spelt correctly or if the punctuation is wrong. This form of feedback can be greatly beneficial to boys whose handwriting can be poor and their spelling even more so. For this reason boys can be better motivated to hand in written work when it has been done using a word processor.

Computers not only exercise literacy skills, they can also allow a student to integrate graphics into their work. Multi-media presentations are possible and this can be particularly appealing to boys who tend to enjoy graphics. It should also be remembered that the vast amount of information made available to students means that information acquisition is now no longer the challenge, but rather it is the synthesis of that information that is the challenge. This means that the use of IT can assist boys to move away from minds filled with knowledge with a limited shelf life, to minds which are adept at critical and creative thinking.

Boys like machines, boys like graphics, boys like independence, and boys like new and interesting things. All these qualities coalesce with the computer. There is the 'fiddle factor'. Boys like to be able to change and

WRITING

Writing — do you remember when we had to do it, when the application of pen on paper could affect the communication of ideas, facts, opinion and foster creative thought? It is, of course, an art form that seems inexorably destined to join the pogo stick and mobile bathing box as the quaint practice of a bygone era. But perhaps we should not yet confine writing thus, but seek to promote the written word.

Now, I know that this will be difficult, for writers have ranged against them an awesome arsenal of micro-chipped wizardry that threatens to annihilate our need to write. For example, the ubiquitous telephone has been granted such a presence in our lives that, being now unfettered by cords, it can invade the most inappropriate and intimate of moments and cause us to no longer need to communicate by written word.

I would like to suggest that the omnipresent television is diverting many from writing. The laborious action of pushing pen over paper is abandoned as we become passive receptors, turned on by a coloured screen. We like to watch, and to brave the jungle of turgid soapies, quiz shows filled with white teeth and serials about American families with dreadful children and unlikely parents. We like to hear the warnings every nine minutes that we may be irresponsibly deficient for having failed to purchase the latest irresistible, labour saving, washes whiter, limited season only, low calorie, at a store near you, commercial or domestic knick-knack.

I am here to suggest that despite all, writing has much to commend it and that the written word can well be worth the reading. I point out that the book is remarkably easy to transport and needs no power source other than the imagination, energy and knowledge of its author. I also point out that the writer is remarkably privileged for he or she is able to achieve a certain immortality by placing prose or poetry permanently on paper free of any bugs and viruses except, perhaps, the silverfish. The reading of written material can also be a remarkable experience for it can be a window into the soul of an author, whose values are portrayed and betrayed in their writing. Writing can also be a catharsis. There is little which is more satisfying than a good 'literary sneeze'.

Source: Hawkes, T F, *The King's Herald*, The King's School, Parramatta, 5 November 1998.

manipulate things on a computer. Self-esteem can be enhanced through self-paced learning which the computer allows.

The embarrassment of having appalling handwriting and poor spelling is ameliorated by an automatic spell check and a range of font options to please the most fastidious of teachers. Even lack of artistic flair can be solved thanks to clip art and a variety of other graphics programs. Rewrites are easy as is the whole editing process, resulting in work of which the boy can be proud.

Using computers allows not only self-paced learning but also collaborative learning. The scrum of boys that can easily form around a computer provides an excellent opportunity for group learning to occur, with enhanced student interaction being encouraged.

Computers also provide flexible learning hours, access to vast amounts of information and can engage a boy's attention in a manner often not possible through other avenues of instruction. There is an activity-based element to the use of computers which can be particularly attractive to boys.

Other points which might be borne in mind as advantages in boys using computers include the interactive capacity of the computer and the possibility of chat lines and correspondence with those outside the classroom to help with learning. Of course, there are real risks of abuse and very clear guidelines need to be given to boys, together with the use of some structures such as web filters.

Computers can give students huge amounts of information. Boys using computers tend to learn quite quickly that the esteem given to the amount of information a student gives a teacher is now significantly diminished. What teachers seem far more interested in is the quality of the information and the appropriate use of information to solve a problem. This ushers in a need for a boy to engage in analysis and synthesis and a whole range of higher order thinking tasks which can appeal somewhat more to boys than the mere reproduction of screeds of information.

Computers are not the educational panacea for boys. It is important not only to know what computers can do, but also what computers cannot do and to discover the virtues of the 'off' button.

SCHOOLS THAT GIVE FEEDBACK

All children need feedback but boys, in particular, seem to need regular feedback for they can develop unrealistic understandings about the quality of their work. Given that boys tend to judge their performance is against those of other boys rather than against the teacher's mark scheme, a shift towards 'criterion' referencing as opposed to 'norm' referencing can be useful. The school administration must ensure that feedback is given, not just in terms of school reports, but also through the use of regular reviews and evaluations. Parent-teacher evenings can also be redesigned to include the presence of the boy.

Feedback which is regular, and which is given soon after the completion of the task, is most effective in contributing to a boy's learning.

The concept of report cards being used as part of the feedback process is not new, but what might warrant some consideration is the idea of boys writing their own reports. Before this suggestion is met with enthusiastic

SCHOOL REPORTS

It's school report time for some of our students. School reports bring a spectre of accountability which is not always welcome. True, there will be some whose school report is a joyous affirmation of ability and application. However, for those of us who are rather more fallible, the news is usually mixed. This requires some thoughtful stratagems when the reports are presented.

To appease the disgruntled teacher, the student might try 'You will find that this report is a true reflection of your teaching skills'.

To appease the disgruntled parent, try 'Everyone thinks I am just like my parents' . . . and then try to steer them as quickly as possible to the encouraging comment made by the sports coach, if there is one.

Reports will generally cause fathers to think whether the grades were worth moving to another school, mothers to think whether the grades warrant tutorial assistance and students to think whether the grades are worth renegotiating one's pocket money.

Reports enshrine the principle of accountability. This principle has been present in religious thought, schools and society for thousands of years, but this does not mean that we necessarily like it — indeed, we appear to be in an age that deplores the concept of accountability. 'It wasn't my fault . . . I suffer from middle child syndrome . . . I was born a Pisces . . . I was dropped on my head as a baby.'

Even teachers when writing reports do not enjoy being the purveyors of bad news and thus any hint by them of inadequacy in the report needs to be taken fairly seriously by parents. The comment 'he has grown older this term' needs to be interpreted as a fairly damning indictment. 'He has made satisfactory progress' can sometimes mean the student has hidden himself successfully within the anonymity of the class and not stood out in any major way.

The comment 'could do better' means, of course, that they could do better and I would like to suggest that whether this comment be on your report or not, there is virtue in striving to do so. If you have been getting 60% in a subject, try for 70% this semester. If you have been twelfth in the class, try to be eighth. If you were in the D team last year, try for the Cs this year. If you gain your Grade 3 music examination, try for your Grade 4.

In particular, I would like to encourage students to extend themselves in their thinking and their writing. All too often, boys can find exercises involving literacy quite challenging and can produce written work which can be unimaginative and limited. We need to do all that we can to avoid the dull-witted response devoid of inspiration and depth. We need to encourage imagination and feeling in our essays as well as allowing the zap, pow and zoom that young men like to include in their writing. Some boys can write brilliantly. All boys can write better. No boy should write what is boring. If any need help in this area they have only to notify their teacher.

▶

67

In terms of thinking, some students may be tempted to display knowledge whereas they could profitably be engaged in higher level tasks such as comprehension. Other students may display good comprehension but need to be challenged to extend their thinking to include analysis. Yet again, some students may need to be challenged even further and engage in the even more complex task of synthesis and evaluation.

The sorts of questions we might like to ask ourselves to stimulate higher order thinking, are questions such as 'What would you have done? What do you think caused this? How is it different from . . .? Can we trust the source of this material? Do you agree with this author? Why? What is the most important idea? Could this have been written better?'

We can always extend our thinking skills just as we can extend our writing ability and any other ability for that matter, including being able to produce a better report card.

Source: Hawkes, T F, *The King's Herald*, The King's School, Parramatta, 18 June 1999.

support from the boys themselves, student-generated reports need to be used 'as well as' rather than 'instead of' teacher-generated reports. Finding out what boys think of their own academic performance can be a useful diagnostic instrument particularly when their reports are compared with the teacher's reports.

Another aspect of school reports that may be useful to check is the compulsion given to teachers to give recommendations. All too often school reports give a 'snap shot' of performance. This is of value, but the really helpful picture is the one which tells the student and the parents what needs to be done to improve. Some teachers do try to cover this in their comments, but it can be a very hit and miss affair. A sizeable section of each report should address the 'So what?' issue. The advice on how to improve needs to be compulsory, specific and constructive. Boys need clear, unambiguous advice on what to do and an unsettling pressure to do it.

CONCLUSION

Schools can help boys to learn more effectively through a conscious attention to the learning climate, the curriculum, the educational reasons for study, the use of modern technologies, giving boys regular feedback, the general make up of the class, a later starting age for boys and an unapologetic academic rigour. Having noted this success in terms of having classes full of boys eager to explore the boundaries of their academic potential may not always be evident to the school administrator. This is when a school administrator may need to be reminded that there are many ways for a boy to succeed and not all of them have to be academic. Success comes in many forms as was recognised by Ralph Waldo Emerson when he wrote the following:

WHAT IS SUCCESS?

What is success?
To laugh often and love much;
To win the respect of intelligent persons and the affection of children;
To earn the approval of honest critics and ensure the betrayal of false friends;
To appreciate beauty;
To find the best in others;
To give of one's self without the slightest thought of return;
To have accomplished a task, whether by a healthy child, a rescued soul, a garden patch or a redeemed social condition;
To have played and laughed with enthusiasm and sung with exultation;
To know that even one life has breathed easier because you have lived;
This is to have succeeded.

ADDITIONAL INFORMATION

For those wishing to have further details on some of the points raised in this chapter, the following references may be helpful. Each number in the text of the chapter relates to a reference number below which will give further information related to the topic.

1	Kohn, A (1999)	*The Schools Our Children Deserve*	Houghton Mifflin Co., Boston.
2	Kohn, A	(op cit)	
3	Spurr, B (2000)	'Boys in trouble'	*Sydney's Child*, August 2000, p 20.
4	Details of the work undertaken by The Center for Development and Learning can be accessed via the Internet on: http://www.cdl.org/		
5	Bainbridge, C (2000)	*Middle School Approach — Interest of both boys and girls*	IES Conference, The Gazebo Hotel, Sydney, 22–23 June 2000.
6	Biddulph, S (1997)	*Raising Boys*	Finch Publishing, Sydney.
7	Biddulph, S	(op cit)	p 136.
8	Ruhlman, M (1997)	*Boys Themselves*	Owl Books, Henry Holt and Co. Inc., New York.
9	Biddulph, S	(op cit)	p 129.
10	Dr Colin Davey as Head of Physical Education, Rusden College, Melbourne researched physical activity and its effect on mental functioning.		
11	Oumano, E (1999)	'Music the key at Alpha School'	*Billboard*, 17/7/99, Vol III, Issue 29, p 1.

chapter 4

Teachers who can help boys

'A student is not above his teacher, nor a servant above his master. It is enough for the student to be like his teacher, and the servant like his master.'
Matthew 10:24,25

INTRODUCTION

Whether a school is a positive or a negative experience for a boy will be determined by many things, but one of the most significant is the quality of his teacher. A teacher who can laugh with a boy, who can paint great pictures in the mind of a boy, who can growl while still conveying a sense that the boy is valued, deserves the respect he or she will get from students. It matters little if a school is government run or private, free or expensive, co-educational or single sex, a great teacher can make these things irrelevant. A great teacher can turn a dreary curriculum and even last period on a Friday into something of spellbinding interest and relevance. A great teacher is not necessarily the friendliest teacher or even the most popular teacher. The great teacher is the one who inspires and disturbs until a new level of possibility is seen. The great teacher connects with his or her students and travels with them.

THE IMPORTANCE OF THE TEACHER

The most significant influence on the educational outcomes of school aged children is the teacher. According to Dr Ken Rowe of the Australian Council for Educational Research, variance in educational performance is influenced:

- 5.5% by the school
- 35% by the student
- 59% by the teacher.

Source: Paper presented by Dr Ken Rowe at the Symposium 'Educational Attainment and Labour Market Outcomes', Eden on the Park Hotel, Melbourne, 22–23 November 2000.

A boy's attitude to school, to learning and to himself will be coloured by the qualities of his teacher. For this reason, teachers must do more than grind through course content. They must build relationships and enter the world of the boy. Humour and approachability will help, over-familiarity will not. Some irascibility and even strictness is allowed in a good teacher providing it is transparently clear to the student that he is still valued by his teacher. Perhaps the cardinal rule for those wishing to be successful teachers of boys is that they must enjoy teaching. If teachers do not enjoy teaching, their students will not enjoy learning.

A teacher who has lost the love of teaching will betray this through low energy and low tolerance. At best, lessons will become a stalemate, born of a mutual non-aggression policy. 'I won't disturb you if you don't disturb me.' At worst there will be a sterile learning environment borne of repression or licence. These are the two main ways an ineffective teacher endeavours to control a class. Neither works with boys. The respect of a boy for his teacher will diminish if the teacher is dictatorial and authoritarian and evaporate completely if a teacher is remote and imperious. This is because a relational bridge must first be constructed before any learning can be carried across.

Teachers of boys need to be transformational, dedicated to changing their students, moving them from one state to another. Teachers need to be optimistic, believing that this transformational process is possible. Unfortunately, there still exists the teacher who is the burnt-out cynic who has given up hope and displays this to the students who are only too willing to fuel the emotional capitulation with further evidence of hopelessness.

A boy must be able to respect the person in the teacher before he will accept the knowledge in the teacher. There must be an engagement between teacher and student based on mutual respect. This engagement may be getting harder for many boys, not only because 83% of primary school teachers in Australia are female and 70% of secondary school teachers under 30 are female, but also because the average age of teachers in Australian government schools is 45 and rising by nine months every year.[1]

In terms of encouraging respect in boys, a teacher can help by ensuring that he or she:

- respects his or her students
- knows his or her students by name
- has a sense of humour
- has the gift of 'relaxed control'
- is firm but fair
- is well prepared
- is empathetic and able to know how students are feeling
- is vigilant and chooses to notice things
- anticipates and works proactively rather than reactively
- keeps his or her students busy on meaningful tasks which the students themselves recognise as being of value
- alters tasks within the lesson to keep the students engaged
- has a 'presence' and an aura of authority
- maintains a warm, positive and supportive culture
- continually gives positive rewards for appropriate behaviour
- establishes clear and consistent routines
- reinforces classroom rules and displays those rules so that they give a visual reminder of the code of conduct expected of students
- creates a pleasant classroom environment in terms of decorations, posters and artifacts
- is able to capture students' interest and develop in them a sense of wonder.

Boys behave better:

■ when teachers behave well in class. Students will take their cue from teachers and will use teachers as models in terms of language, attitudes and actions;

■ with teachers who are neither soft and permissively laissez-faire nor hard and oppressively authoritarian. Boys generally feel more secure with a teacher who is firm and consistent;

■ in attractive learning environments where the classroom has:
  – good climate control
  – good ventilation and light
  – good furniture, fixtures and facilities;

■ when they have inherited a culture of mutual respect and are successfully inducted into that culture where there is respect between student and teacher;

■ when there is a clear code of conduct which is consistently reinforced in every classroom by **every** teacher;

■ when there is, within the student body, a culture that respects individual differences and achievement;

■ when students feel accepted and valued by the school. If students feel they are failures they may seek acceptance within an anti-school sub-group;

■ when staff teach in an appropriate style which appeals to the different personalities and preferred learning styles of students.

It takes nine acts of praise to counter a single negative comment.[2] Given the propensity of boys to soak up a barrage of hostile comments from their teachers, a significant challenge presents itself to find ways and means to affirm and encourage boys; to signal to them that it is the sin that disappoints, not the sinner. If a teacher can show respect to a boy for who he is and what he may become, then a positive alliance might form and with it the grave risk of some very effective teaching.

TEACHERS, BLAME AND HOPE

There are times when even the most phlegmatic and tolerant teacher wants to occasion severe bodily harm to a particularly stupid boy. This course of action is not to be recommended, yet it should not be confused with the right of responsible adults to discipline children. It is as well for such adults to have worked out an appropriate range of sanctions well before any confrontation takes place. The capacity for cool and reflective judgment tends to become rare when a teacher is dealing with the emotional fall out from some particularly gross behaviour by a boy.

Despite the image they portray, boys are not immune from the verbal barbs and stinging character assassination witnessed in some episodes of admonition. They are even less immune to assault be it physical or emotional. Not all wounds show. Some wounds may not emerge until adulthood. The number of men convicted of being violent criminals who had themselves been subject to harsh discipline as boys is too high to be coincidental.

When encouraging boys to learn, it is generally as well to avoid coercion. As Steve Biddulph writes in his foreword in Browne and Fletcher's book *Boys in School*, boys rarely change as a result of pressure, coercion or blame even if the criticism is artistically and dramatically delivered.[3] Being 'got at' is an occupational hazard for boys and their defences are such that such assaults are rarely positive in their effect.

The Australian educator David Hores suggests that teachers who wish to influence the behaviour of boys should:

- spend some time trying to identify where boys are at
- content themselves with teaching boys where they are
- actively affirm boys where they are at
- not blame boys if they should fail to learn
- try to connect with boys in some way
- use humour and share anecdotes from their own lives
- make sure that irrespective of their performance, boys feel safe and valued.[4]

These are admirable sentiments but care needs to be taken not to over-state the case. Yes, there is both merit and wisdom finding out where boys 'are at'. But it might also be appropriate for boys to find out where their teachers 'are at'. A consistent capitulation to a child-centred perspective can create the very monster in a boy that the teacher is trying to discourage. The relentlessly child-centred approach was tried in schools in the late 1960s and early 1970s in England with very poor results. The children who did not want to do maths did not do maths and now clog up check-out queues as they slowly analyse whether they have been given the right change.

Not blaming a boy if he should fail to learn is good . . . when the boy should not be blamed. However, as the veteran teacher will quickly advise any gushing ideologist, there will occur the odd moment or two in a teacher's life when a boy might quite properly be told he is to blame. Telling a boy he is to blame only when he really is to blame is the trick. What is also important is that having suggested the blame and diagnosed the origin of the problem, the boy must be left feeling he is valued, safe and possessed of the necessary skill and inclination to avoid making the mistake again.

Teachers do have the right to encourage effective learning in their classrooms by making it non-negotiable that a boy must:

- respect the right of the teacher to teach
- respect the right of the student to learn.

When disciplining a boy it is important that the experience is as creative and positive as possible. The boy must know that there is something to build on. In short, boys need hope.

Engendering a sense of hope in boys is critically important. Hope is, quite literally, a life-saver. Daniel Goleman, in his book *Emotional Intelligence*, describes a study on 122 men who had experienced a heart attack. These men were evaluated on how optimistic they were. Eight years later 21 out of the 25 most pessimistic had died compared with only six of the 25 most optimistic. The best predicator of survival was mental rather than medical.[5]

There is also the ancient Greek story of Pandora. She was a girl who was more beautiful than was good for her. She was certainly too curious and prone to yielding to the odd bit of temptation. So it was that this princess of ancient Greece attracted the jealous attention of the gods, who gave her a mysterious box she was never to open. Well, curiosity killed more than just the cat, for when Pandora lifted the lid for just a 'it will do nobody any harm' peek, she let loose into the world all its afflictions, including disease, sickness and ill-fortune. However, one of the gods was moved by compassion and allowed her to close the lid in time to capture the one antidote that makes life bearable — **hope**.

This was the sort of hope that kept Tony Bullimore alive when his yacht, the *Exide Challenger*, capsized in the freezing swells of the Great Southern Ocean in 1997. Imagine the scene, nice and cosy with his cup of tea in hand (he was an Englishman), when in four seconds, after a terrific noise which signified the loss of his keel, Bullimore's boat turned upside down. He was in bone-chilling water and darkness, clinging to the detritus of a dying boat. It was four days before some kind gentleman tapped on his boat and invited him to resume his cuppa on the HMAS *Adelaide*. Truly an inspirational tale of hope and survival against all odds.

The bruised, abused and used in this world need hope. Not all will be upside down and adrift in the Great Southern Ocean, but they may be upside down, adrift and despairing in homes and in schools. Everyone needs hope and in this age of growing melancholy in the young, it is a virtue that must be pursued with greater vigour. If boys are to be encouraged to learn, they must believe in the future or else there is little motivation to learn. If boys are to be encouraged to learn, they must believe in themselves or else there is little motivation to learn. If boys are to be encouraged to learn, they must believe in their teachers or else there is little motivation to learn.

Research has revealed an interesting factor which can cause a boy's brain to block information. That factor is poor self-esteem. A negative self-image actually hinders learning. The perceptical register in the brain will not allow knowledge to be processed if a boy is not feeling good about himself.[6] For these reasons great care must be taken to avoid the tragic labelling of boys. If a boy comes to school day after day and the constant message given to him is that he has a behavioural problem, then this is likely to have an adverse effect on his learning. The accumulated criticism, particularly when it is centred on notions that the boy is unable to change and is not responsible for this can be especially destructive.

The challenge for parents and teachers is to give as much praise and affirmation as they can within the bounds of factual integrity. If they should stray from these bounds, then the praise and affirmation will quickly be recognised by boys for what it is — an empty and inaccurate analysis. This will prevent a boy from leaning on that person's judgment again.

Adults must endeavour to find at least one positive virtue they can celebrate in a boy, some 'hook' on which to hang the hat of praise. A boy should always be left with a sense that he has been dealt with honestly and fairly and, despite whatever sins of omission or commission that might have been committed, that he knows that he is still a child of God and a miracle of creation.

USE MULTIPLE INTELLIGENCES

Boys are different. Despite the desire of the members of the herd to melt unseen and unnoticed within the shadow of their peers, closer inspection will reveal differences. These differences are part of the magic there is in raising boys. It is important to acknowledge sameness so a boy feels he can identify with the group. It is also important to acknowledge a boy's uniqueness.

Fortunately, schools are becoming aware that students are different and have unique learning styles. Students also have unique strengths.

Some of the impetus to treat children as individuals, rather than as a group, has come from Howard Gardner.[7] Gardner's theory of 'multiple intelligences' initiated some ground breaking approaches to teaching children. Instead of suggesting there was but one form of intelligence, Gardner suggested there are at least seven forms. This list has now been extended to nine forms of intelligence:

1. verbal/linguistic
2. visual/spatial
3. body/kinesthetic
4. logical/mathematical
5. musical/rhythmic
6. interpersonal
7. intrapersonal
8. naturalistic
9. existential.

It is important to recognise the value of exercising all the intelligences within a classroom setting. It is also important for teachers to recognise what personal form of intelligence they are strong in for in all likelihood they will tend to use this form of intelligence a great deal in the classroom. When one considers that most primary school teachers are female and that the verbal/linguistic intelligence tends to be far more obvious in females, it could well mean that there might be an over-exercise of this form of intelligence to the detriment of other intelligences when teaching boys. For this reason teachers need to understand themselves as well as their students. Many boys are strong in the visual/spatial intelligence and would respond well to the use of maps, aerial photographs, guided imagery, active imagination, three-dimensional shapes, and so on. Other boys might be particularly strong in the area of body/kinesthetic intelligence and would learn particularly well through the use of drama, role play, dance, mime and games.

Some boys have advanced interpersonal skills and their high intelligence in this area would lend itself to cooperative learning tasks and collaborative learning. The most endangered sort of boy within our educational system may enjoy a more individual and reflective style of learning and like testing higher order thinking skills through strategies, such as computer games and chess.

In the light of the above it is now no longer acceptable to assume that all students learn alike or that all boys learn alike. Teachers must be aware of the importance of differentiated learning within the classroom setting and seek to exercise all expressions of intelligence.

The exciting implication is that a teacher may be able to use an intelligence a boy is strong in to help develop his intelligences in other areas. For example, a typical case found in boys is that they have a high visual/spatial ability as revealed in the ability to read maps and aerial photographs. On the other hand, their verbal skills may be limited as demonstrated in poor vocabulary, difficulty in framing appropriate answers and verbal expressions devoid of any real creativity.

An example of how this might be done is with the use of the Navigation Board. Essentially, the Navigation Board is made up of two picture frames hinged at the top and splayed out at the base so that it rests as an 'A' frame on a table. A pair of identical maps or aerial photographs are slid into the frames and two students sit opposite each other studying the identical map or aerial photograph.

One student is nominated as the navigator and his task is to direct the other student along a route known only to the navigator. Consider the following scenario with Bert as the 'navigator' and Alf as the 'driver' (see Figure 4.1).

Bert: 'Alf, go that way.' (Bert points to his left with an airy wave of his hand.)

Alf: (Says nothing and goes in the direction indicated, but because Alf is facing the opposite direction, he is already 180 degrees out. The result is some commotion, accusations, denials, realisation of the error and it all starts again.)

Bert: 'Go west up until you know, like . . . by that squiggly black what's-it.'

Alf: 'Strewth Bert . . . make some sense. What's a "what's-it"?' (This is excellent. Bert is getting some all-important peer feedback that his articulation skills are less than adequate. If a teacher had told him he would not have believed it — but he believes it when Alf tells him.)

Bert: 'All right – keep your hair on Alf – go west until you reach the large factory with the white roof on your left hand side and turn right at the next roundabout.'

Alf: (Executes the manoeuvre successfully and recognises that the grunts that usually pass for Bert's conversation are being replaced by reasonably coherent sentences.)

Bert: (Carries on with the navigation task and gathers his confidence and composure while doing so. He remains oblivious that he is speaking far more clearly and accurately, but wonders why he is enjoying the exercise more at the end than at the beginning.)

Of course, the process of language improvement using the Navigation Board is likely to take much longer than is described above but the essentials of the learning exercise can be gleaned from the scenario described. Bert has to interpret the visual clue, a task he does well and easily, which gives him some encouragement. He then converts that information into speech. This is something Bert finds difficult but he soldiers on inspired by the fact that he knows what he wants to say. Alf decodes the speech and seeks to reconcile it with the visual clue but to no avail. He feels he

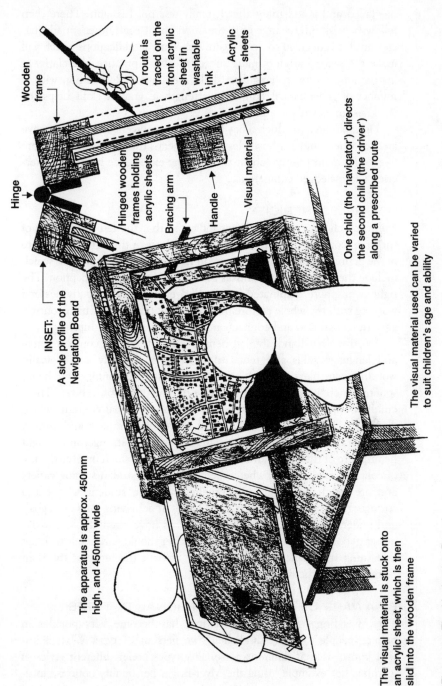

Wooden frame

A route is traced on the front acrylic sheet in washable ink

Acrylic sheets

Hinge

Hinged wooden frames holding acrylic sheets

Bracing arm

Handle

Visual material

INSET:
A side profile of the Navigation Board

One child (the 'navigator') directs the second child (the 'driver') along a prescribed route

The visual material used can be varied to suit children's age and ability

The apparatus is approx. 450mm high, and 450mm wide

The visual material is stuck onto an acrylic sheet, which is then slid into the wooden frame

Figure 4.1 The Navigation Board

has failed and is indignant that it really was not his fault. There then follows a brisk interchange of information about each other's inadequacies until it is decided to do it again with some modifications which will make the second attempt more successful. With practice, the clarity of instruction improves, language skills are improved together with a number of geographical skills. The strength in graphic skills helps the weakness in articulation skills.

Using an area in which a boy has a high intelligence to help improve an area where another boy is less skilled means that both boys are more likely to remain positive about the learning experience because it exercises acknowledged competence.

USE HEMISPHERICITY

Neuro-psychological research has indicated that the left hemisphere of the brain controls different functions from those of the right hemisphere of the brain.[8] Some boys are stronger in right hemisphere functions which include the function that controls geometric and spatial perception. The right hemisphere dominated learner also enjoys creative activities and working with the whole picture. It is the area of the brain which controls pattern recognition and connects non-sequential relationships.

On the other hand, the left hemisphere of the brain controls verbal and language skills and tends to function analytically and logically, working from parts-to-whole using step-by-step reasoning. Left hemisphere functions are a strength in girls and also some boys. These children enjoy learning styles that are strong in verbal content, which deal with abstract situations, involve short term projects and employ clear rules and procedures. Those students who are stronger in the right hemisphere of the brain tend to like learning styles which involve the use of concrete applications, whereas left hemisphere students enjoy variety and are much better at conceptualisation. The student who has a stronger right hemisphericity is often better at achieving long term goals and undertaking self-directed projects. Boys have strengths and weaknesses in both hemispheres and thus a teacher should endeavour to adopt a learning style which involves the use of both the left and the right hemispheres of the brain.

BE AWARE OF DIFFERENT PERSONALITY TYPES

The Myer-Briggs personality inventory has become very popular in helping people to understand their own personality type. What is less well known is that different personality types prefer different styles of learning. For example, using the Myer-Briggs personality options, 'intuitive' people tend to prefer self-paced learning and studying, using their own initiative. They also tend to have high expectations, enjoy essays and can cope with less structured lessons. On the other hand a 'sensing' person may find it difficult to generalise from examples to concepts but will appreciate learning which uses audio-visuals and science/mathematics apparatus. The 'sensing' person tends to find memorising easier.

'Extroverts' will like learning in groups, whereas those who are particularly strong in 'feeling' might find themselves allowing their social lives to interfere with their studies. Those who are assessed as having a 'judging' personality type will be particularly well organised, getting their assignments in on time and presenting their work in an orderly manner. The students who are more 'perceptive' have been shown to be more chaotic in handing in their work and in the organisation of their revision.

Boys will have many different personality types, and once again the teacher and the parent should be aware of these different personality types when setting work for boys. This may require more individualised assignments.

AWAKEN THE INTELLIGENCE
David Lazear suggests that to teach effectively the intelligence must first be awakened. This is particularly true of boys. It is suggested by Lazear that full use needs to be made of the five senses at the start of a lesson for it can help awaken not only the interest but also the intelligence of boys.[9] This also has the effect of triggering the activation of different intelligences and avoids an over-reliance on the verbal/linguistic intelligence.

Teachers who pay particular attention to the start of a lesson make optimum use of what has been known as the 'primacy effect', which is that students tend to learn best in the first 10 minutes of a lesson.[10] All too often teachers can waste the first 10 minutes calling rolls, returning books and dealing with latecomers rather than making this the prime time for learning. Once the lesson is underway, learning may well decline unless there is a significant reinvention of the lesson every 20 minutes or so. Thus the process of 'reawakening' needs to be consciously planned throughout a lesson.

One of the best ways to awaken intelligence is to ask questions in the same way that was undertaken by that great Australian educator Professor Julius Sumner-Miller, who characteristically always asked 'Why is it so?' It is important for adults not to answer the question too quickly and to ensure that the students engage with the question either through interest or relevance. This will result in the boy pursuing knowledge rather than knowledge pursuing the boy.

An example of awakening intelligence in a geography lesson on highland glaciation could well be the use of ice cubes from the fridge, showing slides of glaciated landscapes, reading a heroic description of Oates whose selfless life sacrifice was inspired by a desire to save the lives of Scott's party returning from their fruitless trek to be first to the South Pole. Perhaps even playing *Morning* from Greig's *Peer Gynt Suite* might also serve to awaken intelligence on the topic of highland glaciation.

Another significant learning time in a lesson is at the end of the period and this is known as the 'recency effect'.[11] Once again learning can be made particularly effective in these closing moments when students are made aware of the relevance and implications of the learning they have been engaged in. This can be helped by the transferring of intelligence into the real world situation.

TEACH BOYS THINKING SKILLS

Joan Dalton, in her book *Adventures in Thinking,* writes that if children are to be prepared to meet the demands of tomorrow, they must not be spoon-fed with facts and instruction, for this is an invitation to mental unemployment.[12] Dalton goes on to say that children must learn to think for themselves, to innovate, to create, to imagine alternative ways to get to the same goal, to seek and solve problems. In other words Dalton encourages the teaching of thinking skills.

Can a child be taught to think? Certainly Bryce Courtenay, the author of *The Power of One*, thinks so. The book is an entrancing tale which includes this marvellous description of the impact of two devoted teachers on a young boy's life:

> But above all things, I had been taught to read for pleasure and for meaning, as both Doc and Mrs Boxall demanded that I exercise my critical faculties in everything I did. At 12, I had already known how to think for at least four years. In teaching me independence of thought, they had given me the greatest gift an adult can give to a child besides love, and they had given me that also.[13]

To what extent are boys today taught to read for pleasure and for meaning? To what extent are boys taught to exercise their critical faculties in everything they do? To what extent are boys taught independence of thought? To what extent are boys given love?

The phrase 'independence of thought' is an interesting one for it suggests schooling in moral and ethical integrity and the celebration of courage. It also suggests the development of a certain self-confidence to the extent that a boy is comfortable in expressing a view even if it is contrary to popular opinion. Careful notice needs to be taken of what is being advocated. It is 'independence of thought' not 'independence of ignorance'. A boy belligerently maintaining a point of view based on prejudice and abject stupidity should not be allowed to feel that he is displaying independence of thought. Independence yes, thought no.

Quite what the dimensions are to thinking are not always agreed upon. Robert Sylwester suggests that there are five dimensions which need to be explored to facilitate effective thinking and learning.[14] These are:

1. having a positive attitude towards the task and seeing the task as valuable
2. bringing together thoughts about knowing what to do and linking these thoughts with constructive ideas about how to go about doing it
3. studying the characteristics of the problem and extending and refining one's knowledge about the issue
4. ensuring that the thinking task being engaged upon has a purpose
5. developing habits of mind which are productive and creative.

Many boys are all too acquainted with despair and disillusionment. Too much failure in their lives has left them fatalistic and quite slovenly in their thinking. Some boys are addicted to 'tuning out', and hiding behind lazy phrases like 'I don't know'. It may well be that a boy genuinely does not know. However, there are many occasions when the boy is really saying, 'I don't want to spend the effort in articulating a reasoned response to this question. Far better for me to act vacant and stupid'.

Perhaps the time has come for parents and teachers to say, 'I will not accept lazy statements like "I don't know". You do yourself an injustice using "cop out" phrases like that. You have a good mind, use it and give me an answer which you and I can both be proud of.'

The Pavlovian responses, ('I don't know', 'I can't do this') need to be banned from the vocabulary of boys. Productive habits in thinking need to replace 'don't bother me' responses. Schools have failed to deter these responses enough in their students. Boys should not be allowed to escape thinking duties. Boys might profit from being schooled in responses that are productive. The immediate response to a problem should be, 'There is an answer here somewhere, I'm going to try to find it. If I can't find it, I'll get as close as I can to it.' This is the 'I can do it' mentality which is the trigger for creative and productive thinking.

WHAT THINKING SKILLS SHOULD BE TAUGHT TO BOYS?

The specific thinking skills which might be taught to boys include:

1. The ability to solve problems.
2. The ability to make decisions.
3. The ability to see relationships.
4. The ability to be creative.
5. The ability to judge wisely.
6. The ability to reason.

1. The ability to solve problems

Not all problems are easy to solve. Boys might first need to ensure that they understand the problem. Perhaps it might help to phrase the problem another way, search out the options, look at similar problems in other areas which have been solved that could serve as a guide. This can involve looking at the problem from different perspectives and being audacious enough to consider a really new and weird perspective on the issue. Then some courage is needed to form an hypothesis and to test this hypothesis. A failed hypothesis still provides very useful knowledge. Boys should not be afraid to fail. Thomas Edison failed with hundreds of light bulbs before he found one that would work. If the hypothesis withstands the test, it can then be refined and extended. If the hypothesis fails, boys may need to analyse what has been learned from the experience and consider new alternatives.

2. The ability to make decisions

Making decisions is made unpopular by virtue of both the mental effort required and the dreadful spectre of accountability which haunts any decision maker. For this reason, decision making is becoming an endangered art. The process of decision making involves a searching out of the options, a testing of the appropriateness of each option (the positives and negatives of each) and then selecting the best option and going with it. Some boys are quite unable to make decisions. They have not developed enough confidence in themselves to do so. They have never had to practise the skill. They have only had to look blank for a moment or two and someone has made the decision for them.

If a boy is having a problem making a decision, there might be virtue in getting the boy to participate in decision making exercises for which there are no right answers, such as 'Who is the most significant person born in the last 100 years?' There may be several very valid answers. Practise with such exercises can give a boy the confidence to tackle decision making tasks for which there is but one generally acknowledged correct answer.

3. The ability to see relationships

One of the great wonders of creation is its interconnectedness. This interconnectedness extends beyond the physical world to the world of thought. The capacity to see relationships, to be able to determine cause and effect represents another important domain of thinking.

4. The ability to be creative

Implicit in the ability to be creative is the ability to deal with something in an entirely new way. All too often boys have been hidebound into thinking there is but one way, one answer, one response. This limited thinking may be a product of over-schooling. By over-schooling, what is meant is the incessant presentation of facts. Too much is presented to students as fact when it should be presented as theory. Students can become 'fact fixed', seeing things as black and white, as fact or as fiction, as right or wrong. There is little attempt to explore shades of grey, or to explore other approaches. Thinking is limited to being convergent, of being progressively restricted to the right answer, whereas much of life can be explored far more effectively with divergent thinking, with multiple ideas being generated. The ability to be creative and to be elaborative in thinking is an important mental skill.

> Most people are other people. Their thoughts are someone else's opinions, their lives a mimicry, their passions a quotation.
> Oscar Wilde

5. The ability to judge wisely

It should be noted that this thinking skill does not merely require boys to judge. Anybody can do this. Neither is this thinking skill presumptuous enough to suggest that the mandated task is to judge correctly. Nobody can do this all of the time. What can be realistically and properly hoped for is the ability to judge wisely, to be able to evaluate well. Implicit in this thinking skill is the ability to assess the credibility of an argument. This thinking skill requires boys to know the very real difference that exists between consensus and truth.

6. The ability to reason

This aspect of thinking relates to the capacity of a boy to see logical connections and to use these connections to advance an hypothesis. Reflective thinking is engaged in to help understand the bigger picture, the ultimate purpose. The capacity to link the big picture with the small is not always easy, just as it is not always easy to relate the small picture to the big. Getting boys to expand their thinking in this area may need to start with developing a sense of wonder. Looking at the stars at night and asking boys where they fit into the cosmos, and why, is the sort of challenge that can be given to promote this form of philosophical thinking. The questions asked need to be questions that the boys want to ask, not the questions the teacher wants to ask. Skilled teachers can always cause their students to wonder at the things that are worth wondering at. After creating the wonder, the issue can be explored at different levels, different scales and from different perspectives. An example of how this might be done is using de Bono's 'six thinking hats' technique.[15]

Boys can often be chaotic in their thinking. The synapses of the brain are firing away, but such is the excitement in the brain that there is interference, and a jumble of non-sensical words and illogical statements occur. Sometimes boys can be helped by being taught to calm themselves before tackling an issue in a logical and ordered way. However, the value of a time of chaos should not be underestimated. Order can spring from chaos, as can creativity and a refreshingly new perspective. Nonetheless, after the cerebral storm must come the calm and the articulation of a reasoned response.

Many boys can have a good cognitive grasp of an issue but fail to portray that fact because they may not be able to articulate their thoughts or present them in a logical or sequential manner. For this reason essay planning techniques might well be of particular benefit to some boys, together with the exploration of various logical ways by which an argument can be presented. For example, a logical way to write an essay about Mozart might be to base the essay on time — so, Mozart as a child (born 1756; composed music at five; played for Maria Teresa at six); Mozart's working life (composed, among many works, *The Marriage of Figaro* and *The Magic Flute*); Mozart's later life and death (he wrote the requiem for his own funeral; died 1791, a pauper). Another logical sequence to an essay might be to look at the macro issues, the meso issues and the micro issues, that is, to tackle the essay on the basis of size. Again, it might be useful to tackle an essay on the basis of for and against, using the first part of the essay to present one argument, the second part of the essay to present a counter argument and the conclusion to weigh up the relative merits of both arguments. Teaching the ordering of thoughts in this manner can help boys to attempt an answer to a question which at first glance can be daunting because of its complexity.

DEEP THINKING SKILLS

It has been shown that many boys can become confused by a multi-concept presentation within a lesson and may need to develop their thinking skills through the successful handling of single concepts before tackling multiple concepts. Having said this, it is important to try and move boys on and not merely pander to their limitations, but to encourage them to tackle more complex assignments. This is important because boys can often content themselves with engaging in copying behaviours, in other words merely copying or recording from a teacher rather than actually thinking. For this reason deep thinking skills should be encouraged and boys moved from mere knowledge acquisition through to comprehension tasks and analysis and such activities as evaluative exercises.

Shallow thinking skills	knowledge	(list, recall)
	comprehension	(explain, compare)
↓	application	(apply, demonstrate)
	analysis	(deduce, contrast)
	synthesis	(create, produce)
Deep thinking skills	evaluation	(judge, assess)[16]

One of the ways to stimulate deep thinking skills is to use questions such as:

- What would you have done?
- Can we trust the source of this material?
- What do you think caused this?
- What other ways can this be done?

Deep thinking can sometimes mean breaking down a big question into a series of smaller ones. The astute solving of these smaller tasks in the right sequence can result in the larger problem being solved. Learning these sorts of skills takes a boy on a journey of 'meta cognition' — of learning how to learn.

Effective learning requires students to engage in reflection. All too often boys are bouncing around like a pinball, setting off alarms, and flashing lights in their quest for an ever increasing score of knowledge. But what does it all really mean? 'Time out' is needed to ponder, to reflect on a question, to look beyond the superficial and to explore the issue from a different angle. Sometimes teachers may need to be free of the debilitating effects of having to impart a set amount of facts and be given time to savour the learning moments with their students.

All too often schools become places where creativity, wonder and optimism succumb to an oppressive ritual designed more to control than to create. This may be particularly true of boys-only schools because their energies are such that boys impose a threat to the established order. The objective is to keep boys busy with menial tasks because to have boys less busy is far too dangerous. There is sometimes a need for more danger and uncertainty in schools for this can be the catalyst for deep thinking.

DEVELOP REFLECTIVE THINKING

Children can have a fast and a slow response system. Many boys seem to have a well-developed, fast reflexive system which helps them to deal with danger and is triggered by strong emotional impulses. The other impulse is the slower 'reflective' system which permits a more rational consideration of alternatives. The fast reflexive system helps to ensure survival in difficult and uncertain times. The slower reflective system may be useful in deciding what tie to wear but is not quite so useful escaping the clutches of a 'home boy' gang intent upon taking a few teeth for souvenirs. The trouble is, boys tend to use reflexive thinking and reflexive behaviours when they should be using reflective thinking and counting to ten. Most prisons have people in them who wished they had improved their counting skills. Given the prison population is dominated by males, the challenge is to teach boys how to engage in more reflective responses rather than exercise the reflexive response so much.

One method of helping in this regard is to teach boys the 'traffic lights' system. When they feel themselves emotionally charged up, boys should be encouraged to visualise a set of traffic lights and, on seeing red, to stop whatever they are doing or saying. When the last vestiges of reflexive emotion are gone, the lights are then allowed to change colour to allow some cautious and controlled thinking. Wanting to thump another with a half-brick would show a certain lack of readiness to move off the red light. On permitting oneself to see the yellow, boys are allowed to think of the various options and to endeavour to put themselves in other people's shoes to get a different perspective on the situation. Finally the green light allows boys to go ahead with a carefully thought through and appropriate response. Simple mental pictures such as these can be particularly useful for those boys who often have a propensity to act first and think later.

There is a tide in the affairs of men
Which, taken at the flood, leads on to fortune;
Omitted, all in the voyage of their life
Is bound in shallows and in miseries.
On such a full sea are we now afloat,
And we must take the current when it serves,
Or lose our ventures.
William Shakespeare, *Julius Caesar*, Act IV, Scene III

LEARNING WINDOWS

There is a tide in the affairs of boys as well as men which, taken at the flood, leads on to fortune. There are opportunities which emerge when the heavenly constellations are such that an appropriate tide is formed that allows a voyage of learning to be possible. These are magical moments, not to be missed. It is not often in the natural order of things that one finds in constructive alignment, a boy, a momentary sense of interest, and someone who can develop that interest.

Often one finds boys. They are found frequently in schools. Often one finds teachers. They are found lurking behind newspapers in common rooms. Somewhat rarer are those moments of interest, for schools are consumed with teaching curricula thought important by people who have long since shed their childhood passions and with it the capacity to devise anything that will capture the imagination of a boy. Fortunately, there exist special teachers who recognise the magic of a 'learning window' as it materialises out of the humdrum business of every day life. The moment is recognised, an idea is presented, a question posed, a challenge given that lights up a boy and he is away on a journey of knowledge. There are some parents who also have this gift.

Teachers who recognise a 'learning window' are rare. Even rarer are teachers who can create a 'learning window'. These are gifted educators who can turn the teaching of quadratic equations to Year 9 into a wide-eyed journey of wonder.

The slightly less gifted often need props like a field trip to the zoo to generate the 'learning window'. Other teachers who are slightly more gifted can take their students on a virtual journey. With language rich in imagery these teachers can transform the classroom into a steaming tropical jungle. 'The light switch is an epiphyte — how can it live on the side of a tree like that? The desk is a giant buttress root, be careful not to trip over it — why must these trees have roots like that? Good grief, that's a flying snake. How can a snake fly from one tree to another without wings?' And so the lesson progresses.

Parents and teachers need to recognise when a learning window arrives and to make sure they use that opportunity well. Even more challenging is learning the art of creating a 'learning window'. This is not impossible and before the advent of the dishwasher, could even be done at the kitchen sink. 'Why are bubbles round?' 'How big a bubble can you blow?' 'Why do bubbles sometimes look coloured?' 'Check out the size of the bubble in the *Guinness Book of Records*. It's enormous, nearly 20 metres long! How did Alan McKay do that?' 'That's interesting, Alan McKay chose a day when it was clear and frosty. Why would that have helped?'

Care is needed that adults do not confuse what they find compelling with what boys find compelling. The successful teacher is able to get into the mind of a child and to rearrange the furniture so that new fixtures can be added.

USE CLOSED TASKS

Many boys feel more confident when dealing with 'closed tasks'. A closed task is one the student can say with certainty has been totally finished. 'Do the maths questions 1 to 10' would be an example of a closed task. On the other hand, an open task is one which could be reasoned to never be fully completed, such as writing an essay on the horrors of war. There is always likely to be further information which could be included. Many boys like the security of having completed a task. This should not necessarily be interpreted that teachers should give open-ended tasks. In many ways it is important for boys to exercise the skills associated with completing such tasks. On the other hand, the discerning teacher is often able to disguise an open-ended task by turning it into a series of closed tasks, and this can sometimes lead to boys feeling more secure.

WATCH YOUR SPEED

Australian researchers Kathy and Ken Rowe suggest that many boys flounder because parents and teachers give verbal instructions that are well beyond the capacity of boys to cope with. About 20% of six-year-olds cannot process information in an eight-word sentence. Boys often respond well to shorter verbal communication, good eye contact and slower instructions. Hyperactivity and distraction from the learning task may also be caused by problems with literacy rather than by ADHD. About 80% of children at risk of under-achieving in the area of literacy are boys and this is not helped by using texts, tasks and topics which do not interest boys or which are too advanced.[17]

USE SHORTER LEARNING TASKS

Boys seem to respond better to shorter learning tasks for they are somewhat prone to daydreams and distraction when engaged in longer learning activities. This should not translate into long learning activities not being given to boys. It is just that the teacher may need to give conscious attention to breaking down the large task into smaller subsidiary tasks. Thus a lengthy project on Captain Cook might well be broken down to a series of smaller tasks involving such areas as Cook's upbringing, Cook's early years at sea, Cook's voyage to Australia, Cook's later years at sea, his death and finally an evaluation of Cook's major achievements. In the same way that the proper way to eat an elephant is a mouthful at a time, a large task might be reduced to a series of smaller manageable tasks for boys.

USE TASK-BASED LEARNING

Boys respond particularly well to the introduction of verbs into learning tasks. They will often find themselves engaging well in a learning task if it requires them to run, measure, collect, draw, pace or time. Once again, this preference for task- and action-based experiential learning is something a teacher of boys may use to advantage, particularly when it is remembered that learning tasks practised by actually doing something tend to lead to a much better rate of memory retention after a 24-hour period (see Table 4.1[18]).

Table 4.1 Memory retention

Activity	Average retention rate after 24 hours
Lecture	5%
Reading	10%
Audio-visual	20%
Demonstration	30%
Discussion	50%

Learning by doing makes use of an acknowledged strength with most boys, and that is they like to be active. Thus a project on 'My Garden' could well be tackled from a literary point of view, with a descriptive essay on the garden and what happens in it. However, a boy might be rather more enthusiastic doing a number of tasks like:

- measuring the circumference and the height of trees;
- photographing and sketching the garden;
- doing bark rubbings and leaf rubbings;
- working out the size of the garden and the proportion given over to lawn, flower beds, patio and so on;
- pressing a few examples of the weeds and flowers;
- rubbing wet soil on to paper to record its colour;
- putting soil in a jar of water, shaking it and leaving it to settle to work out the constituents of the soil;
- using a quadrant to do a vegetation study;
- collecting, sketching or photographing the fauna found in the garden;
- mapping the area in shadow at 9.00 am, midday and at 3.00 pm, and seeing if this shadow affects the garden;

■ doing tests to examine the effectiveness of fertiliser on lawn growth, or weedicides on the quality of the lawn.

The options are endless, but enough examples are listed to give the sense that an open-ended writing project can be undertaken quite successfully by converting that project into a series of short, closed tasks which involve the boy **doing** something.

KINESTHETIC TEACHING STRATEGIES

Boys like to be physically involved, they like to explore, they like to do, they like to touch. For this reason, kinesthetic teaching strategies can be particularly useful with boys.

An example is the use of three-dimensional models as an introduction to the development of mapping skills. The ability to read and understand topographic maps requires a boy to understand abstract symbolism. A boy must realise that a little black cross on a map, for example, represents a church. If one is to agree with Piagetian stages of development in a child, the ability to cope with abstract symbolism may not emerge until a child is over 10 years of age.

If apparatus were made that appealed to the boy's innate desire to touch and fiddle with things, then this frustrating trait can be used to great educational advantage. Taking the example of teaching mapping skills, the author has advanced the age whereby children can interpret topographic maps by over five years, with five-year-old boys being able to 'read' abstract maps quite successfully.

A visual and kinesthetic teaching approach was used which involved a variety of pieces of apparatus including a series of wooden models which could be arranged on white paper to make a village (see Figure 4.2). Boys would do navigation exercises using a Matchbox car and driving it along roads drawn on the paper to the various buildings and other features that made up the village.

After a while, the boys would unclip from the base of each model a little tray on which there was an aerial photograph of the model, and the navigation exercises would continue in a two-dimensional way using the aerial photographs on the trays. The final stage of abstraction would come when the tray with the aerial photographs on was replaced and the rubber stamp with the abstract map symbol correlating to the model would be used. As this rubber stamp was stuck to the base of each model, each time the model was grasped and used as a rubber stamp there would be kinesthetic reinforcement as well as visual reinforcement of the meaning of the abstract map symbol. Using the various rubber stamps, a topographic map could actually be created by boys resulting in them

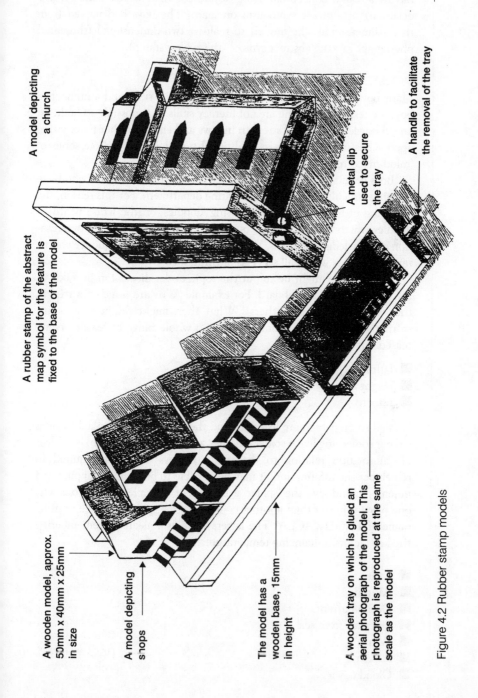

A model depicting
a church

A rubber stamp of the abstract
map symbol for the feature is
fixed to the base of the model

A metal clip
used to secure
the tray

A handle to facilitate
the removal of the tray

A wooden model, approx.
50mm x 40mm x 25mm
in size

A model depicting
shops

The model has a
wooden base, 15mm
in height

A wooden tray on which is glued an
aerial photograph of the model. This
photograph is reproduced at the same
scale as the model

Figure 4.2 Rubber stamp models

having a sound conceptual 'grasp' (quite the right word to use on this occasion) of abstract symbolism on maps. The boys had moved from three-dimensional (the model) to realistic two-dimensional (the aerial photograph) to the abstract symbol (the rubber stamp).

VISUAL TEACHING STRATEGIES

Many boys are strong in the area of visual/spatial skills and a number of boys are less strong in the area of literacy skills. It is possible to build on an acknowledged area of strength in boys and employ rather more visual approaches to such things as traditional note taking. A whole series of 'mind-mapping' techniques exist.

Boys generally respond well to diagrams, particularly those who have learning difficulties in the verbal/writing department. For this reason, the exploring of topics can be done using 'doodles' on the white board — doodles which are not chaotic but which are forms of graphic organisation of knowledge and ideas. Venn diagrams, topic webs, sequence charts, ranking ladders would all serve as illustrations.

An example might be to put the topic under discussion in a box in the middle of the blackboard. For example 'Why are some countries in the world hotter than others?' What then might follow is a brainstorming session which could result in a whole range of reasons being teased out:

■ latitude
■ height above sea level
■ seasons

. . . and so on, which are listed around the topic box and linked by lines so that something like a spider emerges with the topic body linked to legs of information relating to the topic. If boys are then required to remember the information, it may be possible to link mind mapping to a mnemonic and give the 'spider' a name. For example, the reasons why one place is hotter than another could lead to a spider with the unusual name of 'LAODWACLA'. The letters serve as a means of remembering the key factors influencing temperature:

■ Latitude
■ Altitude
■ Ocean currents
■ Distance from sea
■ Winds
■ Aspect
■ Cloud cover

■ Length of day/season
■ Amount of dust, etc. in the atmosphere.

DEVELOP THE MEMORY

Mention has just been made of the use of mnemonics to assist boys with the recall of information. The need to develop the memory, as with many of the learning skills discussed so far, is not the exclusive need of boys. Nonetheless many boys might benefit from being helped with memorising, as memory skills are tested a great deal in classrooms in the western culture. There are two types of memory:

1. **procedural**, such as might be used in remembering how to swim;
2. **declarative**, such as might be used in remembering the seven times table.

Many boys are stronger in procedural memory, that is, knowing how to do things, and are relatively weak in declarative memory. For example learning a foreign language has often been shown to be more difficult for boys than for girls as it makes a great demand on declarative memory.

Given that all boys have about 100 billion neurons in the brain, each with thousands of memory transmitting dendrites, one would think that memory should not be a problem. However, activating a memory trace in the brain involves crossing the synapse gap between neurons and latching the dendrite spines of one neuron to another. Causing the effective crossing of the synapse can be assisted through repetition. There is truth in the ancient observation:

> Repeat again what you hear; for by often hearing and saying the same things, what you have learned comes complete into your memory.'
> From the *Dialexeis*, 400BC

A method which is particularly helpful with many students is the use of mnemonics. For example 'every good boy deserves football' can be a useful way of remembering the notes on the treble musical stave.

Memory retention is assisted if the brain has been given enough time to make sense of the material. Research in the USA has suggested that when teachers ask a question, they are waiting only about one second before providing an answer to that question.[19] Such a short wait punishes those students who are 'slow retrievers' and they will merely stop the retrieval process with the result that learning becomes less effective. Students also need time to make sense of their learning and to see the connections. The amount of content covered in each lesson needs to be monitored carefully and limited if necessary.

Prompt, specific and corrective feedback assists memory, as does the interest generated in the learning material and the sense of relevance of the material to the student. Choosing learning tasks which are particularly interesting to boys, and relevant to boys, is important. Combustion engines, dissecting rats and the maths associated with marking out an athletics track might serve as examples.

Anxiety can be both helpful and harmful to memory recall. Some stress can be good but distress is bad. Generally a moderate level of stress optimises learning, with the brain learning best in a state of relaxed alertness. However, some subjects such as mathematics and languages tend to be learnt better with lower stress. Anxiety and stress might be reduced if boys were able to give immediate feedback as to whether they understand what is going on. Some teachers have had success with using coloured cards whereby boys put a small green card on their desk if they understand, a yellow card if they are just about understanding the material, and a red card if they are totally 'at sea'. This feedback occurs throughout the lesson and enables the teacher to see at a glance just how well the class is following and whether there might be some need for reinforcement.

With boys, the transfer of knowledge needs to be made as positive an experience as possible. One might imagine that announcing to a room of boys that they are about to study a Shakespearian play could well be met with some ambivalence. On the other hand a teacher who was to show a number of extracts of *West Side Story*, including one of the fight scenes, could excite a great deal of interest. This could then be translated into an introduction to *Romeo and Juliet*, which is essentially the same story. It is the practice of such pedagogy, often natural in the gifted teacher, which can be so effective in making learning meaningful and attractive to boys.

Getting boys to reflect on their performance in the light of being given examples of good work can also be very useful. Boys can even be invited to mark their own work, or indeed each other's work, and to provide reasons for the marks they give. Boys often have an unrealistic appreciation of the standard of their work, thinking more highly of their work than they should. Giving examples of quality work is important but this must be done with some care, for one must avoid discouragement.

One of the key elements to effective learning is to provide adequate time. For example there are two ways to handle knowledge. One is to learn it by rote and to store the information exactly as it entered the memory, and the other is to engage in elaborative learning which is to make sense of the information and to explore its relevance. If a boy is given very little training in the exercise of thinking skills, or if a boy is not given much time then the boy will often resort to rote learning rather than elaborative learning. He will often resort to lower order thinking skills and such things as prepared answers, rather than engage in higher level thinking skills and exercise evaluative and analytical judgment.

DISCIPLINE AND ROUTINES

Perhaps it was the rise of the children's rights movement; perhaps it was just a capitulation to the unceasing challenges of boys against authority. For whatever reason many have found it hard to discipline children, particularly boys, and to impose upon them quite reasonable routines like going to bed and doing homework. Parents and teachers are bound by increasingly restrictive legislation as to what they cannot do. Although most of these initiatives are to be applauded in every way, there is the fear with some that adults are losing control of their young and that many children lack the basic discipline to succeed as learners. Some boys also lack the ability to work well without supervision, the ability to produce work which reflects their best ability and the capacity to bring the right equipment to class.

Despite living in an age that celebrates individual rights, there is still virtue in making some things non-negotiable with boys in terms of both their behaviour and learning. Academic goals can be set in cooperation with the young, but that is where such goal setting exercises fail. They often fail to detail how these goals are to be met. A useful response to this problem is to get boys to agree to a contract, which they sign, and a copy of which is stuck to their wall. The contract could use the acronym 'GATE':

- G = Goals: What are the academic goals this term/semester/year?
- A = Activities: What specific activities will be done to help reach these goals?
- T = Timetable: Exactly when will these activities be done?
- E = Evaluation: How will I know I am 'on track'?

Parents and teachers should not shrink from establishing routines and from expecting adherence to certain codes. Such rules and guidelines need to be clear, fair, and worked out in collaboration. In the school setting this can result in a classroom poster which proclaims something like 'A Class Act' and under that the actions that are endorsed by the class can be written out, such as:

- It is OK to do well.
- It is not OK to ridicule or 'put down'.
- It is important to consider different points of view.
- It is important not to distract the teacher from teaching.
- It is important not to distract students from learning.

Lists in school diaries, on bedroom walls, stuck behind fridge magnets can be particularly useful to boys for it is a visual reinforcement of standards, and visual reinforcements can be much more effective than verbal reinforcements.

There is always the temptation when writing about boys and discipline to fall into one of two traps: the trap of permissiveness and the savagely authoritarian trap. Somewhere in between is the right balance, but that balance may be just a little more towards the authoritarian side with boys in comparison with girls.

The growing phenomenon of Asian children dominating the school academic honour lists in western countries may suggest that the work ethic is stronger in some cultures than in others. There may well be virtue in having more noses to grindstones, in higher expectations of boys and fewer apologies for adopting the sentiments of that great educator Kurt Hahn, who founded Gordonstoun School, who would compel his boys into the learning experience.

BRITISH RESEARCH ON EFFECTIVE TEACHING STRATEGIES FOR BOYS

Some excellent ideas on effective teaching strategies for boys can be found at the boys and literacy Internet site created by Frater G (2000) at: http://wwwbasic-skills.co.uk/text.html

Other useful British references include:

Her Majesty's Stationery Office (1993)	*The Gender Divide: Performance differences between boys and girls*	HMSO, London.
The Office for Standards in Education (1993)	*Boys and English*	Ofsted, London.
Pickering, J (1997)	*Raising Boys' Achievement*	Network Educational Press, Stafford.
Plackett, E (1995)	*Developing a Whole School Approach to Reading in the Secondary School*	Borough of Lewisham, Education Department, London.
Qualifications and Curriculum Authority (1997)	*Boys and English*	QCA, London.

Another very good resource is:

Hannan, G (1999)	*Improving Boys' Performance*	Folens Limited (ISBN 1 85008 168–9).

CONCLUSION

Practical steps can be taken to help boys to learn. Further advice is offered in the following chapter in the crucial area of boys' literacy. The pall of gloom can settle rather too readily on common room conversations about boys' learning. There are answers, there are practical pedagogical tricks that can be used to help. It may well be that success will not be experienced in enhancing every area of a boy's learning, but there should be success in some areas. Many will have heard the tale of a navy commander's experience during maritime manoeuvres. There was a heavy fog when the look out reported a light dead ahead. The Captain ordered his signalman to send the message, 'On a collision course. Change course 20°.' The reply came back. 'I advise you to change course'. The next signal said, 'I am a Captain, you will change course 20°.' The unapologetic reply came back, 'I am a Seaman Second Class, you must change course.' The Captain, now furious, sends back, 'I am a battleship. Change course 20°.' The reply was not long in coming. 'I am a lighthouse!'

Even with the best will in the world, it is the adult who must change course if a boy is positioned in a place from which he cannot move. It is sometimes the adult who must accept that a boy who will not change probably should not change. To visit upon some boys totally unrealistic expectations that they must alter course can be extremely discouraging. However, not all boys are lighthouses.

ADDITIONAL INFORMATION

For those wishing to have further details on some of the points raised in this chapter, the following references may be helpful. Each number in the text of the chapter relates to a reference number below which will give further information related to the topic.

1	Rodgers, J (2000)	'Changing boys' self-esteem and self-image'	IES Conference, The Gazebo Hotel, Sydney, 22–23 June 2000.
2	McMullen, J (2000)	'Boys' values, behaviour and peer relationships'	IES Conference, The Gazebo Hotel, Sydney, 22–23 June 2000.
3	Biddulph, S quoted in Browne, R and Fletcher, R (1995)	*Boys in Schools*	Finch Publishing, Sydney.
4	Hores, D quoted in Browne, R and Fletcher, R	(op cit)	
5	Goleman, D (1995)	*Emotional Intelligence*	Bloomsbury Publishing, London, p 177.

6	Sousa, D A (1995)	*How the Brain Learns*	National Association of Secondary Schools Principals, Virginia, USA, p 20.
7	Gardner, H (1995)	*Frames of Mind: The Theory of Multiple Intelligence*	Basic Books, New York.
8	Sousa, D A	(op cit)	p 86.
9	Lazear, D (1994)	*Seven Ways of Teaching*	Hawker Brownlow Education, Australia, p xix.
10	Lazear, D	(op cit)	
11	Lazear, D	(op cit)	
12	Dalton, J (1985)	*Adventures in Thinking*	Nelson ITP, Melbourne.
13	Courtenay, B (1998)	*The Power of One*	Penguin Books, Melbourne, p 389.
14	Brandt, R (2000)	'On teaching brains to think: A conversation with Robert Sylwester'	*Educational Leadership*, April 2000, p 73.
15	de Bono, E (1992)	*Six Thinking Hats*	Hawker Brownlow Education, Australia.
16	Sousa, D A	(op cit)	p 117.
17	Rowe, K and Rowe, K quoted in Arndt, B (2000)	'Attention boys'	*Sydney Morning Herald News Review*, 28 October 2000, p 35.
18	Sousa, D A	(op cit)	p 43.
19	Sousa, D A	(op cit)	p 61.

chapter 5

Improving literacy skills in boys

INTRODUCTION

It was Winnie-the-Pooh who confessed that he was a bear of very little brain, and that long words bothered him. Words can bother boys as well, although this is not true of all boys, for in the top few percent of Year 12 Higher School Certificate (HSC) English results in New South Wales, boys are well represented. However, once one has gone beyond the top few percent, the picture is a rather gloomy one, with girls outperforming boys in this vital area of learning.

In the 1999 HSC 3 Unit English exam, which is typically taken by the more able Year 12 students in New South Wales, for every single boy who managed to get into the top 25%, there were four girls. If the results of all the HSC English exam options were melted together, only three boys for every seven girls would be found in the top 25% of the student body.

It should be remembered that poor literacy skills are penalised savagely in the western education system because writing tasks form the basis of the examination system. These days, essays are even being set in subjects like mathematics and science. Added to this is the fact that the New South Wales state government has made it compulsory to include 2 units of English in the calculation of a student's University Admission Index (UAI) score. There is no compulsion for mathematics or a science to be included in that score. Quite apart from the above, poor literacy is likely to impede learning given that the written word is used so much to transmit knowledge and to excite students to learn.

As well as listing a number of rather pragmatic reasons to improve the literacy levels of boys, it is as well not to forget the quality of life reasons. Put simply, if a boy does not read, he will be denied an immense amount of fun. There will be no capacity to enjoy the sci-fi thrill of Asimov, the humour of Dahl, and the fantasy of Tolkien. From a practical point of view, the shopping trolley may have a few surprises if the shopping list cannot be read, and the sports pages of the Friday newspapers will be of little use in helping with the footy tipping competition, if one is illiterate.

POOR LITERACY SKILLS IN BOYS

The evidence is unambiguous — boys in general are not performing nearly as well as girls in the area of literacy. In a national survey of English schools in 1996, it was found that one-third of boys had not learned to read at the approved reading standard during their first three years at school. By Year 5 the figure was worse and, with the move to secondary school, boys fall even further behind in literacy relative to girls. Similar results have been recorded in Canada and the USA.[1]

Literacy forms the core of learning and is a major way by which information is conveyed. The exercise of literacy skills is the basis of educational assessment with essays, project work and other assignments resting heavily, if not exclusively, on the written word. Of the many predictors of poor academic performance, the most accurate is poor literacy levels in primary school.

The spoken word also forms a part of contemporary academic assessment in schools. It may come as a surprise to some boys that the male grunt is somewhat less valued by contemporary society than it might have been in Neanderthal times. Some boys have not quite woken up to this, with their language limited to a cry of derision or triumph on the football field. Meanwhile, girls are scattered about the school in friendship groups engaged in social therapy and chatting. Try asking adolescent sons what their school day was like, and their verbal response is often limited to an enigmatic shrug of the shoulders and a strange sound like a rusty gate being closed. Ask a girl, and one is likely to be treated to a detailed verbal analysis of the social and educational dynamics of a sizeable proportion of the school.

In a survey undertaken in England in 1994 across all school age groups, it was found that reading a really good book was listed as the preferred activity by 17% of boys and 43% of girls.[2]

In an age being dubbed the 'communication era', a primacy is being placed on speaking and writing skills. School examiners rate these skills, employers rate these skills, tertiary institutions rate these skills. Even life partners may tire a little of a lifetime of birthday, Christmas and anniversary cards whose literary content is limited to 'From John to Beth'.

The Victorian Quality Schools Project surveyed 38 000 students from kindergarten age to Year 11. It became clear through the surveys that in reading, writing and language work, boys were not performing as well as girls. It was also shown that boys were not enjoying school as much as girls. Part of this disaffection with school and growing disengagement with things scholastic may well relate to the heavy accent given to prolonged literacy tasks which do little else than reinforce a sense of failure in a boy. There is stigma enough in being a poor reader, but when that same reader is given juvenile books to read, the humiliation is complete and rebellion, together with a rejection of reading, becomes a very real possibility.

Elaine Millard makes an interesting point about the lack of training in reading after the basics of reading have been mastered:

Once children could 'decode print' and had worked their ways through a reading scheme, they were frequently left to develop further reading strategies independently. The general assumption was that children would grow individually towards reading more complex texts. There was little monitoring of their subsequent progress except for asking them to complete the lists of titles and page numbers recorded in diaries along with a smiley face or star rating system. Poor readers often remained on reading scheme books which reinforced their sense of failure and which repeated the same pattern of syntax and narrative structure.[3]

Help for boys in the area of literacy has been both limited and late. This is surprising when it is realised that the relatively poor literacy skills of boys have been documented for some time. In 1996 the Federal Minister for Education, Dr David Kemp, suggested there was 'a cult of secrecy' among schools and a lack of accountability because there was no public revelation of the truth about academic performance.[4] This resulted in the release of figures relating to a longitudinal survey undertaken on children's literacy. When released, it came as no surprise that some would have preferred the results hidden, for despite much trumpeted educational reform and innovation over the 20-year period from 1975 to 1995, the number of 14-year-old boys achieving basic literacy standards did not improve.[5] In fact they became worse, with an increase from 30% with poor literacy standards in 1975, to 35% in 1995. Girls managed to register an improvement over the same 20-year period, but it was only a modest improvement: 26% of 14-year-old girls were identified with poor literacy skills in 1995 compared with 27% in 1975.

Clearly something is wrong. The number of children failing in the area of literacy is disturbing. The figures which show that 35% of 14-year-old boys in Australia failed to achieve basic literacy are alarming. This means over a third of adolescent boys could be denied the rewards of enjoyable literature. This means over a third of adolescent boys are severely handicapped in learning through literature. This means over a third of adolescent boys may well be angry and rebellious in English classes and seek to prop up their damaged self-esteem by audacious anti-establishment behaviour, and why not, for in many cases, the establishment has failed them.

SOCIO-ECONOMIC INFLUENCE ON LITERACY

Research has indicated that a student's socio-economic ranking has an influence on literacy, with those from a low socio-economic background being more likely to suffer lower literacy levels.

THE LITERACY INVASION

In order for students in Grade 3 in New South Wales to complete their Basic Skills Test in numeracy in the late 1990s they needed the literacy competence of a student at Grade 5 level. The demands of greater literacy have permeated every subject, even mathematics.

Source: Rowe, K, 'Educational attainment and labour market outcomes', Australian Council for Educational Research, Paper presented at the Symposium, Eden on the Park Hotel, Melbourne, 22–23 November 2000.

Australian researchers have looked at the effect of socio-economic ranking on the relative performance of boys and girls in the area of literacy and have found an interesting pattern. Girls outperform boys at all socio-economic levels, but the amount by which girls outperform boys actually increases with growing affluence. Some might have expected the difference to diminish because of the 'glass ceiling' effect, but it appears it may not. Even the rich boy is not spared.[6]

Similar findings were reported in Victoria in an article in the *Herald Sun*, 26 January 1996, which showed twice as many boys as girls were represented in the lowest ability groups in literacy across all socio-economic groups. There is no respite socio-economically from the dismal news that boys are not performing well in literacy. Each socio-economic group records the trend that boys are outperformed by girls.

BOOK SELECTION

The ingredients for a good read will vary from boy to boy and from age to age. However, a formula which time and experience has judged to be particularly useful is to choose books which are age and ability appropriate in terms of language and theme, and then make sure the story has action, adventure and that thrill factor which boys find so compelling.

There are, of course, different sorts of thrills. There is the thrill that comes from reading science fiction, the thrill that comes from horror stories, the thrill that might come from pornography, and the thrill that comes from reading about high adventure, to name but a few. Just because a book thrills does not necessarily make the reading material suitable for boys. Not everyone will agree with the Australian author John Marsden that boys should be allowed to read sexually explicit material because boys find the topic so compelling. It is true that getting boys to read such material is unlikely to be a problem.[7] Any plaudits one might receive for improved reading levels by using this type of material are likely to be lost in the cacophony of indignation, outrage and accusations of moral bankruptcy by a large group of very angry parents. This is just one of the reasons this approach is not recommended. However, the principle of searching out reading material which is attractive to boys is recommended.

There is virtue in parents and teachers paying very careful attention to book selection. In choosing a book for boys, a realisation is needed that generational tastes do change and what adults find interesting does not necessarily interest boys. What boys 20 years ago found interesting may not interest boys today. There are some good books which have ageless appeal, but parents should not necessarily expect their sons to be enthusiastic about *The Secret Seven* and *The Famous Five*. Even more recent series such as *The Hardy Boys* may lose their appeal, but each year produces books which are a very good read. The huge success of the *Harry Potter* series serves to illustrate that books which appeal to boys emerge for every generation.

A cartoon appeared in the April 1993 issue of *Education Alternatives* which presented the scene of a student talking to a librarian and saying 'I think I need a book that's ideologically sound, with a proper gender and ethnic emphasis giving due weight to appropriate societal, familial and peer values in a milieu that's iconoclastic, avoids stereotyping or violence, yet remains relatively unsanitised and won't cause irreparable harm to my emerging psyche. But if you don't have one of those, how about a book that's a rattling good read?'

Examples of some books considered a 'rattling good read' for boys are shown in Appendix A on pages 132–139.

BOOK AVERSION

Book aversion does exist, especially among boys. The experience of reading a book can become so negative for some boys, that they do not wish to put themselves through the pain of reading. Sometimes the genesis of the problem is physical such as poor eyesight. Most of these problems can be remedied. Whether boys will seek the remedy is another question. There can be a social stigma attached to boys who wear glasses, and some boys will avoid wearing them. Contact lenses can sometimes help, but not always. Some counselling and reassurance may be necessary for a boy who is prescribed glasses.

For other boys the reading aversion may be due to medical conditions such as dyslexia. Again there are a number of treatments available including medicines, tinted glasses, sound therapy and diet. There have been some new developments using bio-feedback. Desperate parents are seeking some of these new-age treatments. Bio-feedback involves giving students a sound stimulus to 'awaken' parts of their brain. Many of these treatments need far more research before they can be given unqualified support. In some cases, the improvements boasted about may well be due more to psychological reasons rather than the virtues of listening to whales speak to one another. An open mind is needed on these treatments until they have been tested a little more. What is not in question is the importance of appropriate remediation being sought. Without it the task of inspiring a boy to read may well be a fruitless exercise.

A number of boys have just had a bad experience with reading. They may have been developmentally a little delayed, or they may have grown up in a home environment that only 'watches' rather than 'reads'. For whatever reason, the boy may just be a little behind and as he stumbles clumsily over the words when reading aloud, he experiences the exasperation of parent and teacher, the ridicule of siblings and peers, and the whole reading experience becomes so ghastly that he does not want to repeat it, and so he doesn't.

There are lessons and implications here. One obvious point is that whenever a boy reads, there should be support and encouragement, and a sense of success engendered. Critical comment should be muted, particularly in the early reading stages, and as much praise given as possible. Experiences which can lead to the public humiliation of a poor reader should be avoided, as should unfair comparison between generations, between siblings and between boys and girls.

Some boys have a reading aversion because their role models have a reading aversion. One key model is the father. Are sons seeing their fathers read? Are fathers reading to their sons, talking to their sons about what they are reading, hearing their sons read without undue expression of criticism, and with genuine pleasure in the experience? All too often the only evidence of a father in a young boy's life is some half-eaten toast in the morning, and snoring in front of the TV in the evening.

For reading to be associated with pleasure, it may be necessary for adults to remember that time should be set aside for boys where they are expected to read, not just for improvement, but for pleasure. Reading text books is all very well, but for a love of reading to be engendered there may have to be some encouragement given to get boys started on an age- and ability-appropriate work of fiction. The mere reading of school text books can lead to reading becoming synonymous with work, rather than with pleasure. This can be a trap for educators who must seek ways and means to keep the pleasure component in reading, for all too often it has gone missing from schools. The message needs to be given that it is sometimes alright not to read for personal improvement, and it is quite alright to read for personal pleasure from time to time. This is why initiatives like the Drop Everything and Read (DEAR) and Uninterrupted Sustained

Silent Reading (USSR) programs in schools are so important. These programs involve the setting aside of student-directed reading time, with the activity being written into the school day as a priority task and as an enjoyable activity.

SOME WAYS AND MEANS TO ENCOURAGE THE DEVELOPMENT OF LITERACY SKILLS IN BOYS

1. Start young

The Australian novelist James Moloney suggests that by the time a boy is of school age, his fate as a reader has largely been sealed.[8] For this reason it is vital that the infant boy:

- be talked to, encouraged to make sounds and to hold 'conversations' as early as possible even if the sounds are unintelligible;
- hear made up stories which sometimes include the boy as one of the main characters;
- be read to, even if the boy may not fully understand the story;
- be encouraged to read signs and words that present themselves in everyday life;
- be encouraged to recognise simple words using large 'flash' cards with the words printed on them in big letters. By this method, the small boy can build up sight vocabulary;
- be encouraged to expand upon his spoken vocabulary and to move beyond baby words and a restricted language to a more elaborate language;
- have alphabet friezes, posters, big notices on his bedroom wall and his own collection of books at a very early age, even if it only be cloth books;
- be encouraged to engage with the stories being read with good use being made of questions, guessing what is going to happen from the pictures and so on;
- should never be underestimated in terms of his ability to start learning to recognise and enjoy words at an early age.

2. A magazine-led reading recovery

If boys have become book phobic, a useful approach may be to smuggle some reading into a boy's life via magazines and comics. The magazines will need to appeal to boys and may need to be oriented towards action. Unless a magazine has a gratuitous amount of action, even violence, in it, then the risk is that it will be seen largely as a feminine journal. The sorts of magazines that appeal to many boys relate to power (trucks, cars and muscles), relate to competition and games (sporting, guns and IT software) and relate to lust (pornography, and 'chick' pics).[9] Some of these options need to be avoided. Not all magazines are suitable, and care must be taken not to use magazines that do little else than confirm boys in their anti-intellectual stance. However, a regular subscription to a number of well-chosen magazines may prove to be the catalyst in starting to get a boy to read. Manuals related to specific hobbies can be useful in this regard, even if those manuals are on how to fix a car, play better footy, or the key features of the latest bit of IT software.

Magazines and comics are generally much more pictorial than books and this appeals to boys, for whom visual stimulus can be very strong. Clues are given to word interpretation and to the content of the prose by the picture, and this can prepare the mind as it embarks on the task of text analysis. The vocabulary used in some magazines and comics can also be quite advanced and might extend the literacy skills in boys without the normal pain associated with comprehension tasks.

Having recognised that magazines and comics can be a useful impetus to get boys to read, it would be a shame if the literary momentum generated by this initiative did not result in boys moving on to reading books. Some boys may need encouragement to take this final but very necessary step.

The stronger role played by 'visual literacy' in society, in other words the means of communication other than written text, is being recognised in schools with a greater use being made of magazines, TV and interactive computer activities. Yet it is necessary that an appreciation of text is not lost and that proponents of visual literacy are not allowed to marginalise the printed word.

3. Action and critical literacy

Literature liberally scattered with verbs appeals to boys, as can literature which encourages boys to do something. For this reason literacy and articulacy tasks which are linked to action can be particularly effective. Examples on how this might be done include:

- using drama to help boys develop speaking skills as a way to give 'permission' for boys to show feelings and emotions;
- establishing a rap and break-dancing club to develop skills in poetry, rhythm and rhyme;
- setting up a radio station with interviews, prose and news items being prominent;
- creating an Internet book circle allowing boys to review and comment on books;

■ organising camps which require boys to research the trip and to write out schedules. A journal of the camp experience could also be kept;

■ encouraging boys to give PowerPoint presentations.

The possibilities are endless.

Critical literacy is also something which can appeal to boys for it can involve a greater engagement with literature.[10] This translates into boys actively connecting with the written material by asking critical questions about the accuracy, relevance, bias, truth, defects and politics of a piece of writing. The written material is assimilated for it demands a response from the student. It requires tasks to be undertaken which are related to the text.

Critical literacy leads to action. Possible action might be writing back to the author with the students' views, debating the main thesis of the article, writing to others seeking alternative views, taking up a petition and so on. When literacy tasks lead to action tasks, then the appeal of literature can be enhanced for many boys.

4. Reviewing assessment methods

Great care is needed so that what is taught in the classroom is not assessment driven. The assessment task should serve as a diagnostic and affirming experience which is designed to cause the student to reflect on what has been taught. For this reason educators should be very careful in giving support to any 'assessment-led recovery' as it can give a profile to assessment which is educationally unsound.

Having noted the above, it needs to be questioned whether the emphasis placed on extended pieces of writing in many contemporary assessment tasks means that only a limited range of skills is being tested. Girls tend to be somewhat more competent than boys when completing open-ended writing tasks. These are the types of essays that could go on and on chasing different facts and exploring different themes. This skill that girls have is probably enhanced by a vocabulary which has been enriched by a daily delivery of about 20 000 words in comparison to only about 7000 words being uttered by males.[11]

Yet all is not quite as bleak as it might be. Boys tend to do a little better in writing tasks that are more 'closed'. These are tasks that have a definite finish, for example, list five different words that mean 'beautiful'. Other literary tasks completed reasonably well by boys are those requiring some analysis, such as 'What is the author referring to when he writes "the sob and the clubbing of the gunfire"?' Are enough 'closed' types of responses being used within current assessment programs? To what extent is the current method of assessment mitigating against males? Would a different and rather more positive picture emerge about boys' standards of literacy if less open ended tasks were used and more multiple choice methods of assessment used?

Australian research has found that the better performance of girls relative to boys exists throughout the country and in most types of literacy tests. The few exceptions have been in a number of exams which used multiple choice questions and short, structured answers. It was also found that boys could do better, relative to their performance in other areas of literacy, when the questions asked of them were single concept questions. Unfortunately the same study found that short answer questions and multiple choice questions were appearing less and less in literacy tasks for students in Australia.[12]

It is important to recognise that what is being advocated is not a 'rigging' of the assessment experience to the advantage of boys. Rather the suggestion is being made that there should be a balance in the styles used to assess boys and girls in schools. There are clear educational imperatives to use short answer responses, just as there are clear educational imperatives to use longer answers. It is entirely possible to increase the number of short answer tasks, 'closed' tasks and analytical tasks linked to listening and comprehension without compromising the integrity of the learning experience. For this reason some consideration might need to be given to reformatting some English exams and other literacy tasks in order to ensure that a wide variety of response styles is tested.

5. A father-led recovery

While indicating that the father is a key role model for a boy, it is not implied that a mother is less important. In fact, in the earlier years of a boy's life, the mother is probably the key figure in introducing literature. In later years when a boy begins to search for his male identity, he may well look to an adult male on whom to model his reading behaviours. This is where the problem can occur. There is evidence to suggest that it is more frequently the father who may be at risk in not fulfilling his parenting duties as he is frequently required to be outside the home earning the income necessary to support those within the home. Unfortunately some fathers can become so preoccupied with this task that their home-based duties and obligations may not always be met.

One of the main duties of a father is not only the provision of money, but also the provision of security and the creation of the emotional and physical harmony necessary for the family to live in health and peace.

The needs that a father must meet are not just physical, they are emotional, social, spiritual and intellectual. The growing boy needs to learn the craft of manhood from his father and to model himself on his father so that the best traditions of society are passed on, including the value of the reading experience.

With these imperatives in mind and recognising the unique influence fathers can have on their sons, the help of fathers should be enlisted to fight the battle of declining standards in literacy among boys. The failure of many fathers to read to their sons and to hear their sons read has been linked to the underachievement of boys at every age in school. Quite why so few fathers read to their sons is not always clear. Some fathers see this role as a demarcation issue, with the responsibility for this activity being seen as that of the mother. Unfortunately this only serves to convince a boy that reading is a feminine activity and when the day comes that the boy begins to drift away from his mother and align himself more with the father, all things feminine will be abandoned, the cuddles, mother's milk — and reading.

More dads need to read and more dads need to read to their sons. This is not always easy, as a father may leave home early in the morning to catch the 6.45 am from Epping, and not get back until the children have been fed, watered and dispatched to bed well before the 6.25 pm from Wynyard pulls in. It must also be said that the physical and emotional energy levels of a father may not be great after a day working with 'administrivia' in the city or a day wrestling with machinery in a manufacturing plant in the suburbs. Add to this the fact that some fathers carry within them the same hesitancy to read and the same lack of pleasure in the printed word as their sons. It can be very difficult to get some fathers to read for their own purposes, let alone read to their sons.

Despite the difficulty, there remains the imperative to get fathers involved in the education of their sons. All too often fathers only intervene in the formal education of their sons to discipline them. Love is expressed through criticism. Some fathers may need to give more time to their sons and give less criticism of their sons. The sacrifice made in switching off the TV to hear a son read can be negated if all that it provides the son is a lesson in correction. Having noted this, the reverse can also be true. Consider the harassed mother juggling many roles, who has pleaded and directed her son to do his homework which is abandoned immediately the father walks in for a riot of fun and noise which centres on a football and the misuse of great grandmother's crocheted cushions. Meanwhile, the mother transfers her flagging energies to the stove with the accusation ringing in her ears, 'You're no fun, Mum'.

Returning to various initiatives that can be undertaken by fathers other than the use of great grandmother's crocheted cushions for goalposts, there are a number of options to be considered, including:

- Reading to children each night or each morning. Even 10 minutes before the evening meal can be useful.
- Being readers themselves and giving ample evidence of this by sharing the interesting or amusing content of their reading with the family.
- Listening to children read, in a warm and encouraging manner, with a curb put on the natural impulse to correct and criticise.
- Becoming involved with children's written projects and helping to 'conference' written work. Care needs to be taken not to take over the project, otherwise the educational value of the experience becomes lost for the children.
- Being writers. Whether it is just letters or e-mails to friends and relatives, whether it is prose, poetry or letters to the editor, the sharing of this experience with children can help inspire boys to write.
- Paying conscious attention to language and spoken vocabulary. People tend to write rather like they speak. If fathers model a rich and appropriate vocabulary, and are sensitive to the opportunities of explaining any new words to children, the vocabulary of sons is likely to improve as might the written work.
- Sharing with the family something of the nature and content of the written tasks at work. This is not always possible or appropriate, but boys can be inspired to soldier on with the development of their literary skills if they are made aware of the importance of these skills in the workplace.
- Sending to the sons letters and e-mails from work and encouraging them to respond.
- Being involved with the children's life at school, attending parent-teacher evenings and actively seeking to be acquainted with the curriculum, in particular the literacy program being offered at school.
- Assisting in the school by offering to give a talk or a demonstration to students, or even offering to hear some children read. The dearth of male teachers in many primary schools would mean that such offers of help could be very much appreciated.

Within the school setting various initiatives can be undertaken to help fathers to help their children, particularly in the development of literacy skills. Just getting fathers into the school can be a very positive first step and initiatives such as the following can be very helpful:

- father-son evenings
- father-son camps
- involvement of fathers, grandfathers, uncles and older brothers in school based learning projects.

It is of interest to note that a large study was undertaken of over 1000 families in the USA over a 27-year period to help find the main factor in determining the future income of children. The results of this study might surprise some fathers. What was found by Greg Duncan of Northwestern University was that the most influential factor in determining a child's income at 27 years of age was not IQ, education level or parental occupation. It was the attendance of fathers at PTA meetings.[13]

Use can also be made of strong male role models who are sportsmen or engaged in any form of profession which is likely to fire the imagination of boys. If these role models are then used in the school's literacy program, it may improve a boy's orientation to literature. A policeman reading stories about crime, a mechanic reading articles about cars, a soldier reading accounts of great battles or the specifications of the Army's latest tank are all tasks that can inspire: boys love to identify with and imitate men they respect. If these men read, they might read.

Ongoing links with male authors and other suitable role models can be maintained through the use of letters and e-mail. A school might even 'adopt' an author, a politician or a poet.

Men are sometimes used to mete out punishments to boys. Parents and teachers might need to give careful thought to the punishments they award if these punishments involve written tasks. If punitive writing tasks are set then there is a very real chance that the writing of essays may become synonymous with something which is distasteful. The giving of 'lines' is even less defensible. It is a moronic activity which demeans a boy and encourages rebellion, for it is nearly as much an insult to the boy's intelligence as it is to the intelligence of whoever is giving the lines. A review of the sanctions given by a family and a school, together with an understanding of the subliminal messages they send, might be appropriate. It is also important that adult males, as well as adult females, are used as much to reward good behaviour as well as having to deal with bad behaviour.

Schools also need to choreograph opportunities for boys to write and read beyond their normal classroom duties. School newspapers, orations in assembly, debates, reading about the Olympics or other major sporting events, Drop Everything and Read (DEAR) initiatives all serve as examples. As many of these activities as possible should have some input from a male adult, whether it be the general duties person or the sports coach.

The Australian author John Larkin tells a story of the New South Wales Literacy Council approaching a first grade rugby league team based in Sydney to visit some schools to tell the students what their favourite books were. The scheme was not a thundering success, largely because the players had not actually read any books.[14]

Rather more successful was a scheme developed by the teachers in Rangeville State School in Toowoomba, Queensland, who developed a Real Men Read initiative involving a pool of 60 men being used to read to students. Most of the men were fathers of students at the school. They would read extracts from material they liked to read when they were young, or examples of what they were reading and writing now. Photographs were taken to record the event and these were displayed prominently in a Real Men Read display. The program was augmented by father-son days involving activities such as go-karting, indoor rock climbing, flour bomb fights and mud slides.[15]

6. A peer-led recovery

The extraordinary power of the peer group should never be underestimated. Being expelled from the herd is a sentence to a world of isolation, shame and emotional and social ignominy. Parental power is great in the life of a boy, but parental love is biased. It is generally unconditional, it is always there. For a boy to test his true social ability, to test whether he really has what it takes, he must enter the fickle world of his peers. It is here that he will be judged for who he really is, with sentences handed down unclouded by love or family ties. It is here that the boy must find acceptance and even validation. This is the authentic world, the world which he will live in once he is of an age to exercise his independence. This is the world where love and friendship is conditional — conditional on conformity. It is humbling for the devoted and caring parent to find that a few seconds of unfamiliar behaviour by a strange child will negate years of dedicated parenting and become the chosen behaviour for their child in the playground.

Early teen years bring even less comfort to the parent for they must endure at least a partial alienation from their son as he stretches his juvenile wings and flutters to the edge of the nest in readiness for the great adventure of independent flight. Other chicks in other nests have shed their infant down and squawk derisively that they can fly already. The son is ashamed of his reliance on his mother's warmth and his father's food. He tries to tell himself he needs neither, and this works well until he is cold or hungry. But the taunts continue and they drive him to the edge of the nest again and again. One day, he flings himself into space. Sometimes the chick will fly, sometimes the chick will die. It matters little that the bigger chicks the son seeks to please are emotionally bereft of compassion, relentlessly self-absorbed, highly competitive and aggressive. They represent the flock with which he must fly and so he must leap. The parents can do little but hope their boy flies.

To be truthful, there are times when there are a few other chicks which are less derisive, which can form groups and which are very affirming and imbued with a moral and ethical code even the parents can be proud of. The compassion shown by these friends and the sense of mateship and protection for each other can be quite inspirational. However, the shadows of the sociopathic groups are also to be found as are the bullies and those in much too much of a hurry to grow up. The trick is to find the right peer group. Such groups are not common, but they do exist and some of these groups even tolerate reading.

Most boys generally understand and even appreciate clear rules and directives. True, these rules will be tested to see if the adult world values the rules enough to defend them. This should not prevent rules from being established, but if they are established they must be of a quality that deserves to be supported by adults and children alike. Parents and teachers should not flinch from setting rules for boys that support the push for greater literacy. The full cooperation of boys, both singularly and as a group, needs to be sought when establishing rules, such as:

- We will read for at least 30 minutes each day.
- We will not disturb or distract each other during the reading sessions.
- When invited, we will assist each other with reading and as we do this we will encourage and help each other.
- We will allow reading and writing excellence to exist in this classroom without jealousy or 'put downs'.
- We agree that it is not 'cool to be a fool'.
- We will allow the expression of feelings in our writing and our speech.
- We will not swear or use inappropriate language.
- We will not tease or 'freeze out' any who might be different from us in any way.
- We will share good ideas about what is good to read.
- We will work together when asked to do so, to help each other improve our writing.

These sorts of standards are best worked out collegially with boys rather than imposed. Once decided upon they may need to be enforced with some firmness. This should not translate into a savage authoritarian regime but to a regime which is laced with humour, compassion and an understanding of where boys are at. In other words, what is being signalled is that adult capitulation to the worst elements of boy behaviour is not appropriate. Neither is the belief that a boy's peers are always bad news. Guidelines for peers can be established and the strong desire for group identity among boys can be used to the advantage of those wishing to increase the literacy skills in boys.

7. 'Take home' reading schemes

Some educators commend the setting up of 'take home' reading schemes in schools.[16] Such schemes vary but the establishing of such schemes typically involves the following steps:

- The reading age of boys is established.
- A small library of books is collected with boys assisting in book selection.
- The books are graded according to reading difficulty and each 'grade' of books is stored in a separate box.
- Each boy is assigned to a 'grade' of book, and borrows books from the appropriate box.
- Parents are informed about the take home reading scheme. A contract is signed by parents that their son will read for 30 minutes each evening.
- Boys are encouraged to read to their father if at all possible. If not, then any appropriate member of the family hears the boy read.
- A borrowing record is kept and the teacher monitors the reading patterns.
- The program is constantly reviewed, books are changed, and boys are tested to see if they are ready to move up a grade.

8. The home library

A home library can diagnose a household's orientation to reading. If the library is limited and covered in dust, it will tell a child that books are not really worth being read. If a son were to witness an extensive library in the house with well-used and constantly repaired covers of the C F Forester *Hornblower* series, then he might be persuaded to pick up a copy in order to find out just what it is that has given so much enjoyment and pleasure to others.

Even in this microchip age when the computer can provide so much literature, a print library can be an important signal that reading is valued in a household. In saying that reading is valued, it should be made clear that it is valued for the pleasure it gives as well as for the information it holds. Books should not just become synonymous with dreary scholastic assignments. 'Whodunits' and thrillers need to adorn the shelves, as well as the wisdom of the world's best minds, both past and present. It was Charles Lamb (1775–1834) who proclaimed, 'I love to lose myself in other men's minds'.

An audit by parents of their own library at home, together with the reading habits of the entire family, may be diagnostic in assessing whether the home environment is supporting the school in promoting reading and referencing from books. True, the Internet can also be a very real asset in this regard, but it must not be allowed to be the only asset.

9. Literature-based reading schemes

Some educational commentators argue that rather too much use has been made of a phonics approach to reading, and suggest that a 'whole language' approach to reading is better.[17] The phonics approach is very popular in many schools. This approach teaches the relationship between the visual symbol and the sound it represents. For example the 'ea' letter combination is taught as giving an 'e' sound. A few educators are critical of the phonics approach and suggest that phonics may be successful in teaching work attack skills but may be unsuccessful in teaching the meaning, the relevance and the joy of reading.

Educators will be divided on this issue for there is evidence that phonics-based programs such as the Spalding method of reading can be enormously successful. Supporters of the phonics approach will point out that many boys feel much more secure with logic and rules, and appreciate learning how to apply logic to help with reading. There will also be some who argue that word recognition skills such as may be achieved through phonics are the necessary 'building blocks' required by a child before he or she is able to enjoy reading.

What upsets a number of English teachers about a rigid phonics approach is that out of context language drills, vocabulary and spelling tests based on material the child is not studying, and artificial grammar exercises, can so overwhelm a boy that the wonder and adventure in literature becomes lost. The same might also be said in the learning of modern languages. The chant of 'je suis, tu es, il est, nous sommes, vous êtes, ils sont' does little to excite many about French, whereas cooking up some French onion soup using directives in French might elicit a rather more positive response from boys.

To be fair, teachers' energy levels, creative juices and, significantly, their departmental budgets may be such that they cannot cope with cooking French onion soup or engaging in these types of activities every lesson. Yet a virtual journey through the Louvre using the Internet may be possible. For this reason, 'whole language' advocates try to employ a broad range of strategies to help boys learn to read which extends beyond decoding exercises, and centres more on the meaning of a word and its relationship with other words.

As with many solutions in education, some techniques for teaching reading will work better for some boys than with others. It is the job of the skilled teacher to use whatever method is most appropriate for each child. There are alternatives in trying to make reading enjoyable for boys. If a phonics approach is not working, a 'whole language' approach may be an option.

10. IT-based reading schemes

Boys enjoy using computers and there is now a wider range of software packages available which are designed to encourage reading. It is best to seek advice before purchasing any software, with teachers often being the best source of help in this area.

Some IT reading schemes, such as 'i Read' by Scholastic, grade all their reading material according to a level of difficulty. A boy is tested then given books to read which are appropriate to the boy's ability. Some schemes grade books according to a reading difficulty which is measured in 'lexiles'. A higher lexile indicates a book which is more difficult to read.

11. Using emotions

One way to smuggle good literature into boys' lives is to capture their interest by choosing literature which is going to touch their emotions. Despite the feigned bravado and the overt display of emotional sterility, boys cannot entirely rid themselves of their humanity, of their capacity to feel, of their capacity to be greatly moved.

Good literature exists that can engage a boy's emotions and might even encourage the boy to sprinkle an increased number of references to emotion in his own writing. Literature can be found which can stir a boy's emotion, which can encourage a boy to be emotive and feeling in his own writing. The trick is to find the right stimulus. The hunt is worth it. Suitable literature can even be found in that form most despised by boys, the poem. For example:

> Faire wraithes ye skip and play
> And capture sunbeams through the day.
> E're darkness comes, they must away
> For moonbeams bringeth disarray . . .

is unlikely to inspire the average boy. On the other hand if a teacher was to describe the horror of the battle of El Alamein which led to many dead being washed up on the Mediterranean beaches and read them Kenneth Slessor's poem Beach Burial, a boy's interest and a boy's emotion is likely to be stirred.

> Softly and humbly to the Gulf of Arabs
> The convoys of dead sailors come;
> At night they sway and wander in the waters far under,
> But morning rolls them in the foam.

The imagery of corpses in the water is strong, with the tides and eddies moving their limbs in the deep water before they are washed up as flotsam on the beach. The first verse captures boys through vivid, even grotesque imagery.

> Between the sob and the clubbing of the gunfire
> Someone, it seems, has time for this,
> To pluck them from the shallows and bury them in burrows
> And tread the sand upon their nakedness;

The distant battle is still raging with the muted sound of gunfire sounding like 'the sob and the clubbing' — powerful words of hurt. Yet in this madness there is compassion, for the dead are buried, not by relatives but by an unknown. These are sentiments boys need to reflect on.

> And each cross, the driven stake of tidewood,
> Bears the last signature of men,
> Written with such perplexity, with such bewildered pity,
> The words choke as they begin —

The burial parties, possibly men, are emotional people. They choke; they are perplexed by the waste; the carnage. Boys need to be emotional beings; to be moved with such pity that their words get choked.

'*Unknown seaman*' — the ghostly pencil
Wavers and fades, the purple drips,
The breath of the wet season has washed their inscriptions
As blue as drowned men's lips,

Human mortality is reflected on in the lines above. This is something boys rarely do, to their own detriment, for very few realise that boyhood is but a stage in the journey to the grave.

Dead seamen, gone in search of the same landfall,
Whether as enemies they fought,
Or fought with us, or neither; the sand joins them together,
Enlisted on the other front.

Source: Beach Burial by Kenneth Slessor from his *Selected Poems*. Reprinted with permission of HarperCollins Publishers Australia.

And so the poem finishes inviting discussion on the cost of war and its ultimate futility. Such a discussion might help to neutralise the glorification of combat which is all too often found in a boy's world.

As indicated above, boys may be encouraged to read if the right literature is found — literature which has action and which stirs the emotion. If that literature has been written by a man, then so much the better, for boys make heroes of men they admire and seek to be like them.

It seems a pity that the natural gravitation of some authors, when writing for boys, is to make the material lewd, rude or crude. When objections are raised, these same authors defend their offerings as contemporary and attack their critics, suggesting that their books are not written for moral watchdogs but for boys.[18]

What sort of message is this? Is it proper that authors are made immune from criticism and the requirement that their books conform to basic standards of civility because boys will only read books with crude pictures on the cover and swear words within? This is as insulting as it is inappropriate. It is entirely possible to write engaging literature for boys without pandering to a boy's natural fascination with bad taste. Boys and bad taste are becoming dangerously synonymous as it is without being reinforced by authors.

12. Helping boys to express their feelings in literacy tasks

The contemporary socialisation of boys does not encourage boys to express their feelings, to admit to inner turmoil, doubt, fear, insecurity or affection. The stoic male is advanced as the acceptable model so that feelings must be buried, the tears held back, and their written expressions devoid of the depth and complexity that the true expression of feeling can bring. Written work and spoken words are limited to functional expressions. When pressed to make their writing rather more compelling to read, younger boys will often increase the number of 'baddies' being killed and crank up the 'zap' and 'pow'. When girls are asked to make their writing more compelling, they tend to draw a pretty flower in the margin and then write a thesis. What is more, the thesis is usually both readable and laced with the expression of feelings and emotion.

THE OPINION OF A 13-YEAR-OLD BOY ON BEING ASKED ABOUT HIS FEELINGS, OPINIONS AND VIEWS

My English teacher wants me to write about my *feelings*, my history teacher wants me to give my *opinions* and my science teacher wants me to write on my *views* about the environment. I don't know what my *feelings*, *opinions* and *views* are, and I can't write about them. Anyway, they're none of their bloody business! I hate school! I only wish I could write about the things I'm interested in like sport and military aircraft.

Source: Quoted in Rowe, K J (2000), 'Schooling performances and experiences of males and females: Exploring "real" effects from evidenced-based research in teacher and school effectiveness', A background paper for the Australian Institute of Political Science and the Department of Education, Training and Youth Affairs, Australia, Eden on the Park Hotel, Melbourne, 22–23 November 2000.

A characteristic of subjects like English is that they can demand reflection, an analysis of feeling and the frequent expression of emotion. The undertaking of literacy tasks can often mean the engagement with emotion, for so much of literature is about joy, pain, love, challenge, trial and triumph. This requires students to connect with their emotions and to be sensitive to the emotions of others.

Getting boys to take the first tentative steps in expressing feeling and emotion in both written and spoken form is not easy, but a few suggestions are advanced.

Use third-party emotions

Some boys may feel more comfortable about expressing emotions in tasks by inviting them to describe the likely emotions being felt by someone else. This disassociates boys from having to confess to the emotions themselves and helps the boy to preserve something of the aura of expressionless indifference. The third-party approach can be a useful starting point. The bridge between describing the emotions felt by someone else and describing one's own emotions is not particularly large, and the latter should be attempted at some later date when boys are feeling much more comfortable with the general expression of emotion and feeling.

Use sporting emotions

Boys do get emotional. There are a few occasions where society allows males to be emotional. Sport is such an occasion. There can be an overt display of strong feeling without contravening the male 'code'. Allowing boys to watch the final 10 minutes of the 1999 Australian Rugby League Grand Final, and getting them to describe the feelings of the St George Illawarra players when they lost to Melbourne Storm in the dying minutes of the game, after having what seemed to be an impregnable lead, might serve as an example. The viewing of the reaction of the players after the final whistle will show men in tears. It will show the St George Illawarra Chaplain, the Reverend Stephen Edwards, talking quietly to the broken hearted losers. It will show the unbridled jubilation of the Melbourne players. Such experiences can offer rich opportunities to the discerning teacher who is faced with the task of getting boys to write and speak with feeling. Persuading boys to record their own feelings and the feelings of the sportsmen they venerate can help introduce many to the language of emotion.

Use anonymity

Boys may need to be afforded some anonymity when they are initially invited to write with feeling. The discerning teacher might allow anonymous written descriptions about feelings which are then edited by the teacher and read back to the class with much praise and encouragement.

Use role models

Boys in school need to see other boys, older boys and men who are unafraid to express their emotions and who do it well both in written and verbal form. The example given by other males can be of great assistance in giving boys permission to express feelings themselves. A senior student who spent some time helping flood victims, or a past student doing missionary work in slums, reporting on their work with passion and compassion can be very effective in making boys more comfortable expressing such feelings themselves.

Use professionals
There are men who are skilled orators and skilled writers. Inviting such men into the school should only be done if the material they share is appropriate to boys, and if such men have the ability to fire the imagination of boys with their words. There are great male actors, writers and speakers who are available to speak to boys and who can demonstrate their literary and articulacy skills, and their capacity to express feelings.

Use justice
One of the things that can elicit passion, indignation, outrage and hurt in boys is a sense of injustice. The young often have a passionate sense of justice and will show great tenderness to their own if they feel they have been victims of injustice. 'That's not fair' is a cry which is all too familiar to adults and this sentiment can provide opportunities for teachers to get boys to record their feelings in a passionate way. Describing a great injustice, either real or imagined, and helping boys to visualise and fully engage with that injustice, through multi-media presentations, can cause very powerful feelings in boys which can then be translated into words.

Use drama
Drama can be useful to boys as a way of exploring their emotions. Some boys may not be strong writers, but may feel much more comfortable displaying emotion and feeling in drama, particularly if the boys can identify with a character in the play. For this reason considerable care may need to be taken by the teacher in 'cueing' the boys to the character, to highlighting the tensions and the issues that are in the mind of a character before inviting them to assume that character. Showing video excerpts of passionate orations by great male actors can also help to break down some inhibitions that might exist among boys before they 'tread the boards'.

Create trust
Perhaps the most important task before teachers or parents who wish to encourage the free expression of emotion and feeling in a boy, is to create a culture of security and trust between themselves and the boy, so that the boy knows there will be acceptance and encouragement even with his initial stumbling forays into sharing his feelings. This trust can only be built up over time and can be destroyed so quickly by insensitive comment or derision. The fragility of a boy who is brave enough to transgress the 'macho code' and confess to feelings and emotions must be both realised and respected. Immediate encouragement from adults should be given, for it is unlikely the boy will find it in his peers.

Use films

Boys like to watch. Not for nothing have contemporary youth been labelled 'screenagers'. This love of film can present teachers with a powerful means to explore emotion, for most films are redolent in emotion. Thwarted love, sinking ships, and erupting volcanoes create emotional scenes in movies which can be explored by boys, particularly if the characters being studied are male.

Use compulsion

There are times when teachers and parents can get rather apologetic about making quite reasonable demands on boys. If done properly, the simple directive of requiring boys to record feelings in their essays should not be rejected. It is true that such directives are likely to be more effective if the reasons have been carefully shared with the boy beforehand. Many boys desire to please, to do well. Some boys also have a slightly mercenary streak and wish to do particularly well in a subject because this will open up great rewards for them in the future. This gives some leverage to teachers in saying that boys must record feelings and emotions in their written work if they want good grades. The value of working out marking schemes with boys beforehand, and highlighting the percentage of marks to be awarded for the effective recording of feeling and emotion, should not be underestimated with some boys.

Use parents and teachers as models

There is truth in the Biblical principle that society 'reproduces fruit after its own kind'. If boys see their parents and their teachers as being people who express their feelings well, who are not afraid to be honest and open about how they feel, then this will serve as a powerful example. An audit on the home and the school can be taken to see if there is an empathetic environment which gives boys the right to laugh and cry, an environment in which parents and teachers can express their emotions and admit to their humanity.

13. Collecting vocabulary and phrases

Boys' use of vocabulary is somewhat more limited than that of girls. This may result from a predisposition for action rather than conversation. A casual glance at a school playground at lunchtime will bear witness to boys charging around doing things and girls sitting around saying things. As a result, the vocabulary of girls is both exercised and extended. Boys, on the other hand, have a mental dictionary that is somewhat thinner. Boys may need to be encouraged, even compelled, to engage in both written and spoken tasks that exercise and extend them. Descriptors like 'nice' should be banned as should sentences that start with 'then'. It was Walter de la Mare who wrote:

> Until we learn the use of living words, we shall continue to be wax works inhabited by gramophones.

With 'nice' being taken off the menu, other words can be offered for consumption such as 'delightful', 'agreeable', 'pleasant', 'lovely', 'endearing'. It might be a while before a boy can graduate to 'elysian', 'paradisiacal' and 'congenial' but a journal of 1000 pages starts with a single word.

Quite apart from word collecting, boys might also be required and requested to collect interesting phrases. Rather like a stamp collection, these phrases can be collated not so much under countries but under themes such as anger, pleasure, concern, love, disappointment and so on. When the album is opened up to the heading 'anger', the boy might be able to see that he has collected the following phrases:

- a deep and disturbing displeasure
- an acid bitterness that erodes his soul
- a fierce fury
- hot under the collar
- incensed and indignant
- heart-burning
- kindle one's wrath
- stir one's bile
- smouldering with indignation.

The boy may also have located a quote:

> He spoke with a certain 'what is it' in his voice and I could see that, if not actually disgruntled, he was far from being gruntled.
> P G Wodehouse, *The Code of Woosters*, 1938

Any interesting expression, either heard or read, could be entered and the personal collection of interesting phrases should grow to the extent of genuine usefulness.

Now, of course, all this sounds rather idyllic. The compliant boy earnestly dashing around collecting words is just not going to happen — at least at first. One method by which parents and teachers can demonstrate the worth of such a collection of words and phrases is to find something which is really bothering a boy, which is really frustrating him and then giving him some hints about what he can write down, such as some phrases he might use, some words that could be appropriate to the situation.

An example of this 'problem solving' approach to vocabulary enrichment might be a son admitting to some frustration at being teased for being so quiet. So, filed under 'Q' for quiet or 'T' for teasing might be a few attempts at humour to extract the venom from the teasing. Not all of this will work and not all of the words would be appropriate to every situation but this should not necessarily prevent recording of ideas such as:

- In saying little I can think more.
- In drawing on my fine command of language, I'm saying nothing.
- I like quiet; quiet can be good.
- I'm saving up to spend my words at some other time.
- You are saying it so well for me.

Then there might be some phrases to help cope with the panic of not knowing what to say:

- Hang on a moment, I want to think this through.
- I'm just engaging my brain.
- I'll get back to you on that one.
- Interesting question. Why do you ask?
- Can you put that another way?
- I haven't the faintest idea, but what I can say is . . .
- Do you really want to know?
- Why?

Perhaps a few 'openers' might be written down to help initiate conversations:

- How are you travelling?
- What's up?
- Are you OK?

Then some details might be recorded in the same book on favourite topics of the peer group which could be sprinkled into a conversation.

Boys are pragmatic. If their personal diary of words and phrases can be shown to be helpful and can be shown to solve some of their problems, then it stands a chance of working. Such a diary will have to be very boy-centred and if it should contain an exquisite list of insults to hurl at other boys, a Nelsonic eye might have to be used by adults when reading it.

14. Collecting the tricks of effective writing and effective speaking

There are skills that can be taught to boys to help them enrich their writing and speaking. Books abound on this topic and they can be seen cluttering the self-improvement shelves of airport book shops. Most of these books are for adults. Any self-respecting boy is unlikely to apply himself to any such book anyway, even if a suitable one should be found. The reality is that parents may have to become teachers themselves and be prepared to share with their sons the tricks they have learnt to make writing more accurate and interesting. Society may need to recover the claim that children learn best from people rather than books. This is not to say that books are not important, it is to say that people are even more so.

What are the tricks? What is the literary wisdom that lurks hidden in the human content of a household that can be shared with its sons? This will vary from family to family, but examples of the sort of homespun advice that could be given to boys engaged in writing tasks that might emanate from a home include:

1. In an essay, try to argue a point from different points of view. Evidence both for and against should be submitted.
2. Try to get a mark with the first sentence. You only have one shot at a first impression, don't blow it. Capture the reader at once.
3. In the introduction to the essay, clearly define the main words and ensure you understand the essence of the question by paraphrasing it and writing something like: 'Essentially, this question is asking whether . . .'
4. Ensure that the body of the essay has a logical sequence and that it remains central to the question being asked.
5. Demonstrate knowledge. Do not fill the essay up with facts that everyone knows and expect to be rewarded marks. Include information which is only found through careful and diligent research. Make sure specific illustrative data (SID) are present.
6. Make good use of the odd quotation but not too many. Acknowledge all quotes, do not be tempted to plagiarise. Include references and/or the bibliography at the end of the essay in the correct manner.
7. Leave the reader on a high. The conclusion should not be a tired repetition of what has already been written. The conclusion should involve higher order thinking. It should be evaluative, and contain phrases like 'of all the reasons listed above, perhaps the most important is . . . because . . .'
8. When writing, avoid dogmatic and sweeping statements. Words and phrases such as 'no one', 'everyone', 'always' should be used with

great care. Far better to temper statements with words like 'usually', 'often', 'sometimes'.

9. Enjoy and use interesting words and phrases, but do not overdo it to the extent that one is long-winded and flowery.
10. Do not be boring. Try to display creativity.
11. Do not be overwhelmed by the opinions of others; form your own. Sometimes it is as well to be open-minded on a topic. At other times it is important to arrive at a point of view and to be able to defend it.
12. Alliteration can sometimes work well in an essay: '. . . her eyes were baleful black beads'.
13. Repeated negatives can be useful: 'There is neither pride nor pleasure in . . .'.
14. Opposites can be effective: 'She became alive to the possibilities his death would bring'.
15. Repetition can strengthen a point: 'He was never drab, he was never stale, he was never prim'.
16. Humour can be refreshing but take care not to trivialise the written work: 'Professionals built the Titanic; amateurs built the Ark'.
17. Interest can be generated by the use of slightly less common paragraph commencements: 'Curiously . . .'
18. Adjectives and adverbs should be used to enrich a piece of writing: 'He was spectacularly drab in his presentation'.
19. If the topic and subject allow, do not be afraid to write with feeling, emotion and passion. With increasing age comes decreasing reward for English essays limited to a litany of action. Feelings need to be explored, described and included. Wherever possible, try to move beyond the boring, safe description of action to the raw, dangerous and transparent recording of feelings, for this is what can make an essay so interesting.
20. When you have written something, read it through again. When you think you have done this, do it again, but this time do it properly.

The advice shown above is by no means complete, neither is it advice that all parents and teachers will necessarily be comfortable with. Good. Each family should author its own advice. What is written above is only indicative of the type of collective wisdom that can be passed on to a boy by a family. Some might be tempted to think that these are tasks that should be the preserve of teachers in school. It is not, for it takes a village to educate a child.

CONCLUSION

Western society has tolerated the growth of a culture which seems to support a crude anti-intellectualism in boys. This anti-intellectualism is to be found particularly in the area of literacy. Generations have passed on to generations totally inadequate skills and totally inadequate models in many areas of literacy.

No one can afford to point the finger of blame. Society is complicit in its tolerance of poor literacy skills in boys. There is evidence of indifference to the problem at the government level. Education systems and their schools have been party to a feminisation of both curriculum and assessment. Teachers have been involved in a tragic labelling of boys and have perpetuated the ideal student as being the student with feminine characteristics. Parents, particularly fathers, have not involved themselves enough in their sons' education. Boys as a group seem content to cultivate the image of the rather dim sporting 'jock' as the preferred male and individual boys have had neither the inclination nor the courage to seek an alternative definition of 'male'.

Of course, these are sweeping statements. There are exceptions. There are real innocents, but if as much energy was spent finding solutions as it was in voicing denials, then the poor literacy problems in some males might now be solved. Yes, there are good and effective politicians, school administrators, teachers, parents and boys who are faithfully and even effectively tackling the problem of literacy problems in boys. However, more must be done to break the cycle which seems to be handed from one generation to another. A concerted effort by government, media, schools and families must be made to allow a boy to be bright, to allow a boy to have feelings, and to allow a boy to read. This will require a multi-faceted approach at the macro, meso and micro levels.

At the macro level, government must research the matter of boys' literacy much more, with a view to improving education and teacher training and to putting some controls on media images of boys. It is not just a question of allowing 'the academic dork to have his day'. It is about allowing other expressions of maleness, particularly the reflective academic and the boy who enjoys literature and music, to be portrayed as something other than desperately unattractive and 'wet'.

At the meso level, schools must be honest in their audit of themselves as to whether there has been a feminisation of curriculum, pedagogy and assessment. Ways and means need to be established to help boys engage positively with learning. Real questions need to be asked about school organisation, role models and whether something needs to be done about the value systems to be found within a school.

At the micro level, the family and ultimately the boy himself should accept responsibility. The great tradition of blaming others must stop. Boys are no innocents. Just as they are a party to the problem, they can be a party to the solution. They can be directed to change, they can be encouraged to break out of the culture that 'it's cool to be a fool'. Society must be sensitive in its handling of this issue, but not so sensitive that a paralysis occurs and nothing is said by parents in guiding a boy to develop better literacy skills.

APPENDIX A

RECOMMENDED READING FOR BOYS

Please note that the appropriateness of each book must be determined independently by a responsible adult. What is shown below is indicative only. Not all the books may be suitable to the ages shown, as judgment in this area is very subjective. Parents and teachers must satisfy themselves that a book is appropriate before obtaining it for a boy.

6-8 years

Author	Title
Brown, J	*Flat Stanley*
Browne, A	*Willy the Wimp* (and other titles)
Carroll, J	*Billy the Punk*
Clement, R	*Just Another Ordinary Day*
Clement, R	*Grandad's Teeth*
Dahl, R	*The Magic Finger*
Dahl, R	*The Twits*
Dahl, R	*Fantastic Mr Fox*
Denton, T	*Gasp*
Denton, T	*Zapt*
Denton, T	*Splat*
Fienberg, A	*Tashi* (several titles)
Fienberg, A	*Minton* (several titles)
Fienberg, A	*The Hottest Boy Who Ever Lived*
Fine, A	*Diary of a Killer Cat*
Harvey, R	*Dirty Dave the Bushranger*
Jennings, P	*Gizmo* (several titles)
Jennings, P	*Singenpoo* (several titles)
Legge, D	*Bamboozled*
Tulloch, R	*Cocky Colin*
Tulloch, R	*Rodney's Runaway Nose*
Tulloch, R	*Mr Biffy's Battle*
Viorst, J	*Alexander and the Terrible, Horrible, Not Good, Very Bad Day*
Whatley, B	*Tails from Grandad's Attic*
Whatley, B	*Magnetic Dog*
Also:	The *Solo* series
	The *Aussie Nibbles* series
	The *Colour Jets* series

8–10 years

Author	Title
Ball, D	*Selby* (numerous titles in the series)
Bates, D	*Bushranger* series
Bernard-Waite, J	*The Riddle of the Trumpalar*
Bernard-Waite, J	*The Challenge of the Trumpalar*
Blume, J	*Tales of a Fourth Grade Nothing*
Blume, J	*Superfudge*
Blume, J	*Fudge-a-mania*
Dahl, R	*Charlie and the Chocolate Factory* (and others in the series)
Dahl, R	*James and the Giant Peach*
Eldridge, J	*Warpath* series
Gates, S	*Beware of the Killer Coat* (and other titles in the series)
Honey, E	*Don't Pat the Wombat*
Honey, E	*45 and 47 Stella Street*
Jennings, P	*Freeze a Crowd*
Jennings, P	*Duck for Cover*
Jennings, P	*Spooner or Later*
Lewis, C	*Narnia* series
Lurie, M	*The 27th Annual Hippopotamus Race*
Macleod, D	*Sister Madge's Book of Nuns* (poetry)
McNaughton, C	*There's an Awful Lot of Weirdos* (poetry)
McNaughton, C	*Who's Been Sleeping in the Porridge?* (poetry)
Metzenthen, D	*Brocky's Bananagram*
Rodda, E	*Bob the Builder*
Rodda, E	*Rowan* series
Rodda, E	*Deltora Quest* series
Stephens, M	*Eddy the Great*
Stephens, M	*The Prince of Kelvin Mall*
Weldon, A	*The Kid with the Amazing Head*
Winton, T	*The Bugalugs Bum Thief*
Also:	Any of the *Aussie Bites* series
	Greek myths and legends
	Take a look at the Percy Trezise *Aboriginal Legends*, including the series *Journey of the Great Lake*

10–12 years

Author	Title
Applegate, K	*Animorph* series
Banks, L	*The Indian in the Cupboard* (and series)
Dahl, R	*Boy*
Dahl, R	*Going Solo*
Deary, T	Any title in the series *Horrible Histories*
Fisk, N	*Mindbenders*
Gleitzman, M	*Toad Rage*
Gleitzman, M	*Blabber Mouth* (and others)
Griffiths, A	*Just Stupid* (and others)
Harris, D	*Cliffhanger* series
Jacques, B	*Redwall* series
Jennings, P	Any titles
Kelleher, V	*Taronga* (and others)
King-Smith, D	*Magnus Powermouse* (and others)
Marsden, J	*Tomorrow, When the War Began* (and series)
Paulsen, G	*Hatchet* (and others)
Pullman, P	*The Northern Lights* (and sequel)
Rowling, J	*Harry Potter* series
Rubinstein, G	*Space Demons*
Simons, M	*Totally Weird* (and others)
Tolkien, J	*The Hobbit*

Also:	True adventure, war and escape stories are popular, particularly short stories in these genres as they are short to read and are less daunting for many boys.

12–14 years

Author	Title
Adams, R	*Watership Down*
Applegate, K	*Animorphs — The Invasion*
Baillie, A	*Wreck*
Becker, S	*When the War is Over*
Blacklock, D	*Pankration*
Carmichael, C	*Virtual Realities*
Carmody, I	*Obernewtyn*
Caswell, B	*Mike*
Clark, M	*Body Parts*

Clark, M	*Web Watchers*
Clark, M	*Famous for Five Minutes*
Crew, G and O'Mara, M	*The Island*
Crichton, M	*The Andromeda Strain*
Cross, G	*Wolf*
Deary, T	*The Truth about Guy Fawkes*
Dejong, M	*The House of Sixty Fathers*
Disher, G	*The Bamboo Flute*
Duncan, L	*Locked in Time*
Fine, A	*Madam Doubtfire*
French, J	*Dancing with Ben Hall*
Gleeson, L	*Dodger*
Gleeson, L	*Refuge*
Gleitzman, M	*Water Wings*
Harrison, M	*It's My Life*
Hathorn, L	*Rift*
Higgins, J	*Eye of the Storm*
Hobbs, W	*Far North*
Holub, J	*The Robber and Me*
Hughes, T	*The Iron Man*
Jinks, C	*Eye to Eye*
Johnson, J	*Hero of Lesser Causes*
Kelleher, V	*Parkland*
Kelleher, V	*Earthsong*
Klein, R and Dann, M	*The Lonely Hearts Club*
Konigsburg, R	*A View from Saturday*
LeGuin, U	*The Wizard of Earthsea* (and series)
London, J	*Call of the Wild*
Lowry, L	*The Giver*
Marsden, J	The *Tomorrow* Series
Mattingley, C	*No Gun for Asmir*
McRobbie, D	*The Fourth Caution*
McRobbie, D	*A Little Drop of Wayne*
McRobbie, D	*See How They Run*
McRobbie, D	*Mandragora*
McSkimming, G	*Cairo Jim and the Quest for the Quetzal Queen*
O'Brien, R	*Z for Zachariah*
Paulsen, G	*Hatchet*
Paulsen, G	*Dog Song*
Paulsen, G	*Soldier's Heart*
Pratchett, T	*The Carpet People*
Price, S	*Hauntings*

Rowling, J	Harry Potter Series
Rubenstein, G	Foxspell
Rubenstein, G	Under the Cat's Eye
Rubenstein, G	Space Demons Trilogy
Sachar, L	Holes
Stoker, B	Dracula
Taylor, T	The Cay
Tolbert, S	Escape to Kalimantan
Tolkien, J	The Hobbit
Winton, T	Lockie Leonard Human Torpedo
Winton, T	Blueback

14–16 years

Author	Title
Archer, J	A Matter of Honour
Baillie, A	Secrets of Walden Rising
Banks, L	One More River
Bernard, P	The Outcast
Broderick, D	Zones
Carey, P	Jack Maggs
Carmody, I	The Gathering
Caswell, B	Deucalion
Caswell, B	Only the Heart
Chang, J	Wild Swans
Clancy, T	Patriot Games
Clancy, T	Executive Orders
Clark, J	The Lost Day
Cook, R	Chromosome 6
Cormier, R	I am the Cheese
Cormier, R	After the First Death
Cormier, R	Heroes
Cornwell, N	The Warlord Chronicles: Books 1–3
Courtenay, B	The Power of One
Crew, G	No Such Country
Cussler, C	Inca Gold
Disher, G	The Divine Wind
Douglass, S	Beyond the Hanging Wall
Duder, T	Personal Best
Feist, R	The Magician
Fleishman, P	Seedfolks
Forbes, C	By Stealth

Francis, D	*Twice Shy*
Francis, D	*Field of 13*
Gee, M	*Orchard Road*
Gilstrap, J	*Nathan's Run*
Gleeson, L	*Refuge*
Greenwood, K	*The Broken Wheel*
Grisham, J	*The Pelican Brief*
Grisham, J	*A Time to Kill*
Hamilton, M	*Mister Eternity*
Hathorn, L	*Rift*
Higgins, J	*Flight of Eagles*
Higgins, S	*Dr Id*
Hilton, N	*Square Pegs*
Jinks, C	*Eye to Eye*
Kelleher, V	*Fire Dancer*
Kelleher, V	*Slow Burn*
Klein, R	*Came Back to Show You I Could Fly*
Laird, C	*But Can the Pheonix Sing?*
Le Carré, J	*The Tailor of Panama*
Mattingley, C	*Escape from Sarajevo*
McFarlene, P	*The Enemy You Killed*
Melville, H	*Moby Dick*
Michaels, A	*Fugitive Pieces*
Moloney, J	*Bridge to Wiseman's Cove*
Myers, W	*Fallen Angels*
Noonan, M	*McKenzie's Boots*
Oughton, J	*Music from a Place Called Half Moon Street*
Paulsen, G	*Foxman*
Paulsen, G	*The Transall Saga*
Pratchett, T	*The Colour of Magic*
Riordan, J	*Sweet Clarinet*
Steinbeck, J	*The Grapes of Wrath*
Voigt, C	*Homecoming*
Watson, L	*Montana, 1948*

16–18 years

Author	**Title**
Ballard, J	*Empire of the Sun*
Capote, T	*In Cold Blood*
Conroy, P	*Beach Music*
Courtenay, B	*The Power of One*

Crichton, M	*Airframe*
Fleishman, P	*Whirligig*
Forsythe, F	*The Day of the Jackal*
Frazier, C	*Cold Mountain*
Hansen, D	*Lunch with Mussolini*
Hartnett, S	*Stripes of the Side Step Wolf*
Heller, J	*Catch 22*
Ishiguro, K	*The Remains of the Day*
Le Guin, U	*The Dispossessed*
Ryan, C	*The Kremlin Device*
Schlink, B	*The Reader*
Smith, W	*A Sparrow Falls*
Tan, A	*The Joy Luck Club*

Note: At this age, parents and teachers tend to need to give less guidance and most good quality books read by adults would be suitable. Biographies of sporting heroes can be very popular at this level.

Older boys can still find fantasy literature quite engaging such as:

Brooks, T	*Shannara*
Carmody, I	*Darkfall*
Eddings, D	*Belgariad*
Eddings, D	*Malloreon*
Eddings, D	*Elenium*
Feist, R	*Serpentwar Saga*
Feist, R	*Riftwar*
Gemmel, D	*Drenai Saga*
Jacques, B	*Tales of Redwall*
McCaffrey, A	*Chronicles of Pern*
May, J	*Trillum*
Tolkein, J	*The Lord of the Rings*
West, M	*Proteas*
Williams, T	*Memory*
Williams, T	*Thorn*
Williams, T	*Sorrow*

Science fiction books can also prove popular with some boys, for example:

Asimov, I	*Foundation* (series)
Bradbury, R	*Martian Chronicles*
Clarke, A C	*Rama*
Herbert, F	*Dune*

Perhaps the most successful formula for boys in terms of fiction writing is that of adventure and survival such as:

Clancy, T	*Op Centre*
Smith, W	*Courtneys*
Smith, W	*Courtneys of Africa*
Smith, W	*Ballantyne* novels

ADDITIONAL INFORMATION

For those wishing to have further details on some of the points raised in this chapter, the following references may be helpful. Each number in the text of the chapter relates to a reference number below which will give further information related to the topic.

1	Moloney, J (2000)	*Boys and Books*	ABC Books, Sydney, p 18.
2	Moloney, J	(op cit)	p 39.
3	Millard, E (1998)	'Differently literate — Gender identity and the construction of the developing reader'	*Gender and Education*, Vol 9, No 1, p 32.
4	Jones, C (1996)	'One in three year 9 students lack literacy skills'	*Australian*, 22/10/96, p 1.
5	Arndt, B (2000)	'The trouble with boys'	*Sydney Morning Herald*, 17/6/00, p 34.
6	Davy, V (1995)	'Reaching for concensus on gender equity: The New South Wales experience'	Proceedings of the Promoting Gender Equity Conferences, 22–24 February, Department of Education, Canberra.
7	Tattam, A (2000)	'Let them read sex, says author'	*Education Age*, 31/5/00, p 14.
8	Moloney, J	(op cit)	p 65.
9	West, P (1995)	'Books and bodybuilding: A strategy for boys' education'	*Sydney Morning Herald*, 3/3/95, p 13.
10	Stoessiger, R (2000)	*Improving Boys' Literacy*	Workshop material given at the Training and Development Centre Lewisham, 15/6/00.
11	Teese, R et al (1995)	'Who wins at school?: Boys and girls in Australian secondary education	Australian Government Publishing Service, Canberra, p 94.
12	Teese, R et al	(op cit)	
13	Kindlon, D and Thompson, M (1999)	*Raising Cain*	Penguin Books, London, p 103.
14	Larkin, J quoted in Rapee, W (2000)	'Boys will be boys'	*Classroom*, Issue 6, Scholastic, p 15.
15	Mulligan, D (2000)	'Real men read'	*Classroom*, Issue 6, Scholastic, p 20.
16	Carosi, F (2000)	'Curriculum relevance and diversity'	IES Conference, The Gazebo Hotel, Sydney, 22–23 June 2000.
17	Kohn, A (1999)	*The Schools Our Children Deserve*	Houghton Mifflin Co., Boston, p 161.
18	Rapee, W (2000)	(op cit)	

chapter 6

Boys, friendships and sex

FRIENDSHIP CHANGES OVER TIME

In infancy the gender of a boy's friends does not appear to matter a great deal, with the onset of same gender preference in friendship only becoming an issue when the boy commences school. Even then some good friends from the opposite sex may be maintained as girls in primary school can, by reason of similar strength, interests and ability, engage in the same recreational activities as boys. These friendships will be reinforced by geography (the girl next door), logistics (in the same class) and vicarious associations (the parents are good friends or related).

The pre-adolescent stage and early adolescent stage will often witness the greatest rift between the sexes in terms of friendship. Increasing awareness of the differences between the sexes, and a desire to be successfully identified with a sex through gender-appropriate behaviours, reinforces this polarisation of friendship. Intersex warfare is at its greatest in this 'giggle and tease' stage of life, with a gradual lessening of hostilities only occurring when adolescents become secure in the realisation and acceptance of their own sexuality.

In mid- to late adolescent years, a boy often feels able to reconnect with the opposite sex. There are many reasons, not the least of which is the emergence of the basic instinct to want to procreate. Yet it is important to recognise that the sex 'thing' is not the only reason why boys begin to linger around the girls' lockers at school. The male friendship group has its place and is still enjoyed, but there can be an increasing dissatisfaction in the ability of this group to meet all of a boy's needs. Thus the circle of friends enlarges its circumference to include others who can meet these needs, including girls.

BOYS WANT TO GIVE AND RECEIVE FRIENDSHIP, INTIMACY AND LOVE

Boys have the capacity to hurt themselves and to hurt others in their relationships, but it is as well to remember that the natural inclination of boys is to give and receive love, companionship, support and friendship. Boys may occasionally put on a mask of complete self-reliance, but it is only a mask and in most cases hides a boy who is desperate for acceptance by his family and friends.

There are times when a boy wishes to be independent and self-sufficient. There will be times when a boy may present as unfeeling and without the capacity for care or compassion. In most cases, these conditions are but temporary trysts in a life that prefers to give and receive friendship.

It has been suggested that older boys are driven more by lust than love and interested more in conquest than commitment. While it is undoubtedly true that some sexually active boys in their late teens may be guilty of these descriptors, it is worth pointing out that not all fit this description. Some research among adolescents has found that males value intimacy and socialisation as much as females.[1]

A study undertaken of American college students discovered that boys saw sex as the most romantic element of a relationship whereas girls considered signs of affection such as sending flowers, cuddling and being taken out for dinner as more romantic.[2] Other research has actually suggested that males are more romantic than females. However, the expression of this romance did vary, with females opting for methods that were more expressive, intimate and concerned for their partner, whereas boys tended to be less expressive, less intimate and expressed their romance more playfully.[3]

When one examines research on adolescent intimacy and friendship, at least two main themes seem to emerge. The first relates to 'individuality', the capacity of a person to retain his or her own individual identity in a relationship as opposed to a fusion of identities brought about by an accommodation of the partner's identity and needs. Shulman et al found in their study of adolescent couples aged 17–19 years that males still tried to maintain their own identity in a relationship.[4] Females, on the other hand, tended to stress the interrelatedness of a relationship, the reciprocity of feelings and the sharing of mutual concerns.[5]

The second theme is that of 'closeness'. Boys' friendships with each other tend to be laced with competition which can prevent overt displays of intimacy with their male friends. With girl friends, the issue of competition is removed and boys can become more intimate and disclose more of their romantic feelings. Expressing intimate feelings is something boys will only do once a relationship has developed the trust and acceptance necessary for the removal of the 'cool' facade. Quite apart from a natural reticence to express emotion, a boy is handicapped by a linguistic impoverishment that can hinder the articulation of closeness. Boys can also suffer a lack of social sensitivity and limited observational skills.[6] It can sometimes be days before a boy is made aware that his girlfriend has spent a significant amount of her pocket money on putting highlights in her hair.

Boys have strong feelings, but these feelings are generally kept in check until a relationship is solid enough and secure enough for boys to reveal them. This conclusion flies in the face of those who would have society believe boys to be devoid of feeling or care.

Research also challenges the notion that boys are not romantic. Working with older teens and college students in the USA, researchers have found that more males than females believe in love at first sight.[7]

This is hardly surprising for it has long been acknowledged that for males visual stimuli are very strong, a truth long recognised by girls who purchase short dresses with plunging necklines.

THE GROWING ATTRACTION OF GIRLS

With the gradual withdrawal from the warmth and support of the mother in favour of the companionship of the father, a boy can stop receiving the physical expression of love, the cuddles and the hugs. A boy may also stop hearing the verbal expressions of love, the spoken sentiments of affection which can be so important to a boy's self-esteem. The adolescent boy can lose the affirmation of unconditional acceptance. With mother there was always love, understanding and forgiveness even when a boy was behaving like a complete idiot. With fathers these traits are less common. Fathers can be emotionally more sterile, consumed by work and given to expressing their love by criticising and continually wanting to improve their sons. Compounding the problem are the boys' own friendship groups, the gangs which can have a behavioural code which is rather hard, competitive and unfeeling.

A way of recovering warmth and unconditional acceptance, after having spent a number of emotionally frigid years in male territory, is for a boy to break out of the same sex gulag and seek the companionship of girls. This companionship is not necessarily sexual, but is no less important in fulfilling a deep need in a boy. A boy needs escape from the male conventions of the 'macho' lifestyle and this can be found in friendships with girls.

WHEN DOES CUPID STRIKE?

Boys are able to have strong feelings of warmth and even love from infancy onwards. Developmental theorists have not always been convinced that there is a 'latency' phase through which children must pass before they are of an age to be able to have sexual or romantic feelings. It is being suggested by some developmental psychologists that these feelings can be detected throughout childhood in some form or other, even in infancy.[8] Although there may well be some truth to this claim, the expression of romantic attachment undoubtedly changes. A boy-girl relationship in early adolescence is often more social than sexual with true psychological and physical intimacy occurring in the later teen years.

Perhaps one of the greatest dangers for boys in their initial boy-girl relationships is to move towards a physical intimacy unmatched by a psychological intimacy. The problem can be exacerbated by a desire to keep up with one's peers and the 'leader of the sack' who may be setting the agenda in terms of sexual experimentation. Even if much is hot air and bravado, the effect on others is still much the same: a propelling into physical intimacy for which some boys may not be fully equipped.

From a developmental perspective, a boy's pre-adolescent contact with the opposite sex is rather limited because patterns of play tend to develop which see children playing mainly in sex-segregated settings. In early adolescence, some interest begins to emerge in the opposite sex, but the intimacy of such relationships is kept in check by boys forming platonic friendships and socialising as a group. These can be difficult years. Boys can be frightened about whether they are male enough, and whether they are men enough, to please a girl. There is acute awareness of their own body: its size, the presence or absence of muscle, hair, the depth of voice, strength and, perhaps most frightening for some, their sexual orientation. To be called 'a faggot' or 'gay' can be particularly painful for some boys and, if done frequently enough, can lead to a loss of confidence and depression.

The early teen years are also years when there can be quite dramatic differences in the size and physical maturity of boys. There are also differences in the capacity for intimacy between the sexes which can also complicate the life of a boy. Some researchers maintain that levels of intimacy are greater in females and that the desire for intimacy develops later in males.[9]

Teenagers spend about half their waking hours with each other and only about 5% of their waking hours with parents.[10] Nonetheless, the development of romantic relationships can be problematic for adolescent boys. Previous play behaviours in gender-segregated groups has done little to prepare boys for heterosexual relationships. However, relationships develop and with them the onset of individualism and the daring to break away from the dictates of the group. Boys may need to be warned that some groups surrender the influence of their members very grudgingly, with derision and teasing often signalling the group's sense of grief at losing a member of 'the gang'.

Some boys can remain consumed by winning acceptance by the male group. The desire by some boys to have their sexual or affiliative needs met by girls may not be as strong as their need for acceptance by the male group. This can promote the rather ugly scenario of boys engaging in sex more to be accepted by their peers than to be accepted by their partner.

In mid- to late adolescence some fractionation of the larger group occurs as concern for peer status begins to be subverted by a concern for partner status. The lead up to this has also witnessed an increasing amount of training in the basic competencies of keeping a relationship together. This training has been provided through peer example, and trial and error within the larger social scene.

The typical age at which boys and girls start becoming attached to each other in an intimate sense is not always agreed upon. There are different definitions of intimacy and there are cultural differences and many other variables which must be borne in mind. Montgomery and Sorell tested 186 early to middle adolescent males and 199 early to middle adolescent females in USA and reported the following pattern (see Figure 6.1) of those who stated that they had been 'in love'.[11]

These types of surveys are interesting but problematic, for it is not always easy for an adolescent to distinguish between love, lust or like. Nonetheless, these feelings, whatever they are, should not be dismissed by adults, nor should the capacity for pain as well as pleasure in these relationships be underestimated.

THE STRONG, SILENT TYPE

The expression of a boy's affection has sometimes been limited by a social convention which holds that boys should be free of the disability of emotion. The 'strong, silent type' is reinforced as the preferred male model in many ways, not least in the media. The celluloid response of Bruce Willis and Arnold Schwarzenegger to personal or public disaster is to go out and kill someone. Not for them the inconsolable grief or the choked tears when family and friends have been highjacked, taken hostage, hunted or hurt. They square the chin, steel the eyes, delve into a long forgotten or improvised arsenal and set off to commit some serious carnage. There is usually a hug from the rescued or relieved damsel at the end but it is usually unconvincing and unnecessary. Men don't need hugs, they just need a pump action shotgun and strips of cloth to tie around the wound.

THE DEMAND FOR A NEW MALE

The currency of the 'man without feelings' has recently been devalued. Men themselves are questioning the 'macho' virtue because of an obvious

Figure 6.1 Percentage of girls and boys who have been in love

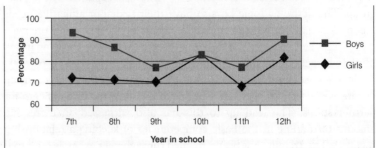

Source: Montgomery, M and Sorell, G (1998) 'Love and dating experience in early and middle adolescence: grade and gender comparisons', *Journal of Adolescence*, 21, p 681.

impoverishment in the quality of their lives, and females are questioning this virtue because they do not wish to be yoked to an emotional eunuch. Society is beginning to recognise that the emotional structures it has placed on its young men have yielded poor returns. The evidence is to be found in marital breakdowns, deliberate acts of self-harm and a bewildered group of males who have found that they do not belong. So they gather in pubs, clubs and sporting venues where their emotional bankruptcy blends with the inadequacies of others, camouflaging their limitations as lovers, fathers, men.

At work, male associations tend not to be emotional, but expedient. Relationships are based on function rather than feeling. There is some mild flirtation in the workplace banter but, save for the furtive affair or adventurous grope, the expression of intimacy is seldom called for by men at work. The anonymity and restrictive hierarchical structure that hinders the development of relationships is only relaxed after five beers at the annual Christmas party and thereafter firmed up for another year devoted to the bottom line.[12]

This is beginning to change and, despite attempts to ridicule the trend through the pillorying of the 'sensitive new-age guy' (SNAG), there is undeniable evidence that emotional transparency is being allowed in boys. However, there is much that still needs to be achieved in this area with Moir and Jessel warning:

> Men want sex, and women want relationships. Men want flesh and women want love. Just as the boys wanted balloons, toys, and carburettors, the girls have always wanted contact, communion and company.
>
> All this, the magazines assure us, is no longer true. This is the age of the new woman, equally capable of, and disposed towards, taking her impersonal pleasures where she finds them and when she needs them. The new man, meanwhile, has rededicated himself at the altar of the greater sensitivity, banishing his sexual brutishness, and is bewitched by his beloved's brains rather than her bosom.
>
> Neither the new age, nor the new man, is likely to last.[13]

HOW BOYS EXPRESS THEIR FEELINGS

Boys display their affections differently from girls. The overt demonstration of love by boys is permitted only in the very young or those targeted by Cupid's arrow. In between, love as a sentiment is ridiculed. Yet within this period of emotional aridity in a boy's life, expressions of love are still present, but they are revealed in 'boy-like' ways. Boys often show their love through doing things for people and through acts of practical service such as weeding the garden, cleaning the gutters or repairing the CD player.[14] It is not a question of actions speaking louder than words, it is a question of actions speaking *instead* of words. Boys often prefer to express their feelings by doing things rather than saying things. The wobbly wooden tray given to mum is not just saying that a boy is yet to discover the virtues of a set square. It is saying that the boy loves his mum and is hugely grateful for her devotion and care. It can sometimes be hard to credit a wooden tray or the washed car as saying these things, but the translated meaning of these actions needs to be learnt by parents and appreciated.

The articulation of feelings by males is not generally seen as strength. This must not be interpreted as a lack of love, but rather as a lack of articulacy, and the remnants of a social convention which would have men mask their feelings. Moir and Jessel write:

> Not for nothing does he 'say it with flowers' — he cannot say it with words. Many men may send their loved one a birthday or anniversary card — that's no problem; the trouble arises when it comes to wondering what to write on the darned thing. Men do not have such easy access to the language of love.[15]

SEXUAL AND PLATONIC FRIENDSHIPS
In cementing friendships, boys use balls, banter and bravado. Girls will talk. Yet the two different approaches are not totally successful in keeping the groups apart. This is not just due to primeval sexual urges but, and this might come as a surprise to some, because it is possible for different genders to enjoy each other without it all degenerating into the mating game.

The sexual friendship can be a beautiful relationship. It need not be characterised by predatory lust and sexual exploitation. A boy and a girl can agree to journey together for a while in exploring the sexual dimension. Sometimes the respect may not be there, with the initial sexual experiences being driven in the boy by a desire for conquest rather than companionship and in the girl by a desire for acceptance rather than a desire for love, but it is not always thus. It should be remembered that both parties are young, inexperienced and will make mistakes.

Adults might also care to remember that both boys and girls are distracted by school, constrained by lack of independence and have limited financial means. This will mean that they are not able to give an adult expression of their love toward each other by living together and thus their sexual liaisons must necessarily be opportunistic and even furtive. These characteristics are not necessarily the characteristics of choice but rather of necessity and adults should recognise this.

The non-sexual friendship can also be a very beautiful relationship with a boy and a girl being able to explore themes and perspectives not available in same sex groups. Platonic friendships serve an important role in the life of adolescents but some would deny them of this and try to interpret such friendships as always being sexual. Parents can do this out of fear. Peers can do this out of envy.

Society must allow the platonic friendship to exist. It can serve a vital function in providing an opportunity to share thoughts, feelings, doubts and insights which cannot be done elsewhere. Such relationships can also serve as a testing, checking and repair centre for the amorous relationship. With the mother unavailable because of the generation gap and the lover unavailable because of complicity, who else is the boy to turn to for female advice on friendship and sex? Where else is a boy going to get empathetic advice that is not complicated by love? The smutty smirks and sly innuendoes which the platonic friendship can attract need to cease.

IDENTITY FORMATION

A boy's ability to form friendships will be influenced, at least in part, by a boy understanding his own identity. Knowing oneself is an advised state before seeking to know others. A boy needs to find out many facts about himself, including his:

- likes and dislikes
- gifts and weaknesses
- goals and purposes
- character and temperament
- values and attitudes
- spiritual orientation and belief.

Erik Erikson suggests that boys can be in one of four states of identity formation.[16]

1. **Identity diffusion** — no real idea of personal identity, unthinking, isolated, aimless, often linked to poor self-esteem and associated problems such as drug use.
2. **Identity foreclosure** — may or may not have some idea of personal identity but allows this to be totally incorporated into a ready made identity such as a gang culture. With the embracing of such an

identity comes some intolerance and inflexibility as the adopted identity leaves little room for individual expression.

3. **Identity moratorium** — searching for identity and exploring all the options. An open mind but not yet committed to an identity. Some people never emerge from this state.

4. **Identity achievement** — this is the stage when a boy has found his own identity and is aware of his character, values, preferences, gifts and beliefs.

HOMOPHOBIA

For boys, the spectre of homosexuality does loom and in the early years of secondary education in particular it can become a real fear. It is at this time that many boys get the most significant clues as to their sexual orientation and manliness. It can be an intensely painful period for boys.

Comparisons are continually being made by boys and teasing dispensed not just for fun but to cover the shame of one's own inadequacy. A number of social commentators such as Peter West suggest that homophobia is rife among boys with the fear of homosexuality driving many boys to prove their manliness through ill-advised sexual liaisons with girls, and through the adoption of a macho style of behaviour and speech.[17] The intensity of homophobia can be increased by a boy's own feeling of sexual insecurity. A boy might fear his weak sexual orientation and as a result might become violently homophobic.

Boys' feelings of insecurity on the issue of gender orientation may be fuelled by the fact that there are probably no absolutes in terms of homosexuality and heterosexuality. There is a continuum with most people oriented towards a certain position but not necessarily 100% so. In an age that is addicted to compartmentalism and categorisation this concept can be hard to accept, but if it were to be accepted there might be greater compassion and understanding.[18] It is worth remembering that even if homosexual liaisons occur among some boys, they may be fuelled more by sexual experimentation and the desire to release sexual energy than by true physical attraction.

One can go even further and say that should a homosexual orientation be confirmed in a boy, the boy is, in all probability, a relative innocent in the situation. It may well be that either through accident of nature or nurture a boy is homosexual. There is little reward for anyone in either denying the situation or blaming the boy. In all probability the boy has had to cope with a huge degree of misery and guilt anyway without this needing to be added to. Compassion and tolerance is needed, not accusation and derision. The thing that makes homosexuality so difficult for homosexuals is not their gender orientation but society's judgment of that orientation. Boys who are homosexual will need extra understanding and acceptance to survive the harshness of the real world, not less.

THE NEED FOR OPENNESS

Establishing a relationship where boys believe themselves to be loved and accepted is a vital prerequisite for open and free discussion on matters relating to friendships, love and sex. Plays, movies and songs proclaim the centrality of these themes in society. They also remind that relationships are society's greatest source of pain as well as its greatest source of joy. Relationships with God, relationships with family, relationships with friends and relationships with enemies are borne better by boys if they can be discussed in an open and honest fashion with someone who is trusted and respected. This trust should never be betrayed because then the boy is condemned to a frightening loneliness of dealing with these issues on his own.

LONELINESS

One of the great driving forces behind a boy wanting to form sexual and non-sexual friendships is to combat loneliness. Humans are essentially social animals and generally prefer to live in communities and forge relationships with each other.

BOYS AND SEXUAL TENSION

Males are maturing earlier and marrying later. Most boys develop the ability to father children in their early teens, yet the average age of marriage for an Australian male in 1999 was 31years. The period between represents the need for a lot of cold showers, for the desire to engage in the act of procreation can be strong enough to over-rule any amount of bromide in the tea. Males also tend to reach the peak of their sexual desire many years earlier than females. The result is a lot of sexual tension in boys.

The sexual tension is heightened in teenage boys by a certain innate wiring which would seem to suggest a stronger orientation to sexual promiscuity. Further inflammation of the sex drive in boys is provided by the media which seems remarkably reluctant to show any real sex scene within the context of marriage. Thus one can begin to understand the attraction of boys to assuage their sexual appetites before marriage.

One of the cruellest things society can do is to dismiss the frustrations boys have in relation to sexual drive. God gives boys the equipment and activates it in their teens, but the necessity to be educated, financially independent and to have found a life partner means a wait of many years

LONELINESS

The good Lord's first diagnosis of the human condition was to judge it vulnerable to loneliness. So . . . Eve was fashioned to provide help and companionship for Adam.

Perhaps there is no coincidence that the spread of secularism in our society has coincided with an epidemic of loneliness. Having no recourse to the support of a Heavenly Father can leave us vulnerable and alone. Having no recourse to spiritual instruction can leave us blundering in isolation, and cause us to become disconnected from ourselves, from society and from our God.

The student when he bullies, spreads loneliness. He spreads the chill of being expelled from the group, of being made to feel inadequate and of being made to feel different. The bullied are often on their own; excluded; pariahs.

Modern technology can also spread loneliness. It can substitute reality for virtual reality; it can substitute social discourse for an electronic mouse and a visual display unit. Although opening communication to an unimaginable host, computers can also isolate.

Dysfunctional families can spread loneliness, for when the place of belonging, the place of security, the place of love is changed to a place of hurt, a place of bitterness, and a place of fear; when the safest refuge in the world fails you, there can be a crushing loneliness borne of insecurity and broken trust. The lonely must then wrap their arms around themselves and rock. There are no other arms to hold them and there is no one else to rock them.

Institutions can spread loneliness. Their hierarchies and rules can isolate. Sharing with subordinates or superordinates can be discouraged. This leaves one's equals, whose sympathy and understanding cannot always be relied upon because of the presence of competition in our society and our predilection to self-centredness and gossip. So we remain isolated, and smile practice smiles. We put on masks like Eleanor Rigby who, according to John Lennon:

. . . waits at the window, wearing the face that she keeps in a jar by the door;
Who is it for? All the lonely people, where do they all come from?
All the lonely people, where do they all come from?

Society can spread loneliness. Nuclear families, broken families, mobile families. Home entertainment systems become a substitute for friends and we hide in individual houses, guarded by six foot fences with intercoms.

I consider loneliness to be one of the greatest threats to our quality of life. As we move into the twenty-first century, our major battles will be not so much with the unwashed masses, but it will be with the unloved individuals. It will come from whose who are disconnected. It will come from those who are lonely.

Source: Hawkes, T F, *The King's Herald*, The King's School, Parramatta, 12 March 1999.

before society will generally smile at the gratification of their sexual desire. Is this unfair? Are current expectations made of boys unrealistic in terms of demanding a repression of sexual energy and celibacy before lifelong commitment to a partner? Individual families will have their own response to these questions, influenced no doubt by parental convictions, religious orientation, the opinion of friends, the portrayal of sex in the media and a whole range of other factors. Irrespective of whatever answers are given, it is important to recognise the existence of a very real sexual tension in boys. It is also important not to dismiss teenage love as 'puppy love' or to judge the sexual urge of a teenage boy as being similar to that of a middle-aged adult.

What can boys do about their sexual frustration? AIDS and STDs combine with convenience to provide a steady market for 'virtual sex', pornography, phone sex and an ever more sophisticated range of sex substitutes for boys. However, there are other answers which may be more wholesome, which may need to be suggested to boys as a legitimate way of dealing with sexual tension. Whatever is suggested must be managed with a genuine understanding of a boy's frustration in this area.

Another source of potential frustration can arrive for a boy when he first engages in sex. The initial experience can be something of a disappointment for both parties, with a lack of experience, guilt and fear of failure often combining to reduce the unbridled joy of initial love making. Kindlon and Thompson warn:

> Because masturbation is such a natural part of an adolescent boy's experience, he is a veteran of sexual pleasure before he ever becomes involved in partnered sex. When he is drawn by his desire for love coupled with mature sex, a boy has to make a precarious crossing over a bridge from that intensely personal, rewarding and predictable fantasy exercise to a real life girl with her own unfamiliar sexual and emotional terrain. From a performance standpoint, it is almost impossible to fail at masturbation. With a girl, what was simple becomes infinitely more complicated, physically and emotionally.[19]

GUIDELINES ON SEX

The vexing question as to what to advise boys on how far they should 'go' with a girl, and when and where they can 'do it' with a girl is a matter for each family to resolve. Some families will want to institute a total celibacy policy and will want the control of unruly passions until marriage. This approach is much pilloried by the media, but conservative

CONDOMS IN SCHOOLS

I am not in favour of condoms being sold in schools. This does not mean that I am against the use of condoms or the promoting of responsible sex. What I am suggesting is that the potential for harm in selling condoms within the school is greater than the potential for good.

I have arrived at this view for a number of reasons. The first is the fallacy that condoms offer safe sex. Condoms do not offer safe sex. Condoms merely offer safer sex. Research has indicated that as many as one in 10 condoms break or are not used properly. It can be argued that it is the school that promotes abstinence that promotes safe sex.

One also needs to be aware of the subliminal messages given by a condom vending machine. Its proponents say that the message is 'safe sex' and 'be responsible'. However, the language heard by teenagers is not always the same. Those who have had some experience with teenage students in schools will bear witness to other messages being heard, such as — 'come taste the forbidden fruit' — 'using this is fun' — 'you should be sexually active' — 'if you're not having sex there's something wrong with you'. The capacity for some teenagers to resist these types of messages is not always great.

One needs to be mindful of the enormous peer pressure to experiment and to identify with the 'coolest' and the 'hottest'. Do our teenagers really need a machine that has the potential to provide them with another arena for ego advancement peer pressure to enter into sexual activity before many would otherwise want to?

I would also suggest that a condom machine in a school is often not so much a symbol of institutional approval of responsibility but rather an institutional approval of fornication. This can be a problem for schools who choose, for spiritual and/or moral reasons, to celebrate celibacy until marriage. Although divine directives are somewhat less attractive these days, society should remember that the general wisdom to be found in our spiritual texts has the alarming habit of being very apposite for today. Having noted this, it is important to acknowledge that some of our students are sexually active. Fortunately, modern society provides many opportunities for these students to acquire the means to practise responsible sex without having to shop at school.

Then there is the image problem. The poor condom has never been able to shed its association with casual sex and sex with multiple partners. This is not always fair but the association should not be surprising. With the use of the condom in this age of the pill, what we are often asking is 'Where have you been?' The latex says 'I don't trust you' and wonders at other experiences and other exploits. Thus, there is a barrier to sensitivity and feeling, both physical and emotional.

The condom machine makes it easier. It caters for the impulse, for the now. 'Here is rubber, what doth prevent us?' I am not always sure that history shows that making things easier for our youth has always paid dividends. The discipline of being able to wait and work towards a deferred reward is an important one and it is a discipline in danger of being lost. There is sometimes virtue in waiting. For example, virginity can be offered only once and some will choose to offer it as a gift to their life partner. Others will choose to offer experience to their life partner. A condom machine may appear to judge the latter as the preferred gift and this may not necessarily be true.

The accusing finger pointed to a vacant toilet wall does not shift the blame for pregnancy or disease. Those who are unable to engage in responsible sex are not going to be saved from their condition by the provision of a condom machine on a school wall. Their condition will be better prevented by a responsible education program taught by responsible educators and responsible parents.

Source: Hawkes, T F, *Newslink*, St Leonard's College, Melbourne, 16 November 1995.

wisdom often has the habit of being proved the best for society in the long run. Self-control, freedom from STDs, AIDS, unwanted pregnancies and the emotional wreckage that can go with having many sex partners is avoided, as is the ageless discomfort of going against the dictates of one's God.

Other families might advise differently, and advocate growing intimacy with growing commitment. This can be an admirable solution providing there is a clear understanding of commitment. Is it being engaged? Is it being 'in love'? These things need to be discussed. It is also worth reminding young men that they are very likely to fall in love more than once. Older boys might also need to consider what sexual experience they want their life partner to have had before having sex together. Often there is an hypocrisy among young men that sees them sewing more than one paddock with wild oats but wanting their wife to be an unsullied garden.

Other advice will also be offered by some families such as, 'make love not lust'. In other words, by all means go 'all the way' but make sure that as a result both feel enriched by the experience. If there is any chance of guilt, betrayal, a reduction in respect for the partner or a decline in a sense of self-worth, then learn to recognise that the moment is not right. There may be worth in reminding boys that the experience should be a giving experience rather than a taking experience, whereby each partner should seek to give pleasure rather than just take pleasure, and where each wishes to ensure that the moment is remembered as a positive experience for the other.

Whatever guidelines are given to boys, they will need to be worked out by consensus rather than imposed. They must be discussed openly and honestly within the security of a loving home, otherwise the issue will be decided covertly in less secure settings.

BOYS AND GIRLS, LOVE AND SEX

Although not entirely accurate, there is some truth that young men give love to get sex and young women give sex to get love. The expectations from a sexual liaison can differ between boys and girls, particularly outside the context of a steady relationship. Moir and Jessel write:

> His relationships are those of power and dominance. Hers are those of interplay, complement and association . . . suddenly, these alien species are thrown together by their biology — a biology which attracts them physically, yet in so many other respects, is mutually antagonistic. No wonder being in love is so confusing . . . Most teenagers receive manuals on how to plug in their respective genitalia, yet none explain the different, yet complementary apparatus of mutual perception . . . below the surface lie two separate submerged continents of appetite, attraction, appreciation and desire.[20]

It is not always true that young men want sex whereas young women want relationships, but there is some evidence to suggest that the need to release sexual energy may be stronger in males with males registering higher irritability when in a state of celibacy.[21] This may explain assertions that boys may be born rather more promiscuous than girls. 'Hoggamus Higgamus, men are polygamous, Higgamus Hoggamus, women are monogamous' may be slightly less true now than when first these words were uttered; nonetheless, parents and teachers may need to remind themselves of the very real sexual tensions that are likely to exist in a teenage boy. Struggling with these tensions is bad enough, struggling with these tensions in isolation, and smitten with guilt on the one hand and frustration on the other hand makes the process of growing up even worse.

TEMPTATION

A boy can often be sexually aroused more quickly than a girl. The fairer sex has known intuitively that a key perceptual sense in males is sight. The pornography industry and the male desire to make love with the lights on, bear testimony to the strength of the sight stimulus for males. This is important for a parent to remember should they see their son completely befuddled at the sight of an alluring girl. The female fashion industry has been preying on the male 'visual thing' for years, as indeed have girls themselves in seeking male attention. Cynthia Heimel in her humorous book *Sex Tips for Girls* writes:

Seamed stockings are not subtle but they certainly do the job. You shouldn't wear them when out with someone you are not prepared to sleep with, since their presence is tantamount to saying, 'Hi there, big fellow, please rip my clothes off at your earliest opportunity'. If you really want your escort paralytic with lust, stop frequently to adjust the seams.[22]

Nothing can excuse boys putting unwanted pressure on girls to engage in sex, but girls must know what power they have over boys, and boys must know what power they have over girls. Both need to be encouraged to use this power wisely. Boys must be aware that it is not just the Achilles heel which can lead them astray. There are other areas of the anatomy which can also leave them vulnerable. Correct behaviour is obvious while waiting outside the principal's office but it needs to be just as obvious in the back seat of the car.

GIVING ADVICE TO BOYS

When dealing with boys it is important to let them know someone understands their frustrations, temptations and biological chemistry. Talking with boys about the tensions they are likely to face, and the choices available to them in how to deal with these tensions, is important. Failure to show

FROM THE GIRL'S ANGLE

Two research projects undertaken by La Trobe University involving 3550 and 1324 teenagers were reported in the *Age* on 17 January 2001. The projects found:

- Twenty per cent of the girls surveyed engaged in sexual intercourse aged 14 years and younger, and nearly 40% before their sixteenth birthday.
- Although some girls felt in control of their sex lives, others did not and felt pressured by boys to engage in unwanted and irresponsible sex.
- Only one in five pregnant girls had wanted to get pregnant.
- Of the girls falling pregnant, half claimed to have been using some form of contraception.
- The girls less likely to have engaged in sex at an early age generally came from one or a number of groups. These groups were:
  - two-parent families
  - church going families
  - migrant families
  - families that talked openly about sex.

Source: Tim Colebatch, 'Sex talks help teens decide when the time is right', *Age*, 17 January 2001, p 4.

empathy can lead to a boy becoming lonely, withdrawn and cut off from the catharsis of discussing his fears and his joys with someone who will understand. One of the reasons boys might talk more readily with their peers on matters relating to sex is that parents have not signalled an approachability on these matters and teachers even less so. As a result, teens will huddle covertly and whisper confessions to each other on telephones, and thank goodness they do, for they must find someone who understands, for the feelings are too strong to be locked within.

Many boys can feel guilty, deviant or odd when analysing their own sexuality. They need to be assured, not once, but time and time again, that the emotional and social battles they fight are the same battles that their parents and teachers fought. They need to be helped to develop coping mechanisms for lust and for love, and to know the difference. They need to be helped to develop appropriate behaviours to express their sexual attraction. They may be shocked to realise that the beery bravado, rough horseplay and endless discourse about their football skills, does not necessarily make them attractive to girls.

VIRGINITY

It might come as a surprise to some adults and even to some adolescents that the average teenager is not the promiscuous person some would have them believe. Australian research carried out in 1997 involving over 3500 students from 118 schools found fewer than 50% of Year 12 students and only 20% of Year 10 students had engaged in sex.[23]

This news might be much needed relief to many adolescents who are being given far too many messages both inside and outside of their ranks that unless they are copulating energetically most nights and on a significant number of days, then somehow they are inadequate. They are not, and by not rushing headlong into the loss of their virginity, they may be displaying a respect for themselves and their prospective life partners that is not being shown by their more promiscuous friends. Figure 6.2 shows the percentage of boys who have not had sexual intercourse.

Society is doing rather too much in fuelling the 'just do it' mentality. The value of sex is all too often measured by what is gained rather than what is given. The value of sex is all too often measured by short-term pleasure rather than by long-term joy. The legacy given to the youth of today by those setting the pace in the sexual experience race needs to be analysed honestly. Yes, there is certainly a very real pleasure to be gained from sex, including the personal reassurance that all the bodily parts can function well. There may also be the sense of personal flattery gained by having a body that is able to excite another person sexually. Adolescent sex can be fulfilling and rewarding.

Figure 6.2 Percentage of boys who have not had sexual intercourse

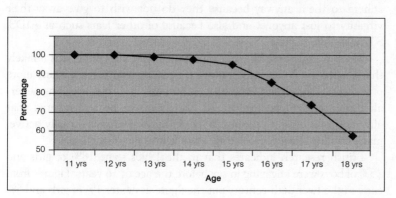

Source: Evans, A (1999), Australian Institute of Health and Welfare, unpublished analysis of survey by Australian Research Centre in Sex, Health and Society, La Trobe University, 1997.

However, teenage sex can also cheapen what can be an intensely wonderful experience and can cause emotional as well as physical wounds which may never heal. There is little one can celebrate about the current generation of young Australian women being the most infertile ever, due to the debilitating effects of STDs. There is probably not much joy in the one-third of Australian teenagers whose first sexual 'all the way' experience was not just under the covers, it was under the influence of drugs either legal or illegal.[24] The offering of one's virginity in such a manner, often to someone relatively unknown and unliked, is hardly something that should be applauded or encouraged. Too many teenagers have convinced themselves that having 'L' plates in a relationship is demeaning. They want to drive like adults even if they haven't quite figured out how to do it safely.

CELIBACY AND PROMISCUITY

Boys may learn that expectations of sex with a girl may not be realised for a number of good reasons. Some girls, and indeed some boys, may be bound by admirable personal scruples or religious principles which mean they wish to offer their virginity to their life partner rather than to a passing passion. In 1 Corinthians, chapter 6 reads:

> The body is not meant for fornication but for the Lord, and the Lord for the body . . . Shun fornication.

Not everyone is going to be persuaded by religious directives, but many adhere to them anyway because they do not wish to give away their virginity to just anyone, and also because of other fears such as AIDS, STDs and pregnancy.

Much is said about the sexual promiscuity of our young. It is unlikely that generation X, and generations Y or Z for that matter, is any more promiscuous than their baby boomer parents, and thus sweeping generalisations need to be avoided. It also needs to be remembered that although a number of teenage boys choose to become sexually active, many do not. Having noted this, some figures are disturbing.

British research indicates that in the 1990s some 18% of girls and 25% of boys were engaging in sex before the age of 16 years. Figures from early in the twentieth century put the figure as nearer 1% of girls and 5% of boys.[25] Before the moral outrage erupts, it is as well to remember that the validity and reliability of these figures needs to be questioned. It would have been a brave person indeed to have ever admitted to underage sex in the early twentieth century. Even so, it would be just as irresponsible to minimise the problems associated with teenage sex.

A huge pressure can be placed on boys by their peers to become sexually active. Much of this pressure is fuelled by a feeling among some tribal groups of boys that unless you have 'done it' you are not a man. Thus the desire to prove one's sexual prowess and one's sexual orientation can be strong. Boys may need to be warned of this and advised that true maturity is not necessarily to be found in keeping up with the sexual 'pace setter' of the group.

Another reason why boys may need to be warned lies in the fact that girls losing their virginity is not just a mental or emotional issue. For a girl there is often a physical change with the rupture of the hymen. This is a change that cannot be reversed even if the girl should wish it. The physical change can remain a permanent reminder of the first sexual intercourse. Thus boys should understand if a girl wants those memories to be particularly pleasant.

Boys need also to consider the unfairness of the judgment which labels a promiscuous boy as 'a stud', and a promiscuous girl as 'a slut'. A girl can make herself vulnerable to social criticism if she accedes to requests for sex, particularly the sort of casual sex which sees the boy doing nothing in the post-coital afterglow except shouting to his mates that he has 'scored'. Not every boy is the predator, the feckless moral bankrupt who will seek 'a fix' for his lust habit before returning to the loud plaudits of his mates. Some teenage boys can even find themselves preyed on by girls who are often physically, socially and emotionally more mature.

For some boys, losing their virginity is not always a triumphant 'rite of passage'. It can be an awkward, unsatisfying affair which leaves them scared and guilty. It must also be remembered that boys can feel trapped between societal codes and peer codes; between adult codes and teenage codes; between religious codes and secular codes; between boy codes and men codes; between heterosexual codes and homosexual codes; between lust codes and love codes. Young men do not necessarily enter the sexual arena brim full of confidence, clutching condoms and flowers.

Society needs to accept its responsibilities towards its sons and teach them properly about sex and friendship. If responsible adults do not supply the answers to questions on sex topics boys may seek answers at 'alt.sex' on the Internet, or in grubby magazines and smutty sessions behind the toilet block.

A PARENTAL CHECKLIST

It is dangerous to suggest what parents should discuss with their sons and even more dangerous to suggest when they might do it. The 'what' and 'when' will need to be decided by the parent, mindful that the time and topic will probably vary for every boy. The best conversations with sons cannot normally be predicted or planned. They occur spontaneously. Nonetheless, it might be useful for parents to think through the sorts of topics that need to be covered with their son about sex. Chats should be relaxed and age appropriate. Examples of the types of topics that might be covered are shown below:

Possible sex-related topics to be discussed with a son
Early and mid-primary years

- The parts of the body and their functions.
- Physical differences between males and females.
- Respect for and care of one's body and other people's bodies.
- Circumcision.
- Stranger danger.
- Good and bad touching, kissing, hugging.
- What to do if approached or spoken to in a way which makes one feel uncomfortable.
- Basic theory of reproduction by animals, plants and humans.
- Elementary discussion on relationships between people and how they vary.

Late primary school and early secondary years

- *As for the above but in greater detail!*
- Good friendships, bad friendships.

- Menstruation, fertility, pregnancy.
- The function of intercourse.
- The biology of reproduction by humans.
- Basic differences between like, lust and love.
- Masturbation, its normality and associated hygiene hints.
- Introduction to the concept of contraception.
- Introduction to the topics of STDs and AIDS.
- Respect for the other sex and appreciation of individual differences in size, shape and maturation.
- Virginity — what it means physically, emotionally, spiritually, socially.

Early to mid-secondary years

- *As for the above but in greater detail!*
- Care of the body, particularly the skin.
- Safe sex.
- The influence of drugs on sex, promiscuity, fertility and health.
- The emotional and social differences between boys and girls and how they might vary on a 'monthly' cycle.
- Identification of STDs and AIDS and treatment for such conditions.
- How to cope with lust as well as love.
- What girls find attractive and unattractive.
- Testosterone and how to cope with it.
- Attitudes towards people with a different sexual orientation.
- Celibacy.
- Responsible dating.
- Looking after a relationship while still having friends.
- Agencies specialising in helping teenagers.
- Guidelines and rules associated with pornography, cyber sex, virtual sex, etc.

Mid- to late secondary years

- *As for the above but in greater detail!*
- Hints on how to 'pleasure' a partner.
- How to cope with love as well as lust.
- Coping with thwarted love and being in love.
- The desirable qualities of a life partner.
- Legal responsibilities and rights associated with relationships including de facto relationships.
- Looking after platonic friendships while still having a sexual relationship.
- Home rules such as where the girl friend sleeps.

Not all will agree with the timing or the topics listed above and undoubtedly there are other themes which should be added. Parents will need to draw up their own 'checklist' and customise it to the spiritual and moral values they wish to honour within their family.

ADDITIONAL INFORMATION

For those wishing to have further details on some of the points raised in this chapter, the following references may be helpful. Each number in the text of the chapter relates to a reference number below which will give further information related to the topic.

1	Lacombe, A and Gray, J (1998)	'The role of gender in adolescent identity and intimacy decisions'	*Journal of Youth and Adolescence*, 27(6):795–801.
2	Cimbalo, R and Novell, D (1993)	'Sex differences in romantic love attitudes among college students'	*Psychological Reports*, 73:15–18.
3	Shulman, S, Levy-Shiff, R, Kedem, P and Alon, E (1997)	'Intimate relationships among adolescent romantic partners and same sex friends: Individual and systemic perspectives'	*New Directions for Child Development*, Winter, 1997, p 78.
4	Shulman, S et al	(op cit)	
5	Moore, S, Kennedy, G Fulonger, B and Evers, K (1999)	'Sex, sex-roles and romantic attitudes: Finding the balance'	*Current Research in Social Psychology*, 4(3):124.
6	Dion, K K and Dion, K L (1993)	'Individualistic and collective perspectives on gender and the cultural context of love and intimacy'	*Journal of Social Issues*, 49(3):53–69
7	Sprecher, S and Metts, S (1989)	'Development of the "romantic beliefs scale" and examination of the effects of gender and gender role orientation'	*Journal of Social and Personal Relationships*, 6:387–411.
8	Montgomery, M and Sorell, G (1998)	'Love and dating experience in early and middle adolescence: Grade and gender comparisions'	*Journal of Adolescence*, 21:677–689
9	Montgomery, M and Sorell, G	(op cit)	p 678.
10	Newberger, E (2000)	*The Men They Will Become*	Bloomsbury, London, p 228.
11	Montgomery, M and Sorell, G	(op cit)	p 681.
12	Moir, A and Jessel, D (1989)	*Brainsex*	Mandarin, London, p 172.
13	Moir, A and Jessel, D	(op cit)	p 107.
14	Pollack, W (1998)	*Real Boys*	Owl Books, Henry Holt and Co., New York, p 66.

▶

15	Moir, A and Jessel, D	(op cit),	p 111.
16	Erikson, E H (1968)	*Identity: Youth and Crisis*	W W Norton, New York.
17	West, P (1996)	*Fathers, Sons and Lovers*	Finch Publishing, Sydney.
18	Pollack, W	(op cit)	p 220.
19	Kindlon, D and Thompson, M (2000)	*Raising Cain*	Penguin Books, London, p 206.
20	Moir, A and Jessel, D	(op cit)	p 102.
21	Moir, A and Jessel, D	(op cit)	p 105.
22	Metcalf, F (1986)	*The Penguin Dictionary of Modern Humorous Quotations*	Penguin Books, London.
23	Donaghy, B (2000)	*The Sixth Trent Long Memorial Lecture*	St Paul's School, Bald Hill, Queensland, 3/4/00.
24	Donaghy, B	(op cit)	
25	Norton, C (2000)	'Teenagers struggling to find ways to express adulthood'	*Education Review*, March 2000.

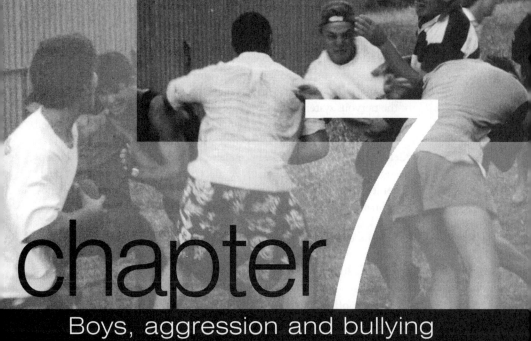

chapter 7

Boys, aggression and bullying

'In brief, we are all monsters, that is,
composition of man and beast.'

Sir Thomas Browne, 1642

AGGRESSION

Aggression is not the sole preserve of boys, although there is more than enough anecdotal evidence to suggest it is a common characteristic, particularly among adolescent boys. Parents wake up one morning and find that overnight their son has changed from a sparkling, fun-filled creature into a morose and hostile young man for whom everything 'sucks' and for whom speech has become a Neanderthal emission of low octave growls. Confrontational exchanges become common, as does the desire to institutionalise the son until the basic social graces are regained to the extent that they are no longer an embarrassment to the family.

Anger in all

Anger is to be found in all people, the triggering of the limbic surge, the quick episodic rush of energy which comes from the release of the catecholamines, the amygdala-driven ripple down the adrenocortical branch of the nervous system. All the above is but the flowery detail of the 'flight or fight' response of bodies when angry, and it is to be found in everyone.[1]

Sometimes it is right to be angry. The Danish philosopher Sören Kierkegaard regarded the great malaise of the young as being its lack of passion, probably a product of minds satiated in too much artificially generated excitement and a general apathy towards the future. The trick of course is to be guided by Aristotle who wrote:

> Anyone can become angry — that is easy. But to be angry with the right person, to the right degree, at the right time, for the right purpose, and in the right way — this is not easy.[2]

On the other hand, it should be remembered that anger, of all the human emotions, is probably the one which is least controlled and, as Benjamin Franklin said:

> Anger is never without a reason, but seldom a good one.[3]

Daniel Goleman, in his book *Emotional Intelligence*, reminds his readers that anger is endemic in society and writes of a general rise in aggression within society with road rage and drive-by shootings becoming common. The contemporary greeting is evolving from 'have a nice day' to the threat 'go ahead and make my day'.[4] While not all may necessarily have the arsenal of Clint Eastwood, that does not mean that the capacity for violence is removed. People still experience self-esteem blown away, ego shattered and confidence destroyed by those loaded with a dangerous amount of aggression. The custodians of decency in society are at risk of being overwhelmed by those who wish to be vulgar, risqué and confrontational. All too often the media promotes the uncontrolled venting of violent anger. Watching virtual anger on the screen can fuel real anger in the streets.

Even the retail and marketing world contributes to the promotion of violence, particularly in boys. Boys' toys are packaged in military camouflaged boxes with names printed on them like 'Intimidator' and 'Shock'. On the other hand, girls' toys nestle in pretty pink boxes with scenes of genteel domesticity on a lid bearing names like 'Mystique' and 'Misty Magic'.[5] Su Langker, in making these points, goes on to describe a TV advertisement for sunglasses which featured scenes of urban ganglands. The advertisement concluded with the sound of a gunshot and the line 'Ray Bans — designed for war zones'. The imagery is not inappropriate, for many boys feel they are growing up in a society which is at war, a society in which they must fight for recognition and esteem. Rewards are given for displays of dominance on football fields and playgrounds, in relationships and work. Like the gun fighter, boys can live a lonely, violent life but do not always have the satisfaction of slaying their enemies and riding off in triumph.

The role of testosterone

Before the finger of accusation is pointed at boys, it needs to be remembered that aggression is a product of many things, including testosterone, the presence of which is largely beyond the control of boys. The hormonal surge is such that there is nearly a 100-fold increase in the testosterone level of a boy during puberty.[6]

While accounting for slightly less than 50% of the population, males perpetrate most of the physical violence and a good proportion of the emotional violence throughout the land. Scientists have sought to find out why. By the simple expedient of subtracting testes from a number of once proud animal subjects, it was found that levels of aggression could be reduced. Thus a major culprit for the querulous nature in boys was found to be testosterone. The clues were there to be found in nature. A prize Brahman bull positively radiant in testosterone does not make for a docile family pet. The clues were also to be found elsewhere. Athletes wanting a little chemical enhancement of performance found that when they injected themselves with the anabolic steroid called 'testosterone' they then started throwing training weights at their coaches in what is now known as ''roid rage'. They also blitzed everyone else in sporting competition.

A young boy about 13 or 14 years of age wakes up one morning with an attack of the grumps which lasts for several years and only begins to dissipate at about 18 years of age. The voice drops an octave, language regression happens with communication limited to a few hostile grunts, bodily hair and muscle definition occurs, together with a belligerent slouch. The once perfect skin takes on the cratered appearance of the moon and confrontation occurs about bed times, clothes, money, hair, homework, manners, hygiene and phone bills with the result that serious thought is given by parents to boarding schools and the rewriting of wills.

Before the chemical culprit is fully condemned, it is worth noting that a number of endocrinologists have put an important caveat on the link between testosterone and aggression: testosterone does not actually cause aggression, it merely exaggerates the aggression which is there already.[7] Monkeys sitting on the branches of a tree display a dominance hierarchy with the obsequious grovellers towards the bottom and the chest-beating conquerors towards the top. Somewhere in between is a group of monkeys who, when pumped full of the androgen testosterone, do not swing their belligerent way to the top of the tree, but stay where they are and terrorise those sitting below them with rather less subtlety. The testosterone did not bring about this aggression, it merely removed the inhibitions in controlling that aggression and exaggerated the innate rage that was already lurking within.[8]

SOME OTHER REASONS FOR AGGRESSION IN BOYS

Maternal responsiveness

Boys do not have to wait long before the social conditioning starts which leaves them prone to emotional barrenness and anger. Some mothers respond differently to their sons than they do their daughters as newborn babes. A baby girl cries and the 'who's a pretty girl then' responses are given. A baby boy cries and the 'big boys don't cry' responses are given.[9] Without malice, without intention, the process of hardening begins for boys even in their first few days of life. Subtle messages are sent that the expression of emotion in boys is not on, whereas rough and tumble is.[10]

Some parents are concerned that they may spoil their children, particularly their sons, if they over-indulge them. Research has indicated that in the initial few months of life, it is virtually impossible to over-indulge an infant. Eleanor Maccoby, in her research, found that responsive mothers who immediately would soothe, comfort and cuddle their infant a great deal in their first three months of life tended to produce children who were socially better adjusted and who were more obedient.[11] This runs counter to the view that over-indulgence produces a less obedient child.[12]

The caresses and cuddles given to a newborn child actually affect brain development in a positive way. Brain chemistry and connection is improved through the expression of tenderness and love in the early months of life. The cooing and cosseting also contributes to building a child who is emotionally secure and intellectually better developed. When a baby has more limited affection in their early months there may be more limited maturation, particularly of their socio-emotional skills in later life.[13]

Paternal deprivation

The father has a direct and indirect role in raising a son and encouraging in the son emotional, behavioural and moral maturity. The direct way is by modelling appropriate behaviour for the son to copy, particularly when the son begins his search for male identity. Without this modelling, a boy will pick up his clues elsewhere, often from tutors of doubtful value. The media has not always celebrated the best images of maleness and peer groups even less so, particularly those whose interpretation of maleness leads to aggression and high-risk behaviours.

The underfathered boy can become hyper-masculine in his orientation, filling life with sport and the walls of his bedroom with pictures of guns, muscles and engines with mega 'grunt'. This can be augmented with an exaggerated masculine posture (the slouch) and exaggerated masculine speech (the growl). The underfathered son may also feel insecure about his own masculinity to the extent there is compensation by acting in what is perceived to be the male way. This male way is often angry, emotionally barren and intimidating. Gays, females and any others of another tribe will have war waged upon them for they are an aberration of the ideal human condition, the 'ocker' male. 'Poofter' bashing, racism and chauvinism are the preferred behaviours.[14]

A father can teach a son rules, a knowledge of behavioural boundaries and a discipline that a boy with a deceased, divorced, distant or delinquent father may not always learn. Knowing how to control anger, competitiveness and aggression can be taught by rough and tumble play with the father. A father is not just having fun with his son in a backyard game of cricket. The father is imparting life skills: teaching a boy how to win and lose; how to compete within the rules and how to repair windows.

The father's indirect role in raising a son is by providing the mother with the emotional and material support necessary so that she, in turn, might have the energy, inclination and will to meet the needs of the son. This vicarious influence should not be underestimated. One of the best ways a father can love a son, is by loving the boy's mother.

Delinquent behaviour in boys is often linked to boys who have not enjoyed the presence in their home of a supportive father. Consider the following:

- Of children presenting with behavioural problems, 85% come from homes without a father.
- Boys from fatherless homes commit rape 14 times more than boys who have had a father figure.
- Ninety per cent of homeless and runaway children are from homes without a father.
- Eighty-five per cent of juveniles in prison come from homes without a father.[15]

With nearly one marriage in two collapsing and with a number of surviving marriages witnessing inadequate fathering, the risk to children in general, and to boys in particular, is significant. Stepfathers and other adult male role models can certainly negate the potential difficulties in fatherless homes as can the dedication and skill of the single mother. But the task can be a difficult one. Substitute fathers often have to deal with anger and emotional scarring brought about by the absence of the biological father.

Parental punishment patterns

Inappropriate behaviours in boys can sometimes be linked to inappropriate parental punishment patterns. Boys who receive from their adult carers punishments that are harsh and inconsistent can become boys who also become harsh and inconsistent themselves. The parent who is physically brutal and who is unable to control his or her emotions will be the parent whose son will probably have the same characteristics.

Sometimes the parent will be fed up with a son playing up like a second-hand lawnmower but the temptation for brutality in punishment must be avoided. The frightening or shaming of a boy by threats or humiliation can do irreparable long-term harm as well as replicate the bully in the son. A boy must always feel that there is a way out, a way to make amends and a way to improve.

Parents might also be reminded that if their offspring should sin, they might need not only to upbraid their son, they might need to examine the reasons why the deed was committed in the first place. Parents might need to look at their own parenting as being a contributing factor to a son's misbehaviour. Don't expect an intelligent or articulate response from a boy to the question 'Why did you do it?' Most boys don't fully understand themselves and, even if they did, the chances of them articulating a coherent response are slim.

The two extremes of permissive and authoritarian parenting need to be avoided. A beaten boy is a dangerous boy, for he will either slide into depression and nihilistic thinking or he will seek to bolster his self-esteem by beating someone himself. An uncontrolled boy is also a dangerous boy as he will continue his destructive ways until he finds behavioural boundaries. If the parents will not show a son where the boundaries are, the police probably will.

The best punishments tend to be punishments which are consistent, that have been worked through beforehand in a cooperative manner and which are uniformly applied not by one parent, but by both. As far as possible, punishments need to be effective as a deterrent, effective educationally and effective in encouraging restitution.

It is important to try and ensure that not too much attention is paid to a boy's negative behaviours without paying attention to the positive behaviours. Carrots need to be used as well as sticks. Parents need to avoid giving physical or financial rewards for behaviours which can quite reasonably be expected of a responsible boy. Keeping a room tidy, completing homework and being well mannered are the types of things a boy should do normally. Sensationalising normal behaviour by giving substantial rewards leaves little room to reward genuinely good behaviour and fails to signal behavioural 'norms' for a boy.

Abuse in the home

Boys from fatherless homes face greater risks of sexual abuse.[16] Father substitutes and other adult male relatives and friends account for a significant proportion of sexual abuse. Father substitutes themselves account for a quarter of child sexual abuse.[17] However, it is important to point out that many father substitutes make outstanding fathers and that some natural fathers, and even mothers, can perpetrate the most shocking forms of abuse within the home.

Quite apart from sexual abuse, there is physical abuse with punishments meted out which are excessive and destructive. There is also psychological abuse where the self-worth of a child is eroded by a policy of embarrassment or shame. Many parents who engage in such approaches are not even aware they are doing it and require the intercession of an external mediator or properly qualified counsellor to help them realise the mind games they are playing with their sons. Abuse by adults in the home will often be replicated by children in society. Breaking the cycle is not always easy but can be done through professional help and through the mediation of other responsible adults.

THE WARNING SIGNS OF A VIOLENT BOY

There is good news and bad news. The good news is that there are signals that can indicate the likelihood of a boy engaging in violent behaviours. The bad news is that these signals cannot be relied upon, for there are many boys with a high-risk profile who manage to live quite responsible lives and there are other boys without such a profile who need to be volunteered to populate the planet Pluto. Having noted the above, Garbarino, in his book *Lost Boys*, suggests that a boy is twice as likely to commit murder if:

■ there is a family history of criminal violence
■ there is a history of abuse
■ there is membership of a gang
■ there is drug or alcohol abuse.[18]

Also signalling a propensity to violence is the boy with neurological and learning difficulties such as ADD or ADHD, ownership of weapons, poor performance at school and prior arrests. To these lists must be added the level of violence in the home, ineffective maternal and paternal care and whether a boy engages in recreational habits such as watching violent movies or playing violent video games.

Other warning signs include:

■ hyperactivity
■ emotional sterility
■ a conscience that has been dulled
■ an incapacity to view a situation from another's perspective
■ a bravado and fearlessness
■ a dislike of oneself
■ an anger towards others
■ an incapability to deal with criticism or threats
■ a soullessness and lack of spirituality
■ a low intelligence
■ a social insecurity
■ a purposelessness
■ lack of emotional and social resilience
■ a hopelessness
■ deliberate acts of self-harm
■ a preoccupation with Satanism
■ an enjoyment of sociopathic music.

DEALING WITH AGGRESSION IN BOYS

> Of all animals, boys are the most
> unmanageable.
> Plato

Many of the ways of dealing with aggression in boys are touched on in other chapters but it is appropriate within the context of this chapter to expand on a number of initiatives.

1. Stimulate empathy

In order to help boys connect with the feelings of others, boys may need to connect with their own feelings. If parents or teachers wish to elicit in-depth sharing from a boy, a trust and confidence needs to be established and this may take some time. A boy will maintain an artificial façade for as long as he feels vulnerable in showing people what lies behind the façade.

After connecting with his own feelings, a boy is better able to connect with the feelings of others. This might be encouraged by giving a boy responsibilities such as caring for a pet, or acting as a mentor or minder of younger children. The giving of responsibility signals a sense of trust and signals a sense of worth. These can be powerful foundations for therapy.

Encouraging 'other person centredness' may be achieved by guiding a boy not to view issues in black and white but to explore shades of grey. Getting a boy to recount an incident through the eyes of different people can be a profitable exercise, particularly if this then leads to a boy describing not just the facts but the feelings of other people.

There may be value in giving boys permission to feel, to show emotion and to be shown that real men do have feelings and that real men have the courage to admit these feelings. Adult males who model emotional maturity should be a part of any program to develop empathy and emotional literacy in boys.

By emotional literacy the authors of *Raising Cain*, Dan Kindlon and Michael Thompson, mean:

> . . . being able to identify and name our emotions . . . recognising the emotional content of voice and facial expression, or body language and . . . understanding the situations or reactions that produce emotional states. By this we mean the link between the loss and sadness, between frustration and anger, or threats to pride or self-esteem and fear.[19]

Kindlon and Thompson suggest that while girls get this training, many boys do not for they are not encouraged to be expressive in their feelings or reflective about the feelings of others. The cost of this emotional illiteracy is high, and when adolescence arrives and with it a peer culture which can be very cruel, the lack of empathy in a boy can be compounded.

2. Stimulate resiliency

There is a growing intolerance of the bully. There is a growing intolerance of hurt. There is a growing intolerance of injustice. All this needs to be applauded. Yet it might be as well to be reminded that life cannot be expected to provide a constant stream of undiluted fun, praise and success. If a boy is going to crumple because he does not get his hourly fix of adulation, then he may not have been well served by those who have raised him. Self-esteem needs to be built up but never to a stage that ordinary performance is exalted as extraordinary. Warm fuzzies are good, but so too are the words of admonition if they are shared with love and understanding.

What boys think of themselves should not depend entirely on whether or not they have been fed a constant diet of praise. Disappointment happens, discouragement happens, distress happens and thus a modicum of intestinal and physical fortitude is required.

Paul Kropp writes:

> In the past, self-esteem was attached to the idea of good and ennobling behaviour, not whether Mum and Dad were going to applaud you for finishing your soup at dinner. We don't want our children to become praise junkies, entirely dependent on their parents, a boss or lover for verbal strokings to make them feel good.
>
> In schools these days, praise-junkie kids have become a real problem. These children are invariably the offspring of parents who slather praise on their children with a verbal spatula, whether it's merited or not.[20]

Some boys might need to learn that if the world didn't suck, they would fall off, and that some resilience is needed against 'the slings and arrows of outrageous fortune'.

This is not to condone a callous indifference or to promote a tolerance of abuse or injustice. It is to remind boys that life will inevitably bring trials and tribulations. It is incumbent that coping strategies be learnt rather than retreating to petulant rage, or defeatist withdrawal or escapist denial.

The gods play with all and cause us to laugh and cry. Some emotional and physical courage is required. As it is said, we are all born naked, wet and hungry and then things get worse. Fortunately, things also get better for most people, with life being a constant journey through high points and low points.

The foundation of resilience rests in:

■ a realistic understanding of oneself
■ a realistic understanding of others
■ an ability to cope with the strengths and weaknesses in oneself
■ an ability to cope with the strengths and weaknesses in others.

The capacity to cope can be increased by a boy having:

- faith in God;
- someone with whom he can share his deepest thoughts and his most personal feelings. More than one person is needed for there is wisdom in having someone:
  - within the family
  - outside the family
  - who is older
  - who is a similar age;
- a knowledge that he is unconditionally loved by at least one other person;
- skills at dealing with:
  - failure and success
  - threats and fear
  - rejection and disappointment
  - anger and hurt;
- good intrapersonal skills and good interpersonal skills.

The capacity to cope is not helped by:

- over-protection
- denial of inadequacies
- aggrandisement.

Some boys may need to be encouraged to see their glass as being half full rather than half empty and to recognise their blessings as well as their bruises.

3. Stimulate hope and spirituality

Linking hope with spirituality is not accidental. A future oriented and positive disposition is only ever likely if one has hope. Hope can be fostered by the divine encouragement that even the 'hairs on one's head are numbered'. Periodically one may not like oneself, but a faith in God can persuade a boy he is liked by God, particularly if he should obey God's precepts. God is usually:

- a being of power
- a being of justice
- a being of love.

All of these qualities can inspire hope in a boy who feels angry, frustrated and volatile.

The psychologist, Andrew Weaver, found that spirituality in children led to:

- less suicide
- reduced depression
- a reduction in casual sex
- reduced substance abuse
- greater resilience to trauma.[21]

VIDEO GAMES

Many games played in arcades and on visual display units require the player to blast an enemy using an awesome range of fire-power. The figures destroyed are often human, as testified by their internal organs being splattered all over the screen when a 'hit' is registered. Some researchers are worried that virtual carnage may be creating the wrong impulses about weapons and the wrong values about people.

An interesting study was undertaken by David Grossman who found that in World War II only about 20% of American regular riflemen were able to shoot an enemy with a gun. An inner revulsion at taking a human life prevented many triggers being squeezed and many rifles being aimed accurately. In the Vietnam War, 90% of American riflemen could shoot to kill. One of the big differences was the training. In World War II, soldiers would shoot at black circles on targets. In preparing for Vietnam, soldiers shot at human-shaped targets.[22] Many boys are shooting at a large number of human targets today and not all of them are restricting the targets to video screens.

UNDERSTANDING THE MESSAGE BEHIND THE ACTION

It is important to get boys to understand the reasons for their anger, to try and understand that their anger, like acne, is as much a product of infection as it is of age, that under the skin there is an unhealthy germ. A regular regime of cleansing through helping boys to articulate their feelings and frustrations in a non-judgmental environment can help. Getting the boys to understand the messages behind their actions can also be useful.

The boy who is aggressive may be saying:

- You are not as good as I am.
- I am stronger than you.
- You and your feelings do not deserve respect.
- Strength is the only currency worth having.
- My image is more important than your safety.
- Your pain does not bother me.

The one who puts down others may be saying:

- Your humiliation is something I enjoy.
- I have social power and you do not.

■ You are not allowed to make mistakes.
■ You are not allowed to be different.

If boys understand the messages they are sending through their behaviour, they may be less motivated to behave in the way they do. It is not easy to take much pride in these messages. However, this tactic does not always work and shaming boys into compliance does not always bear fruit.

THE MESSAGE BEHIND LITTERING

An example of analysing the message behind the action can be found with something as trivial as littering. Littering is a form of violence for it despoils the environment. If a boy is led through the messages he is giving when dropping litter, he may be less inclined to do so. It could be pointed out to him that litter is the dandruff of society — unsightly, indicative of poor health and despite 'do the right thing' shampoos, is difficult to remove.

What is it that has caused the boy to litter, particularly when facilities are provided for rubbish? Is it an act of pure laziness, of not being prepared to inconvenience himself by walking to a bin? In so doing, a clear message is sent that the boy does not care about the rest of society having to suffer by putting up with his litter. Thus selfishness is diagnosed and a view of the universe proclaimed that it should revolve around him.

Is it that the boy's conscience might be seared to the extent that he doesn't really think it is wrong to litter? The rhetoric in school assemblies asking for consideration when disposing of litter is dismissed as the prattling of anachronistic authoritarian figures. Far stronger role models in their lives exist, and these drop litter, in fact everyone does . . . don't fight it, run with the pack, the very messy pack.

Is it because of anger? Society has given some boys too little esteem, love, employment or worth. So they hit back at that society, colour it with spray cans, desecrate it and rubbish it.

When a teacher sees rubbish being dropped, he or she has every right to get upset because of the message behind the action. 'But it was only a plastic wrapper.' No, it wasn't just a plastic wrapper, it was an indication of either selfishness, a warped morality, or anti-social tendencies. If a boy is punished for littering, it is not the act of dropping the litter that should worry, it is the testimony of a sick values system, a values system which the world cannot afford. It is no use a boy 'tree-hugging' in the local forest, sewing up holes in the ozone layer with threads of anti-CFC legislation, or whingeing when he cuts his feet on glass at the beach, if his lunch is decomposing in the classroom and his wrappers are decorating the school fence.

Source: Hawkes, T F, Newslink, St Leonard's College, Melbourne, 6 June 1991.

DEALING WITH ANGER

When dealing with anger in boys one needs to recognise that rational and well-reasoned logic does not always work. A cooling off or 'time out' period may be required. This is stage one. The next step is to signal unconditional love and acceptance so that boys feel that they are able to talk about the episode. The preparedness to talk may take time. Boys may need to brood awhile and to chase their mental demons. They will do this until quieted by acceptance or exhaustion whereupon they will open up seeking justice, understanding and absolution.

This is not an easy process to manage for there can be anger and high anxiety not only in the boy, but also in the parent. However, an angry parent or judgmental teacher may close down any chance a boy might have of experiencing the soothing balm of reflective analysis. The boy may just get angrier and more withdrawn. Having noted the value of holding back the reforming rebuke, it is important that adults not present themselves as people without values or without emotion. They have a right to feelings as well.

HOW TO DEAL WITH ANGER

- Do not brood on anger with mental reruns of the incident. Learn the lessons, get on with life and allow the indignation to cool. The perpetrators have no right to compound the hurt they have caused by highjacking the senses so there is emotional hurt as well.
- Try to put the incident in perspective by examining why it happened and by trying to tease out the causal factors. Then try to see the incident through the eyes of the perpetrators. See if another interpretation is valid.
- Recognise the anger signs and have an antidote ready which consists of controlling the impulse to say or do anything. Seneca recognised that the greatest remedy for anger is delay and it is a truism which should be recognised today. Writing, speaking and doing things when angry is seldom wise. The options include a diversionary stroll, moving away from the situation and walking the dog, meditating, praying, relaxing in a bubble bath.
- Avoid those situations which one knows can cause anger. This may not always be possible but it may be possible to minimise contact with the aggravating agents.[23]
- If confronting the person who is the source of the anger, try to work through to a 'win-win' situation. Send 'I' messages rather than 'you' messages, reduce the volume of speech and pay conscious attention to the inflammatory messages that might be sent through body language.
- Recognise that life is not always fair and that true character results not from knowing how to deal with comfort and success, but knowing how to deal with hurt and failure.[24]

There are many books with impossible titles that deal with the topic of anger but most seem to agree that the advice above is helpful when dealing with anger.

Not all agree on any singular remedy for anger. Daniel Goleman suggests it is a myth that there is catharsis in allowing a boy to vent his rage, and suggests it will generally have the reverse effect and leave the boy more angry. On the other hand, William Pollack suggests there can be healing when a boy is given permission in a safe and private environment to vent his spleen and rage against his circumstances. One should not signal to boys that unchecked emotions are always acceptable, yet the Japanese report great success in putting in place 'boss-bashing rooms' complete with straw effigies of people and big sticks to hit them with, as a means of expurgating their emotions.

Perhaps one of our most urgent tasks with boys is to get them to develop their intrinsic (internal) resources for dealing with anger rather than relying purely on extrinsic (external) resources. Sticks break and carrots rot but an inner disposition towards tolerance and empathy will last a lifetime. Browne writes:

> The difficulty is that boys frequently behave as if the only valid form of power is *power over* others, or domination. This can be contrasted with *power with* others, or cooperative and representative forms of power. A third form is *power within*, which describes a personally-centred sense of individual power found for example in some martial arts disciplines.[25]

If a boy is at peace with himself, he is more likely to be at peace with others. If a boy's inner soul has been fed by noble values and appropriate examples, particularly by parents, then 'cope-ability' is improved. This represents a level of emotional quotient (EQ) in a boy that will need to be nurtured as much as his intelligence quotient (IQ).

Spurning co-efficient variables and IQ measures, Daniel Goleman, in his book *Emotional Intelligence*, talks of soul, of character, of inner peace, and a new imperative to encourage emotional well-being and the repair of a fractured and alienated society. While schools churn out knowledge on the causes of the World War I, the properties of H_2SO_4, the value of X and the curse of the split infinitive, they are ignoring a key element in preparing boys for the future. Goleman suggests that IQ contributes only about 20% to the factors that determine a successful life. Despite the popular mystique of IQ and UAI scores, they are singularly ineffective in predicting success in life.

Empathy is the ability to identify with, to have compassion for, to know the unspoken feelings of, and is a gift which the post-modern world is threatening to make a rarity. An increasing number do not have this quality — the sociopath who causes pain without remorse; the cold hearted manipulator; the psychopath who is unable to feel another's hurt. These are they who suffer some form of disruption between recognising signals and attaching feelings to them, who are unmoved by the cries of a baby or the joys of another's achievements. Put in scientific terms, the neural pathways between the verbal cortex and the limbic brain are damaged, making a person immune to parasympathetic arousal.[26] In less scientific terms, these people become a liability, blundering through life causing harm to themselves and to others.

Implicit in having a high EQ is the ability for a boy to put himself in another person's shoes, to be able to step back from a situation and to view it from a different perspective. This 'other person centredness' is an important skill to develop in boys and may be achieved in part by asking them to pretend to be someone else and to ask what they think someone else would be thinking and would be feeling.

This should not necessarily translate into a total subjugation of one's own feelings or an invalidation of one's own perspective, but it can encourage greater understanding and fewer black eyes.

BULLYING

> Man, biologically considered . . . is the most formidable of all beasts of prey and, indeed, is the only one that preys systematically on its own species.
> William James

Bullying is selective and uninvited behaviour which causes harm. It is psychologically or physically perpetrated by a person, or indeed a group, who has greater power, and is often repeated. Bullying may be motivated by a desire to gain status and control, or to foster a reputation for power. At other times bullying, such as extortion, can be motivated by the hope for material gain. Other causal factors of bullying can include boredom, jealousy and revenge.[27]

With boys it is often difficult to determine where rough play ends and bullying starts. Boys can be aggressive but not actually bully. Some guide is given by the intention. Was it to cause hurt or discomfort? The severity of the hurt must also be taken into consideration as must its frequency. The 'collectivisation' of hurt is also worth bearing in mind. This relates to a group situation where each contributes just a little bit of pain or derision which by itself does not amount to much, but collectively can be devastating to the victim.

Most parents have been tortured by the anger and helplessness that comes from one of their children falling victim to the playground Mafia or classroom Triads. The bullies are the children weaned on the infant pastime of removing wings from flies and frying ants with a magnifying glass, the children who gain a peculiar pleasure in making another child miserable by removing their friends and frying them with ridicule and rejection.

When trapped by parental instincts to protect and nurture, and entertaining thoughts of dismembering the offenders and boiling all their soggy bits, discerning parents realise with shock that they bear the very same impulses of the bully in their own genes.

Bullying in some form or another is endemic in society. Parents bully children with threats; children bully parents with sulks; partners bully each other physically, sexually, mentally and emotionally; lawyers bully each other; and advertisers bully everyone. Thus it is not surprising that bullying should be found in schools, not because it is a school problem, but because it is a societal problem. Meanness, destructiveness and maliciousness do not stop outside the school gate. Inside the school gate one finds boys inflicting pain, often physically, and one finds girls inflicting pain, often verbally, through gossip, ostracism, indirect vendettas and passing little folded notes saying 'I hate you'.

The Options Project, a joint project by the Mental Health Foundation of Victoria and the Victorian Council for Civil Liberties, studied over 350 schools and concluded the following:

- US, English and Australian studies are indicating that about 10% of school children are being bullied frequently, that is, about once a week.
- Boys tend to bully others more than girls do.
- There is more bullying in primary schools than secondary schools.
- Most bullying in secondary schools is in the first two years.
- There tends to be less bullying in co-educational schools.
- Boys tend to perpetrate more physical bullying whereas girls tend to engage more in social and emotional bullying through such activities as verbal abuse and exclusion.
- The most common form of bullying is teasing and taunting.
- Some bullying is long lasting, that is, going on for over a month. This longer bullying was reported by 7.5% of girls and 4.1% of boys.[28]

Bullying appears to be spread across all sectors of schooling. The first few weeks of 2000 saw the Australian press reporting parents suing a state school because of the bullying experienced by their daughter. Hodge, writing in the *Sydney Morning Herald* at the same time, was reporting on boys being bullied in elite private schools. Hodge suggests that these last bastions of genteel society and *Flashman* characters need to rethink their values. He writes that some of these private schools need to do rather more to remove violence and extortion within the school grounds and to re-evaluate just what sort of citizens they are producing.[29]

Another reporter, Gerard Noonan, was writing at much the same time about 15 private schools in New South Wales engaging the services of lawyers to help deal with the issue of bullying. Noonan writes:

> Twenty-five thousand students from 60 schools around Australia have been surveyed on bullying, which is seen as different from other aggressive acts such as fighting or quarrelling between equals. A third said they had never been bullied while another third said they had been bullied 'for a day or two' at school. But a disturbingly high 19% of boys and 18% of girls had experienced bullying for more than a week. And more than one in 10 boys reported being bullied for anywhere between months and more than two years. Slightly fewer girls faced such extended periods of bullying.[30]

For students, acceptance by peers is absolutely vital to their happiness and well-being. If a child is excluded from friendship groups, teased for being different or for lacking certain physical, mental or social skills, then great hurt can occur. Often it can be the sort of hurt that expresses itself in later years when that person in turn hurts others, and so the vicious cycle continues.

The current societal mood is such that a student who engages in physical assault is going to end up in significant strife. This has required the contemporary bully to be rather more subtle; more verbal. Hence a new hyphenated lexicon is appearing including 'put downs', 'pay backs' and 'freeze outs'.

REASONS FOR BULLYING
There are many interesting, and at times contradictory, opinions as to the reasons for bullying. Some evidence suggests that bullying can be learnt behaviour. One does not need a PhD in psychology to see the causal link when an overbearing parent looms menacingly over a school principal and booms 'I'll teach you to suggest my son is a bully!'

Table 7.1 Why boys bully

Reason	8–12 years	13–18 years
They were annoying	69.5	77.1
Need to get even	66.7	73.2
For fun	19.0	30.5
Copying others	17.3	23.7
They were wimps	13.4	17.9
Demonstrate toughness	12.1	16.5
Gain possessions or money	7.0	9.5

Source: Rigby, K (1998), 'The Technical Manual for the Peer Relations Questionnaire (PRQ),' 2nd edition, The Professional Reading Guide for Educational Administrators, Point Lonsdale, Victoria, Australia. With permission from Dr Ken Rigby, University of South Australia.

An interesting observation has been made by some educators that the contemporary bully is not always the child who is from a troubled home, has low self-esteem and is desperately looking for some sort of status within a school. The bully can be a child with high energy levels, who is travelling quite well academically but who has the leadership and inter-personal skills necessary to get others to collude in making the life of another quite miserable.[31]

With other boys, bullying can be a means whereby a sense of inadequacy drives them to point out the inadequacies in others, in the hope that their personal failings are camouflaged by the failings of those around them.[32] Consider the statistics in Table 7.1.

DEALING WITH BULLIES AND THEIR VICTIMS

Dealing with bullies can be difficult, for bullies are wont to hide within each other's shadows. They often seek to trivialise their own contribution to the pain and pass it off as normal boy behaviour and part of the general code of boyhood. However, boys must not be allowed to disregard the behavioural fences, and if this means running a dissuading current through the wires, then so be it. Boundaries of acceptable behaviour need to be established and enforced.

When trying to do something about bullying, initiatives need to be considered at the individual, family and community levels. At the individual level, both the victim and the bully need to be counselled. A popular approach is the Pikas method which advocates talking to bullies in a non-punitive way, and exploring their value system, self-esteem and the reason for their behaviours. Sanctions and deterrents do have their place, but the Pikas system argues that lasting change can be encouraged more by a diagnostic approach which hopefully will lead to permanent healing.

The victim will also need immediate support and reassurance. They will need to know that justice is being exercised, otherwise a bitterness may ensue which can become both permanent and debilitating.

Those bullied must know that they can talk to someone. Mechanisms need to be put in place which will encourage this to happen, not just in the home but in schools, through the use of peer helpers, monitors, student representative councils, tutors, house coordinators, year coordinators and so on.

The bullies, once identified by adults, should be isolated, informed of the inappropriateness of their behaviour, warned of the sanctions linked to such behaviour and counselled in order to arrive at the cause of such behaviour so that remedial action can be taken to prevent it recurring. It is worth noting that bullies often copy their behaviour from others, that they themselves may be suffering from bullying, and that they may have deep insecurities of their own which must be dealt with.

However, it should also be remembered that some children's interpersonal skills are such that they invite teasing and rejection. Whether this behaviour is learnt or innate is immaterial. They are social misfits to those who have to suffer their blundering attempts to cope with communal existence. Such children will need to be coached on how to get on well with others. When people attract nothing but abuse, it might be worth checking their orientation to themselves and to others. When a person writes 'please kick me' on his or her 'derrière', one should not be unduly surprised if from time to time that the person is kicked in the butt.

All this should not divert from the behaviour of the bully as being unconscionable and the fact that a great number of people are victims through no fault of their own. Bullying can never be condoned. It may be understood but never tolerated. Families, schools and society have every right to commit to the maintenance of an environment where all feel safe, valued and supported, and to take whatever steps are necessary to secure that end.

Bullies need to be confronted and appropriate sanctions used to deter them from such behaviours. Studies suggest about 6% of children are bullies with most bullying occurring in primary school between ages five to eight and in secondary school between ages 11 to 14. The incidence of verbal bullying tends to increase with age. Teachers, parents and the students themselves need to be aware of the incidence of bullying, with researchers saying about 5–20% of children are being bullied. This can help victims recognise that they are not 'the only ones.'[33]

Children also need to know what bullying is, be taught how to identify it, and learn how bullies can 'hide' their behaviour as normal.

Boys need to know that bullying can be physical, social, emotional, sexual or racial, and that bullying may be suffered individually or as a group.

Teachers and parents, as well as children, might require help to recognise the symptoms of bullying such as school phobia, anger, tears, depression, low self-esteem, together with the whole raft of psychosomatic symptoms such as headaches and stomach aches. Bed-wetting and sleeplessness can also be symptoms of bullying, particularly in the very young. Withdrawal and reluctance to 'join in' can be a warning sign as can be truancy, misbehaviour and aggressive behaviour. Cuts, bruising, torn clothing, requests for extra food or money as well as a decline in academic performance can also be clues that a child is suffering from bullying.

Those being bullied need to be reassured that someone cares, and that initiatives can be taken which will stop the bullying. The code of silence which can mute both victim and bully must be rewritten to allow the victim to talk about the bullying. Victims also need to know that they do not deserve to be victims.

BULLYING AND THE CODE OF SILENCE

Adults can find it discouraging when seeking information from some child about an incident that has caused harm to people or property. Enquiries are often met with silence or, even worse, a sullen hostility to the truth emerging. In some obscene way society has allowed this 'code of silence' to become a positive virtue. It is excused as a part of the culture, part of supporting one's mates, part of not 'dobbing'. However it is not always a virtue, particularly when silence is motivated by fear, apathy and a lack of courage.

It may be time that boys realise that in calling for silence, the guilty do nothing other than signal their own cowardice and unwillingness to face the consequences of their actions. The guilty are also signalling that they want the complicity of their friends in supporting them in their cowardice. It is time to realise that the code of silence is a code that must sometimes be broken, and this can take courage, conviction, and a knowledge of what is right and wrong. 'His silence supported sinners' is hardly a label a boy can be proud of.

Although difficult, society must train its sons to speak, particularly when their voice can bring justice and take away pain; when their voice can right a wrong. There is a time for boys to speak. Silence can sometimes encourage reoffence; can encourage the bully to bully again; the thief to steal again; the drug user to use again. When in later life the bully is a person in despair; when in later life the thief is in gaol; when in later life the drug user is dead; society must know that remaining silent allowed actions to become a habit, and habit a character; a character the ruin of those who needed anything but silence. In breaking the silence, the bully can be treated, the thief reformed and the drug user counselled. Boys may need to learn that with the breaking of silence, healing and justice can sometimes flourish.

A zero tolerance policy may need to be proclaimed towards bullying within a neighbourhood or school. Boys will need to be shown the need to see the necessity for change and to move through what Browne and Fletcher describe in Table 7.2[35] as the five stages of resistance to anti-bullying initiatives.

Schools should develop a culture which allows the bully nowhere to hide. The code of silence should be lifted with a school community agreeing that the acquiescent and protective silence is not deserved by the bully. Schools also need to teach that bystanders are not immune from the guilt of bullying if they allow it to occur without comment or intervention.

There is a time when silence does not enrich or edify. Silence can be a terrible thing, for silence is not always 'golden'. It can be yellow, the yellow of cowardice when people see a bully at work causing physical, social or emotional harm, and remaining silent. Cowards are people who hear a cry for help and remain deaf.

Table 7.2 The five stages of resistance to anti-bullying initiatives

	Levels of resistance	Key messages
1.	Denial	It doesn't happen.
		It doesn't affect me.
2.	Trivialisation	It happens but it doesn't matter.
		It doesn't affect me.
		I have no responsibility.
3.	Powerlessness	It happens and it affects me.
		It's not my fault. It's someone else's responsibility.
		What difference can one person make anyway?
4.	Coming to terms/ identification	It happens and it affects me.
		I have some responsibility.
		What does it mean for me if I get involved?
5.	Action	It exists, I'm involved and I want to do something.
		How can I help?

> There is a time for everything and a season for every activity under heaven; a time to be born and a time to die; a time to be silent and a time to speak, a time to love and a time to hate, a time for war and a time for peace.
>
> Ecclesiastes, chapter 3

PEACEMAKERS

A behavioural modification and anti-bullying program that appears to have had some success is a 10-year-old program called Peacemakers. This Queensland-based program appeals to the altruism of its participants and is based on four imperatives:

1. no 'put downs'
2. give praise
3. seek wisdom
4. right wrongs and notice hurts.[36]

ADVICE TO PARENTS

Parents, when reporting bullying behaviours to the school are likely to be upset and at times angry and emotional. It is worth noting that there may be some virtue in curbing some initial choice of words. Hostility can sometimes evoke a defensive reaction by schools. Bullying must be reported as soon as possible, but how it is reported is important. Experience has shown that keeping to the facts is useful rather than giving vent to hearsay and rumour. Likewise it can be helpful not to focus so much on the fault of the bully, but more on the distress to the victim. In other words, the judicious use of conflict resolution skills can be helpful.

Having noted the above, parents should not let the case rest until they have communicated frankly and honestly with the school, and are convinced that appropriate and immediate steps have been put in place to help both the bully and the victim.

'Bully proofing'

The victim can be helped to deal with the bullying through a program of 'bully proofing'. The sort of advice that can be given to a child being bullied might include the following:

■ Try not to get angry, or at least not to show your anger. If anger is shown, the bully has the satisfaction of knowing that he or she has the power to control the emotions of the victim.

- Admit to imperfections. This can have the effect of removing the issue under contention and can send positive messages about having a realistic understanding of yourself.
- Use non-offensive humour. The barbs in the bullying can be blunted by a good laugh. The capacity to laugh at yourself and with others can create a bonding with a group that might otherwise remain hostile.
- Review your own behaviours and body language. If one looks like a victim, one can become a victim. Squared shoulders and an affable smile can do much to deter a bully.
- Avoid trouble spots. There are always places in a school where the shadow of a teacher is seldom seen that can become high-risk zones for bullying. Avoid them.
- Develop your EQ — the ability to read body language, to sense mood, to be intuitive and empathetic can enable a potential victim to see where a situation may be heading. An early detection can provide more options for evasion of bullying.
- Surround yourself with good friends. Those with strong friendships will be less of a target for they are less vulnerable.[34]
- If bullied, try not to retaliate for this can often inflame the situation. Having noted this, protecting yourself is sometimes going to be necessary.
- If you are being bullied, try to remind yourself that it is the bully who has the problem, not you. Try to think through what inadequacies the bully might have that causes him or her to behave this way. It is probably as well not to articulate these thoughts but they are useful as they can help protect your self-esteem.
- There are occasions when it is quite appropriate to identify a person's behaviour as bullying and to ask him or her to stop it. It might even be possible to invite the bully to talk through the matter and to consider what is causing the problem. This should not be done in a precious or imperious way, but in a conciliatory yet firm manner.

ENCOURAGING A BULLY-FREE CULTURE

A 'whole school' approach to bullying can be useful, involving a statement of the rights of every individual and a statement of the responsibilities of every student.

A culture can be encouraged that will not tolerate bullying. Students can be taught what bullying is and how to recognise it. Schools can work on establishing a clear mechanism of reporting and dealing with bullying and on creating a culture of care which discourages the presence of bullying within the school. Many boys will experience bullying either as victims, voyeurs, or perpetrators. It is a practice that is unworthy of any society that should wish to call itself civilised.

ADDITIONAL INFORMATION

For those wishing to have further details on some of the points raised in this chapter, the following references may be helpful. Each number in the text of the chapter relates to a reference number below which will give further information related to the topic.

1	Goleman, D (1995)	*Emotional Intelligence*	Bloomsbury Publishing, London, p 80.
2	Aristotle quoted in Goleman, D	(op cit)	p ix.
3	Franklin, B quoted in Goleman, D	(op cit)	p 59.
4	Goleman, D	(op cit)	p xi.
5	Langker, S (1995) in Browne, R and Fletcher, R (1995)	*Boys in Schools*	Finch Publishing, Sydney.
6	Hall, S (1999)	'Bullying in the mirror'	*New York Times Magazine,* section 6, 22/8/99.
7	Sapolsky, R M (1997)	*The Trouble with Testosterone and Other Essays on the Biology of the Human Predicament*	Simon and Schuster, New York, pp 147–159.
8	Sapolsky, R M	(op cit)	p 154.
9	Garbarino, J (1999)	*Lost Boys*	The Free Press, Simon and Schuster, New York, p 78.
10	Pollack, W (1998)	*Real Boys*	Owl Books, Henry Holt and Co., New York, p 42.
11	Maccoby, E and Martin, J (1983)	'Socialisation in the context of the family: Parent-child interaction'	In Museen, P H, *Handbook of Child Psychology, Vol 4, Socialisation, Personality and Social Development,* 4th edition, Wiley, New York, pp 1–101.
12	Garbarino, J	(op cit)	p 78.
13	Pollack, W	(op cit)	p 57.
14	McCann, R (2000)	*On their own*	Finch Publishing, Sydney.
15	McCann, R	(op cit)	p 47.
16	McCann, R	(op cit)	p 42.
17	McCann, R	(op cit)	p 42.

18	Garbarino, J	(op cit)	p 10.
19	Kindlon, D and Thompson, M (1999)	*Raising Cain*	Penguin Books, London, p 4.
20	Kropp, P (2000)	'Is your child addicted to praise?'	*Reader's Digest*, June 2000, p 161.
21	Weaver, A quoted in Garbarino, J	(op cit)	p 156.
22	Grossman, D quoted in Garbarino, J	(op cit)	p 114.
23	Goleman, D	(op cit)	p 180.
24	Kindlon, D and Thompson, M (1999)	(op cit)	p 234.
25	Browne, R and Fletchner, R	(op cit)	p 180.
26	Goleman, D	(op cit)	p 109.
27	Browne, R and Fletcher, R	(op cit)	p 11.
28	Watkins, S (1996)	'Half State students are bullied . . . survey finds'	*Age* 5/3/96.
29	Hodge, A (2000)	'Trouble in private school of hard knocks'	*Sydney Morning Herald*, 18/1/00.
30	Noonan, G (2000)	'Schools battle bullies by unleashing lawyers'	*Sydney Morning Herald*, 29/2/00.
31	Browne, R and Fletcher, R	(op cit)	p 14.
32	Pollack, W	(op cit)	p 338.
33	Jackson, A (1999)	*The King's School Policy on Bullying*	Unpublished policy document, The King's School, Parramatta, NSW.
34	Pollack, W	(op cit)	p 357.
35	Browne, R and Fletcher, R	(op cit)	p 86.
36	Healy, G (2000)	'Bullies aren't forever'	*Australian*, 30/10/00, p 13.

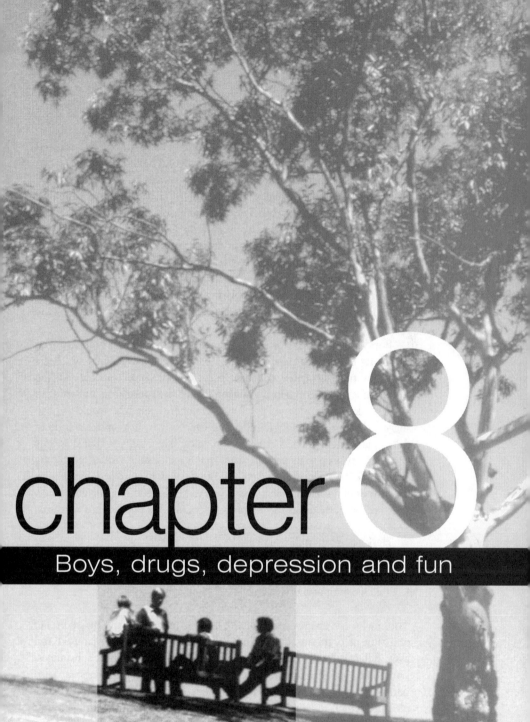

chapter 8

Boys, drugs, depression and fun

INTRODUCTION

It is not just the alliteration that joins depression with drugs, it is the tragic frequency with which one finds an alliance of drugs and depression in boys. In the western world, society is becoming more and more burdened by drug dependency, substance abuse and mental health disorders.[1]

Alcohol abuse in 12- to 24-year-old Australians in 1999 rose to 11% for males, and 7% for females, and the use of illicit drugs like cannabis, heroin, amphetamines and ecstacy also increased. Linked with this trend has been a 70% increase in the suicide rate for young Australian men over the last 20 years. The coordinator at the Centre for the Advancement of Adolescent Health at the New Children's Hospital at Westmead, Dr Michael Booth, suggests that Australia is going backwards in controlling drug use with there being no really effective interventions. The suggestion that Australia is the lucky country is not borne out by the number of people suffering depression.[2]

Boys do not have a drug problem, society has a drug problem. The launching of the Australian anti-drug campaign, Operation Noah, bears testimony to drugs being endemic in society. Like the Noah of old, the operation is a rescue mission, a mission to stop the young from drowning in a rising tide of drug induced psychosis. There are some who would want to suggest that it's not really raining, and even if it is, just smoke a little of this . . . and then you will enjoy the puddles! The reality is that it is only when society is up to its neck in water that it realises the virtues of building an ark and it is only when society is up to its neck in trouble does it realise the virtues of a society that is dissuading its students from drug abuse.

Used properly drugs have a place in society. As one wit has written:

> Hark the Herald Angel's sing
> Beecham's pills are just the thing
> Peace on earth and mercy mild;
> Two for man and one for child.

Those who have sustained sporting injuries may know the blessed relief of a shot of pethidine in the rump. However, drugs can be abused and even household items are now being used as mind-altering substances. Drugs can heal and lead to independence from pain, but drugs can also harm and lead to a dependence on their pleasure. Unfortunately it is a pleasure which does not last, and neither do the solutions drugs might bring. Escapism through chemicals solves nothing. The chemicals wear off, the problems do not. A society conditioned to the avoidance of reality lacks integrity and a society that seeks shallow answers to deep problems lacks wisdom.

The highs that boys should enjoy are those of an epic sporting tussle; the thrills that boys should enjoy are those related to learning new truths; the daring that boys should enjoy is that of abseilling down 30 metres of horizontally bedded sandstone in the Pokolbin State Forest or in the tree-ferned canyons of the Blue Mountains. The real world can provide excitement aplenty; there is no need to escape from reality through the use of chemicals. The real world can give satisfaction, pleasure and purpose if one looks hard enough and if one tries hard enough.

In saying this, it is important not to trivialise the problem and pain having to be borne by some boys or to ignore the nihilistic feelings and anger that is the fruit of abuse, prejudice and rejection. Non-chemical solutions to these problems can be found even if one cannot get to the Pokolbin State Forest or the Blue Mountains. Answers can be found in friendships, counselling and various help agencies. Personal problems can be put in perspective, when brooding on one's own misfortunes is replaced by helping others with their problems.

IS MY SON ON DRUGS?

There is in most parents an innate pride in their offspring and a reluct-ance to believe that the fruit of their loins could ever engage in irrespon-sible or self-destructive behaviours. There can be genuine disbelief when parents are presented with irrefutable proof that their son has been using drugs. Denial is the only way some parents can cope, but it is a reaction which is neither appropriate nor constructive. Parents need to be honest, and aware of the potential for substance abuse in their family.

Although by no means conclusive, a parent may be forgiven a slight frisson of fear that their son may be 'doing' drugs if the bedroom wall is plastered with pictures of *cannabis sativa* and there are blackened spoons littering the floor together with cigarette papers and strange bottles with funny tubes protruding. In all likelihood, a boy is not going to be quite this transparent about his predilection towards drugs. Not wishing to incur parental wrath, a significant reduction in pocket money and the ability to have unbridled freedom on Friday night, the drug taking will generally be hidden from parents.

It may not be particularly well hidden. There is among some adoles-cents an 'in your face' attitude which can quite brazenly proclaim that they could be into drugs. Call it a proclamation of independence; call it rebellion against authority figures; call it disillusionment with the estab-lishment; call it whatever one likes, some boys will 'do' drugs. Other boys will wear the uniform, adopt the speech and take on the demeanour of the drug user but may not necessarily be into drugs. This is signalling anger and a predisposition to do so. A parent has a right to be worried by these signals. Unfortunately, the parent who does not see these signals cannot be entirely free of worry either, for some boys are very adept at disguising or minimalising their significant involvement with drugs.

SOME OF THE TELLTALE SIGNS OF SUBSTANCE ABUSE

1. Academic

- a decline in academic performance in school
- a growing anti-school sentiment
- behavioural problems in class ranging from listlessness, apathy and inattention through to anger and defiance
- truancy
- increasing vagueness and memory problems
- short attention span, difficulty in concentration

2. Social/emotional

- moody, resentful and prone to secretive behaviours
- rapid changes in temperament; intolerance to criticism, either real or imagined
- growing delinquency
- shortage of money which can lead to involvement in theft or in selling drugs

3. Physical

- reduced resistance to colds and flu
- changes in eating habits and weight
- pallid, unhealthy appearance
- sleep problems, both too much and too little[3]

Care should be taken in putting too much emphasis on the telltale signs listed above for they should be recognised for what they are, and that is signs, not proof. It should also be remembered that there are many other conditions which can lead to the symptoms described, and it will need the intercession of professional medical help to decide the matter properly. Tests do exist which many doctors and other properly qualified people can administer which are simple and non-intrusive in their detection of substance abuse. Having noted this, a simple test devised by Dr Forrest Tennant from California can be used by parents to help indicate whether their son is using marijuana.[4] It involves the boy recounting what he did, in detail, hour by hour the previous day. If the answers are vague then this might mean that the tetrahydrocannabinal (THC) in marijuana has caused the clogging of the brain's neurotransmitters and has interfered with the neurochemicals to the extent the boy just cannot remember. This test should be seen as indicative only, rather than as positive proof that one's son is using marijuana. It also is important to remember that substance abuse is not limited to marijuana, with each drug having different presenting disorders.

SMOKING

Jean Nicot lent his name to the alkaloid now known as nicotine found in the leaf of the tobacco plant. Nicot was an enthusiastic supporter of the plant and ascribed to it many medical and social virtues. One might forgive Nicot given that Portugal in the 1560s was not alive to the health risks associated with smoking.

Research has now found that nicotine is a toxic, addictive stimulant. Cigarette smoke is poisonous and carcinogenic, promoting premature ageing of the skin, respiratory problems, heart disease and circulatory problems.[5] It is not good news.

There is evidence to suggest that fewer boys may be smoking relative to girls, but nicotine still remains one of the most popular social drugs for boys. The sublime optimism in boys together with the strong desire to be accepted by the group will generally mean that anti-smoking videos and lectures may not always be effective. Some may stagger out and have to have a cigarette to calm their nerves, but most will not be greatly affected. Most boys know that smoking is not good for them, but this will not stop many of them from doing it.

Imparting knowledge about the health risks associated with cigarette smoking is important and should not be underestimated in its ability to turn a number of boys from wanting to smoke. However, logic and knowledge are not terribly effective when a boy is feeling socially vulnerable on a Friday night and in the presence of peers who are smoking. Add to this the allure of the opposite sex, many of whom may be smoking, some brain-deadening music and the erosion of inhibitions brought on by a half-empty bottle of Jim Beam, and the Quit campaign rhetoric is lost.

Four approaches which can work well with boys are:

1. the deterrent approach
2 the fitness approach
3. the emotional approach
4. the 'I don't need it' approach.

1. The deterrent approach

Although lacking a certain sophistication, the threat by a parent to curtail a son's freedom or expenditure does sometimes work. A few

SMOKING

Why do boys do it? Why do boys smoke when evidence is overwhelming in terms of its harmful effects? It not only yellows fingers, and wallpapers lungs with tar, it can bestow upon the smoker an ashtray breath, a thin wallet and a carcinogenic wheeze. Even more appalling is the preparedness of smokers to allow themselves to be enslaved. While laughing at wowsers and speaking of freedom, the shackles of addiction snap tight around their lives.

Some boys do it to experiment. This is vaguely defensible, for it has a nice educational ring to it. Unfortunately some experiments are dangerous, and before the smoke has cleared another boy has surrendered part control of his life to Benson & Hedges.

Others do it to grow up. The socially fragile feel they must augment their aura of maturity by sticking white sticks in their mouth. It often takes some years to realise that true maturity is not found in the decision to smoke. Indeed there is evidence to suggest that the more mature will probably say 'No thanks . . . I don't need it'.

Many smoke because of peer pressure. The desire to be accepted by friends is so strong it will dictate what you wear, what you speak, and even what you breathe. Control is given to the group which determines the chemical which should be lived with.

Some smoke out of rebellion or daring. There is a thrill factor — will I get caught and get punished? Will I get caught and get a cancer?

Too many of our young are sending smoke signals asking for help; smoke signals that confess to some personal inadequacy; smoke signals that they don't like society or themselves.

Tragically, smokers are dying out . . . sometimes painfully and slowly. The pathetic, emaciated features of those in the oncology wards of hospitals are reminders that the final days of a smoker are not filled with careless abandon, fun and devilment, but rather in wrestling with gurgling tubes, pain killers and bitter recriminations.

Often boys find it difficult to believe they are mortal . . . and accordingly take unacceptable risks with their lives. There is a need to blow the smoke away and give them a clear indication that smoking is not worthy of them.

Source: Hawkes, T F, *The King's Herald*, The King's School, Parramatta, 19 March 1998.

parents have turned the deterrent approach around and offered financial inducements and even such rewards as a car if the son furnishes clear evidence of not being a smoker up to the age of 18. Care needs to be taken with these approaches for it may do little else than drive smoking 'underground'. Then again, it can be argued that underground is better than above ground. Another potential problem is developing a mind set among the young that sees them being rewarded for normal behaviours which can properly be expected by parents. Not smoking is normal and should not necessarily be rewarded lest the dependency is transferred from nicotine to rewards. Neither is good for a boy.

The deterrent approach can be enriched by regular reminders of health risks associated with smoking. Lung cancer and respiratory diseases will not only be 10 times more likely, there is a litany of other medical problems which can be drawn to a boy's attention such as heart attack, blood circulation disorders, stomach ulcers and premature ageing of the skin. Again, it is as well not to pin too many hopes on the factual deterrent approach for many boys have developed a world-weary cynicism and immunity to facts, and even if they were to believe them, many find a certain pleasure in daring the gods. There is a thrill factor in playing Russian roulette with a smoking butt; a daring; a risk taking which boys mistakenly see as courage.

2. The fitness approach

Sport is the mainstream religion for many boys and they like to see themselves as athletic and as being fit. This is not true of all boys, but it is true of enough to make the fitness approach worth considering. The supportive data is simple enough. To be successful in sport, one needs a body that is able to function efficiently. Smoking reduces the capacity of the blood to carry oxygen and can bring about many other performance limiting problems ranging from respiratory problems to gangrene. It is not just sport that might be adversely affected: everyday functions and even the capacity for rewarding sex can be reduced by smoking.

3. The emotional approach

Abstract reasoning does not always work well with a boy. It is too divorced from reality for many boys to take seriously. However, the testimony of a relative or friend who has been a smoker and who is now having to battle a smoking related illness, can have a strong impact on a boy. Failing this, a trip to the cancer ward of a local hospital can be effective, as can the viewing of a number of powerful anti-smoking documentaries.

4. The 'I don't need it' approach

Somehow or other, society has failed to capitalise on the opportunities to discredit the smoking experience by ignoring the fact that many start smoking to gain peer approval and social acceptance. Is a boy's social standing so fragile, his capacity to be accepted so unlikely, that he has to advance his cause by burning nicotine between his lips? Perhaps it is now time for the non-smokers to take some ground and to say to those offering a cigarette 'No thanks . . . I don't need it'.

Such a response implies pity for those who do need a cigarette. Good. There are very few forces more potent than pity in goading a boy to want to regain his pride. If the sense can be engendered that the smoker must have a problem, then perhaps some ground can be won. 'You poor thing, I can see why you smoke, you need every social crutch that is going' may be the sort of uncharitable sentiment that might have to be fostered in this battle against smoking.

Smoking and other drugs

Parents whose sons smoke can be forgiven for thinking that drugs other than nicotine may be a feature of their offspring's lives. British surveys in the 1990s found that half of all tobacco smokers had tried illegal drugs. Among non-smokers, the figure was only 2%. This is a non-trivial difference.[6]

ALCOHOL

Some alcohol can be good — even Saint Paul urged his protégé Timothy to take a little wine for his health's sake. Jesus' first miracle was to make some high-quality wine at a wedding, and a not inconsiderable amount of it either. More contemporary authorities have recognised the benefits of the antioxidants in red wine and the improved blood flow and brain functioning associated with the imbibing of limited amounts of alcohol. Unfortunately, boys need to be reminded that if a small amount is a good thing, a large amount it not necessarily a better thing. Getting 'rat-faced', 'maggotted' and 'wasted' does not create in a person a feeling of radiant health.

Just when does alcohol use become alcohol abuse? This question is not particularly difficult to answer — even for a boy. The body sends out very efficient reminders of the line having been crossed. It's called a hangover. Having noted this, boys may need to be reminded that the line is getting pretty close when the stimulation ceases and the sedative effect begins to take over. Also worth noting is the fact that the capacity to make sound judgment as to the near presence of a line tends to become less as the line is approached.

For some teenage boys, there is the necessity to get drunk rather than to drink. It seems an occasion is more special only if it cannot be remembered; with the only clues of the evening activities being nausea, a pair of pink knickers in the pocket and some vomit on the shirt. It is even more odd that such drinking binges seem to take place on those occasions one rather hopes will be remembered, such as eighteenth birthday parties. Twelve per cent of Australian adolescent boys have a serious problem with alcohol.[7]

When young, boys are less able to metabolise alcohol than when a little older. Alcohol is absorbed more quickly when young, but not processed more quickly. The capacity to cope with alcohol varies from boy to boy and is influenced by a variety of factors including the amount of body water. For this reason the generally accepted formula of the body being able to process one alcoholic drink an hour needs to be treated very carefully. Drinks vary in size, as does the size of the liver and the presence of many other factors which can make nonsense of such general guidelines.

Perhaps the greatest menace associated with alcohol is not so much the direct results of acetaldehyde poisoning but rather the capacity alcohol has to reduce sound judgment. Alcohol plus testosterone plus a minor irritation can lead to violence. Alcohol plus fast cars can lead to a road carnage which is frightening.

By day, all boys are mild-mannered reporters, but on Saturday night they don't so much go into phone booths and emerge as supermen, they get into the grog and become invincible. True, a few will get depressed and moody, but most will be tempted to engage in feats of valour that would not be believed in the sober light of dawn — picking a fight with Slugsy (the fist) Jones and picking up herpes from Suzi (I will) Smith, to name but a few.

Drinking by boys is seen as the social gesture needed to be admitted into the ranks of manhood. Not being allowed alcohol can be a growing irritation for a boy. The irritation arises from each reinforcement of prohibition being a reinforcement of the boy's immaturity. When a boy is desperately wanting to be considered mature and fully male, these messages become increasingly irksome and so the quest for alcohol begins. There is shame associated with childishness; there is pride associated with manliness and a demonstration of manliness is made even more convincing if the adolescent boy doesn't just drink, he gets 'swilled to the back teeth' drunk.

Adolescents are less practised at drinking, are less aware of the dangers in mixing drinks, have bodies less able to process the alcohol and are more prone to 'binge' drinking. After a while drinking is not engaged in just to signal manliness; drinking is engaged in because the adolescent is wanting to experience the drug effect of alcohol. Getting drunk is:

■ **Exciting** — inhibitions are lowered with some very interesting results.
■ **Bonding** — loneliness disappears as does the male code of emotional neutrality. When drunk, boys are allowed to hug each other, to stagger with arms around a friend's shoulders, become sentimental and enjoy intimacy albeit an artificial intimacy.

- **An analgesic** — for pain is dulled, at least for a time.
- **Releasing** — people become understanding and even tolerant if the stupid things a boy does were done while the boy was drunk.

Given the prevalence of alcohol in society, it is unlikely that most boys will escape at least one hangover in their teen years. Quite what can be done about this is not always clear. However, the following advice might be considered useful for a boy.

- Do not drink and drive. Appoint a designated driver.
- Be wary of drinks when you do not know for certain what is in them.
- Do not mix drinks.
- Observe the one drink an hour rule.
- Match each drink of alcohol with one glass of water.
- Develop a 'buddy' system whereby a small group undertakes to look after each other.
- Do not be too proud to drink light beer.
- Have an emergency plan in place in case something goes wrong.
- Do not mix alcohol with drugs for the effects can be very dangerous. Marijuana, for example, can suppress the body's natural defence for over-indulgence by making vomiting less frequent. This can allow the alcohol to stay in the body when it would otherwise be expelled.
- Do not drink on an empty stomach.
- Try to determine the maximum number of drinks allowable before going out.
- Be careful of sweet alcoholic drinks. The sugar content can disguise the alcoholic content.
- Never arrive at a party thirsty. Drink plenty of water before arriving at a function.
- When returning from a function, rehydrate by drinking plenty of water.

Rather than just stating this advice, parents will also need to model this advice and look at their own drinking habits.

MARIJUANA

The signs are not good. *Cannabis sativa* is about as hardy a plant one can find, producing a strong fibre which has been used for centuries to make rope. Yet if the resin from this plant is injected into its root system, it will die. The same resin will also kill boys, who seem more prone to smoking marijuana than girls.[8] Nine per cent of Australian boys have a serious problem with cannabis.[9]

The price paid for the euphoria and relaxation induced by marijuana can be a reddening of the eyes, anxiety and even paranoia, dry throat, hallucinations, increased appetite, poor concentration, impaired short-term memory and reduced ability to drive or operate machinery very well. The longer term problems make even more depressing reading and include addiction, respiratory disease, permanent memory damage, schizophrenia, leukemia, weakened immune system, reduced ability to have children, premature ageing, and respiratory tract cancer.

Marijuana comes in many forms — as dried leaves, dried resin and even as oil extract — from the flowering tops and leaves of the *cannabis sativa* plant. It is also called many names — weed, grass, hash, dope, pot, hemp, to name but a few. None of it is particularly beneficial except for those suffering from some select medical conditions where marijuana can be used under medical supervision as part of the treatment.

The potency of marijuana has increased over the years so that a joint smoked today is likely to be far more dangerous than a joint smoked 20 years ago.

The advice that parents can give their sons in the matter of marijuana, is simple . . . don't use it. No responsible form of compromise can really be countenanced, just don't have anything to do with it.

OTHER ILLEGAL DRUGS

There is a plethora of illegal drugs in contemporary society and the ease by which they can be obtained has reached a stage whereby traffickers and pushers seem to be able to operate quite brazenly. Not only is it marijuana on offer, but so too are:

- amphetamines
- barbiturates
- cocaine
- hallucinogens
- inhalants
- opiates/narcotics
- steroids.

Added to the drug list are the legal substances such as caffeine which is the world's most popular mood-altering drug. It is present in coffee and tea, and also in cola drinks and high-energy 'rage' soft drinks designed to empower youth to dance into the not-so-small hours of the morning.

Space constraints prevent a thorough exploration of all such drugs but information is readily available to parents and teachers through your local doctor and through government drug agencies.

MARIJUANA

Some boys choose to smoke marijuana out of curiosity, daring or peer pressure. Some boys choose to smoke marijuana because of some personal inadequacy or to make some socio-political gesture. Some boys choose to use marijuana as a means of punishing those who love them. Other choose to use marijuana as a means of punishing those who hate them. Whatever the reason, marijuana is unworthy of them and has no place in the lives of our sons.

Deterrent alone is not enough. Schools need to put in place a drug education policy and a general program of education that is designed to reduce the need for students to experiment with illegal drugs.

There will be some who might suggest that marijuana is no more dangerous than alcohol or cigarettes. This may or may not be true, but this should not prevent schools from dissuading their students from experimenting with marijuana. There are a number of reasons for this attitude but not least because there is mounting evidence to suggest that marijuana has been linked to schizophrenia and psychosis. It has also been linked to depression, low self-esteem and violence. Unlike alcohol which is generally removed from the body within 24 hours, cannabis is attracted to the fatty tissues such as those in the brain and can remain there for up to five years. It is interesting to note that Sweden, which has a strong tradition of liberalism, has dramatically altered its policy towards marijuana from that of a very relaxed attitude to one of strong legal sanction. This is because studies undertaken using over 50 000 military conscripts indicated a strong link between cannabis consumption and schizophrenia, suicide, intravenous drug use and violent crime.[10]

A further problem with marijuana is that it is generally packaged in an anti-establishment culture; in an alternative values system which can be damaging to the individual and to society.

There should be no apology in asking boys to break their silence in relation to drugs and those who supply them. Boys should be asked to support the anti-drug campaign Operation Noah. Boys should break their silence, for there are some who do not deserve their protection; who do not deserve the accolade of mateship. Those who distribute their packages of pleasure are often predators, for they distribute the very real risk of drug dependency. So it is that we must have the courage to speak out and act against dealers and distributors of illicit drugs. There is no place for them in society; there is no place for them on the ark.

Source: Hawkes, T F, *The King's Herald*, The King's School, Parramatta, 4 June 1998.

The figures in Table 8.1 are disturbing but must be kept in context. The same survey found that 61% of males and 74% of females did not engage in the use of heroin, cocaine, amphetamines, cannabis or any substance abuse whatsoever, excluding the social use of alcohol or tobacco.[11] It is important to remember that most boys avoid illegal drugs, just as it is

Table 8.1 The proportion of Australian youth aged 14–19 years who have used drugs in the last 12 months

	Male	Female
Alcohol	63%	61%
Cannabis	35%	20%
Tobacco	18%	19%

Source: Commonwealth Department of Health and Family Services 1995, National Drug Strategy Household Survey. Commonwealth of Australia copyright reproduced by permission. For further information which is rather more up-to-date, a useful resource is Moon, L, Meyer, P and Grau, J (1999), 'Australia's young people: their health and wellbeing 1999', Australian Institute of Health and Welfare, Canberra, http://www.aihw.gov.au

important not to minimise the problem of drug abuse in the youth of today. The average boy is not an addict. The average boy may use social drugs and may experiment with illegal drugs but will not be drug dependent. There are many levels of drug use:

1. no use due to ignorance
2. no use due to choice
3. experimental use
4. occasional recreational use
5. regular use but no addiction
6. dependent use and addiction.

A boy using a drug does not necessarily mean that he is dependent on the drug, but counselling is still warranted as early intervention is best.

One of the most effective ways to reduce drug use in children is to reduce drug use in the home. When parents smoke and when parents drink, children watch; children who are in a hurry to grow up and be just like mum and dad.

Girls often smoke more than boys. However, boys appear to be engaging in more 'binge' drinking than girls. From the 'rum rebellion' to the '6 o'clock swill', drinking has been a feature of the Australian male. This country has produced cricketers who can drink a slab of beer on a flight to London and a prime minister who held a world drinking record. Changing individual drinking habits is one thing; changing national drinking habits is another.

Whether one adopts a zero tolerance policy or a harm minimisation approach in regard to drinking and other forms of drug use, will depend upon the personal convictions of the parents and school. However, it could be suggested that, particularly in the case of alcohol, the modelling by parents of how to drink sensibly can be useful to boys, particularly the example given by fathers.

RANDOM DRUG TESTING IN SCHOOLS

Some schools take a zero tolerance policy approach to drug use within a school and will expel any student caught experimenting with drugs. This policy has been shown to be effective in a few schools — but not many. An approach which is rather more constructive, yet more controversial is to undertake random drug tests on students in schools. This option has outraged civil libertarians who point to abuse of power and erosion of personal freedoms.

A responsible compromise might be for the school principal to meet with the accused student and his parents and to agree that within six weeks the student must produce a medical certificate to say his urine is free from the trace of drugs. If all parties agree, then a positive outcome is probable, with the student stopping his involvement with drugs to achieve the 'all clear' certification from his doctor. Behaviour modification has occurred in a positive and constructive manner.

If the student or the parents refuse to allow the test, or if the test should come back still indicating drug use, then the school will need to examine other options including further counselling or expulsion. Generally, parents would be supportive of a school taking the drug test initiative as they are probably very anxious that their son should stop involvement with drug abuse and are looking for any initiative that will work.

Once the 'all clear' has been established, the school, with the agreement of parents and student, might ask the student at any time in the future to repeat the test in order to ensure that he remains motivated to keep clear of drugs.

Initiatives such as these need to be explored. Those who shout loudly about personal freedoms being violated are not nearly so vociferous in their suggestion of other options that might be taken to rid society of the menace of drugs.

PARTIES

Given that parties often provide opportunities for boys to involve themselves with drugs, the scope of this chapter has been widened to include a few thoughts and advice for parents about parties.

Many boys are the very model of sobriety most of the time, but come unstuck at parties. There is no simple solution but the guidelines on pages 206–208, based on advice by the Association of Heads of Independent Schools of Australia, can be useful.

Boys need to recognise that it is quite possible to have fun without engaging in something that is either immoral, expensive or illegal. Preaching abstinence from parties is as unhelpful as it is inappropriate. We have a God who partied and who told stories of redemption that concluded with a fatted calf being killed and eaten . . . 'for this my son was dead and now is alive; but he was lost and now found. And they began to be merry.' (Luke 15:24)

Unfortunately the contemporary party often fuels its merriment with things other than fatted calves. Recreational drugs are common, as is teenage inquisitiveness, resulting in the need for some guidelines. Boys know the rules when they are stone cold sober and in the presence of parents or school principal on a Monday morning. They must seek to ensure they remember the rules at 11.30 pm on a Friday night when music, friends and a variety of beverages may have clouded their ability to do so!

I like a good party, but not quite as much if I'm invited to it! This is probably because I am out so much; a night at home is bliss. You might have to pay for your own drinks, but at least you can choose the music. Nonetheless I do find some parties pleasurable, particularly when they are full of interesting people who are not intent on trapping me for three hours in order to share their personal insights into how the school should be run.

As one wit has noted, 'Nothing is more irritating than not being invited to a party you wouldn't be seen dead at' . . . so keep the invitations coming, for the parties that worry me are the ones I wouldn't be seen alive at . . . and in truth, that's not many for I enjoy people and the carefree camaraderie that the party spirit can bring.

I've decided to pen a few thoughts about parties, at the invitation of several parents who have suggested that they would value the school setting some guidelines on this matter. This request has probably arisen from conflicting policies and practices among parents and the loneliness associated with parenting; a loneliness exacerbated by such isolating manoeuvres from our sons as:

- 'You are the only parent who rings up beforehand.'
- 'Everyone else's parents allow them.'
- 'Don't you trust me?'
- 'It's all right. I'll be with my friends.'

For this reason there may be some virtue in reaffirming some common guidelines that parents can retreat to and use in the face of hostile protest. The value of these guidelines is increased enormously if we are consistent in our implementation of them. Keep the guidelines on the fridge door next to the dial-a-pizza, and other emergency information.

▶

Students' behaviour at social functions — guidelines and suggestions

The issue of whether the school should be involved in students' out-of-hours behaviour is always a contentious one. School principals will continue to involve themselves in this area for the following reasons:

- Education is a collaborative process between parents and school that continues beyond school hours.
- The school offers support and guidance to school families.
- What happens outside school hours — in public places, on public transport and in homes — affects people's perception of the school.
- When students enrol at a school, they take on a commitment to the values and standards of that school. These values and standards cannot be shed simply by removing the school uniform.
- Our pastoral care of students goes well beyond the normal school hours of teaching and co-curricular activities. This is true of day boys as well as boarders.
- When students get into trouble outside school hours, the first port of call for the police is often the school. Inevitably, we are drawn into matters of discipline by the police and the general public.
- This is not an attempt by the school to tell parents how to run their homes. It is an expression of shared experience about what might be termed reasonable standards for students' social behaviour and it is supplied in response to requests for some guidelines on this matter. Guidelines for students' social behaviour proceed along the lines of a gradual transfer of responsibility and freedom of choice.
- Students need to be educated in the use of their freedom.
- Students appreciate it when there are reasonable limits to liberty and when these limits are clearly designated and reinforced.
- It should be remembered that the determination of limits by parents and school allows the student to experiment and initiate behaviour within those limits and this can be a constructive and worthwhile experience.

Guidelines for parties
Invitations

- Invitations should be written and distributed to guests well in advance.
- Invitations should give information about times of starting and finishing, location of the function and a contact telephone number.
- Invitations should include details of supervision and the names of supervising adults.
- Where possible, replies to invitations should also be written. In any event, the acceptance or refusal must be communicated to the parents of the host.

Alcohol

The consumption of alcohol at parties, even by senior students, should be discouraged. If the host parents take on the responsibility and risks of serving alcohol to their own or other people's children, then:

- Parents of invited guests should be made aware that alcohol is to be served.
- Guests should always be offered ample quantities of attractive, cold, non-alcoholic drinks as an alternative.
- Guests should not bring alcohol to parties unless agreed to by parents. Parents should be aware of concealed alcohol (especially spirits), in bags, mixed in bottles of soft drink or left outside in cars.
- If guests consume excess alcohol during a function, their parents or teacher should be contacted and asked to collect them.
- The host should ensure that guests who are 'over the limit' do not drive but have alternative transport home.

Videos

The popularity of the video recorder has led to the ready availability of 'soft' and 'hard' core pornographic and violent films (X-rated, R-rated and even M-rated). Host parents should be aware:

- of the increasing use of videos at parties
- of the videos their children are watching
- that the responsibilities for providing appropriate entertainment extend to invited guests as well as to their own children.

Recommendations
Host parents should:

- encourage other parents to assist at parties or organise appropriate alternative security if numbers require it;
- be present, vigilant and mobile at all times;
- be firm about excluding gate crashers;
- ensure that no alcohol is brought by guests, unless by prior agreement with parents;
- ensure that any videos to be screened at the party are appropriate to the age group;
- ensure that the party finishes at the indicated time;
- ensure that all guests remain at the party throughout and, if a guest is missing, advise the guest's parents;
- not be intimidated by claims that standards at other parties are more liberal than suggested by these guidelines;
- ensure that guests are accompanied home by a responsible adult;
- have emergency phone numbers on standby.

◀

Host students should:

- ensure that guests are welcomed and introduced to the host parents;
- ensure that all guests remain at the party until they are accompanied home;
- comply with the standards of entertainment and behaviour agreed upon with parents before the function.

Parents of guests should telephone and check with the host parents:

- the times of the start and finish of the party;
- whether alcohol will be served;
- whether the host parents will be present;
- the transport arrangements;
- a telephone number where the host parents can be contacted if they will not be at home.

Guests should:

- answer invitations;
- arrive on time;
- meet and greet the hosts;
- remain at the party venue;
- treat all hosts' property with respect;
- thank the hosts on departure;
- dress and behave appropriately, recognising that it is all too easy to engage in activities within the heat of the moment which might be bitterly regretted in the long run;
- have a good time, but not at the expense of anyone else having a bad time;
- seek to look after each other and their hosts.

Source: Hawkes, T F, *The King's Herald*, The King's School, Parramatta, 4 June 1999.

RAVES AND RAGES

Many older boys engage in 'raves' and 'rages' such as the 'Big Day Out'. The psychology behind involvement in such activities is not always easy to understand, although Malcolm Knox makes the following insight:

The Big Day Out is itself a celebration of space, a privileged zone from which adults are barred by the unspoken apartheid of not fitting in. By taking ecstasy, or marijuana or amphetamines, the multitudes are seeking to open out universes of inner space in which they can romp to exhaustion. The adult contexts of drug use — as a crime, as a health risk — are irrelevant to the thousands of young people who explore their own territory through the use of drugs each week. Ask them for a context and they will place drugs on a continuum with issues of independence, experimentation and discovery — of finding their own space.[12]

'SCHOOLIES WEEK'

The last few years have seen a dramatic escalation of 'Schoolies Week', a period of unofficial celebration by students completing their Year 12 examinations. There is growing concern that Schoolies Week seems to be limited to neither 'schoolies' nor to a week. A large number of other people seem intent on joining school leavers, and there have been instances where some of these people seem at best opportunistic and at worst predatory. The celebrations also seem to be going on for much longer than a week, fuelled by a tourist industry which is highly motivated to extend the celebratory season for as long as possible.

Whereas it is entirely understandable for students to want to celebrate the end of one set of responsibilities before taking on a new set of responsibilities, some growing concerns have been identified in relation to Schoolies Week. These include the high costs and the behaviour by some within the tourism and hospitality industry, such as landlords failing to return bond money for no reason, and providing sub-standard services.

The heady cocktail of freedom from the strictures of both home and school, and the excitement of travel to a location specialising in the pursuit of pleasure, needs to be handled with care. To this must be added the extra synergy of being in a large group; a group which has time on its hands and money in its pocket; a group in the athletic prime of life; a group with minimal responsibilities and in celebration mode.

It is difficult to mitigate against all potential problems without curtailing the enjoyment of Schoolies Week, but experience gleaned from a number of schools has identified the following guidelines as being useful.

Guidelines for Schoolies Week

- Be prepared to stand up for what you want to do in Schoolies Week rather than merely following the crowd.
- Explore all options for Schoolies Week, including low budget options, local options, holidaying as a family, travelling, and getting a job.
- Establish a Schoolies Week budget before exploring the options.
- Book facilities only after checking them.

■ Read the small print and undertake commonsense precautions such as publicly recording any deficiencies in rental property before handing over bond money.

■ Be very careful about possessions and security, as communal or shared living can greatly increase the danger of items being lost or stolen. Possessions should be kept to a minimum, and be named or engraved and properly insured.

■ Appropriate limits need to be set for credit cards. Withdrawing from ATMs should only be done in the company of trusted friends.

■ Behavioural norms need to be established such as insisting on a nominated driver who will not consume alcohol.

■ Adopt responsible behaviours in relation to sex, drugs and the consumption of alcohol. Be aware of stranger danger.

■ Avoid 'trouble spots' and have in place support systems such as phone cards/link-home telephone access systems. Establish 'safe' houses owned by friends or relatives which might act as a refuge if needed. Put in place contingency plans.

DEPRESSION

> What you think of yourself is much more important that what others think of you.
> Seneca

Suicide rates in Australia have increased by 71% between 1979 and 1997 with the Australian Bureau of Statistics indicating in the 15–24 age group in 1998 that there were:

■ 82 female suicides
■ 364 male suicides.

This translates into eight suicides a week in Australia by people in this age group.[13] Some 60–90% of these suicides have been linked to depression, with the incidence of depression increasing 10-fold from 1995–2000. Those involved in drug use are three times more likely to commit suicide.[14]

Some 10–17% of young people in Australia think about suicide. Both depression and suicide are strongly linked to families in which there is discord. There are very real implications here for parents. Whatever the pain parents suffer, parents must seek to minimise strife and stress in the children for it can, quite literally, be a killer.

Dr David Brent of the University of Pittsburgh suggests that 3–8% of adolescents suffer depression with the incidence of depression increasing with each generation.[15] It is becoming apparent that the joyful exuberance of youth is being invaded by the dark cloud of depression, with its occurrence being recorded at ever younger ages.

The nature of the disease is that it is repetitive. This is because the causal factors keep reappearing because they were not fully resolved or dealt with the first time around. There is typically a 40% recurrence of adolescent depression within two years and a 72% recurrence within five years.[16]

Drugs can be linked to low self-esteem and a need to escape from reality. If one does not like oneself, one has no qualms about engaging in deliberate acts of self-harm. For this reason drug use is often linked to depression. However, there are other signals that might indicate depression including:

■ relationship problems and an alteration of sexual behaviours
■ difficulty controlling emotions and anger
■ denial of pain and an inability to cry
■ low self-esteem, deliberate acts of self-harm, and self-loathing
■ difficulty with concentration and sleep, and eating disorders including rapid weight gain or weight loss, and fatigue
■ demands for independence and autonomy and a self-absorbed orientation
■ problems at school, incomplete work, low grades, and behavioural problems ranging from withdrawal to attention seeking behaviour
■ high-risk behaviours
■ compulsive behaviours which can include over-indulgence in such things as work or sport
■ a morbid interest in suicide and death.[17]

While more girls attempt suicide, boys are more than four times as likely to succeed in killing themselves. Dr Erica Frydenburg's research at the University of Melbourne found that when boys were confronted with major difficulties, they tended to take an action-oriented strategy such as diverting themselves from the problem by playing a game of football. There is tragic evidence that this strategy does not always work. On the other hand girls tended to engage in group dynamics and talk to one another about the problem, therein experiencing some catharsis and healing.

Boys can be prone to significant fluctuations in self-esteem, and although not all will require Prozac and a psychiatrist, they may require empathy and support from a loving adult or friend. It is important not to await the full-blown diagnosis of clinical depression before offering remedial attention. Bouts of depression, although not officially labelled 'clinical', can be very painful and will need early medical intervention to head off major depressive illness and even suicide.

Establishing a means whereby boys can articulate their fears, insecurities and thoughts about their self-worth is the vital prerequisite to any healing. Parents, peers, psychologists and psychiatrists can all help. However, preventative options are always better than reactive options. The creating of a home and school environment where each child feels valued and loved, where opportunities are choreographed that enable a boy to succeed at something, become very important in reducing the incidence of depression and drug use by boys. If a boy likes himself, he will take care of himself. He will feel he is worth preserving. He will be less likely to inject, swallow or smoke things that are bad for him.

Abuse is often a product of poor emotional quotient. Parents and teachers may need to build coping skills into boys; may need to address their emotional and social well-being as much as their intellectual and physical well-being. In so doing the incidence of drug abuse and depression in boys might be reduced.

BOYS AND MOBILE PHONES

There was a time when the warble of a telephone would summon a member of the fairer sex. Well not now. The gender of those piling up the phone bill is now less predictable.

It is not exactly clear why this change has come about although a number of reasons present themselves. The first is that the mobile phone, rather like the credit card and the fourth-hand Mazda 323 with its dodgy muffler, is a symbol of independence for a boy and a coming of age. The corded phone quite literally ties boys to the home. The mobile phone does not. No longer do conversations have to be whispered or parental ears alarmed. Chats over the mobile phone can now be unhindered and uncensored.

Added to this boundless freedom is the sheer pleasure of being able to accommodate the impulse. Contemporary youth are not good at waiting. A lunch must be cooked and served in a bun in less than a minute or else the fidgeting starts. A call must be dialled and answered or else the same frustration is manifest. The mobile phone is perfect for the instant age.

Then there is the 'fiddle factor'. A phone is not just a phone. It is a complex instrument that can be programmed to sing countless tunes. The message can be sent in either verbal or text form; music can be played; and e-mails and computers accessed. The mobile phone can be an amusement arcade as well as a mobile office.

Boys love toys, particularly interactive microchipped complex toys which grant access, not only to friends but countless other diversions. The mobile phone has much going for it and may be obtained absolutely free.

Unfortunately the generosity does not usually extend to the calls. This is but one of the shadows that threaten the bright world of cordless communication. Boys need to be aware of:

■ The real costs of having a mobile phone. The best way for boys to learn what these costs are is to require the user to pay the bills, or at least a proportion of them. There is little more effective than a thinning wallet to drive home the economic reality of using a mobile phone.

■ The possible health risks associated with using mobile phones. The lack of conclusive proof of health dangers associated with using mobile phones should not be confused with there being no possibility of a health risk. This is particularly true of the young, whose brains are still undergoing significant development in their formative years. For this reason young boys may be more susceptible to permanent harm through prolonged use of mobile phones unless protective measures are put in place.

■ Many mobile phones offered for sale outside of the normal retail outlets are stolen. Some phones are offered for sale by those who claim to be 'upgrading' and no longer needing their old phone. In some cases this may be true, but in other cases it is merely a front for fencing filched phones.

■ Being small and valuable, mobile phone security can be a problem. Security can be enhanced through responsible behaviours including secure storage of the phone, engraving the phone, recording the serial number, using a security code to access confidential information and so on.

Despite the above the mobile phone is not all bad news, particularly for boys. Any device that is going to encourage articulacy, connectedness and a range of useful e-skills cannot be totally condemned. The connectedness is particularly important, not only from a physical point of view but from a psychological point of view. The propensity for boys to play close to the edge in life can mean that a helpline is often needed. If hurt or in danger a boy can ring for support. The mobile phone can give access to physical help and can give access to emotional help. All too often the boy that slides into depression, despair or self-destruction does so out of loneliness and isolation. The mobile phone is no panacea but it can erode that isolation and loneliness and give access to those whose friendship, love or training is such that they can bring support and healing.

However in allowing a boy to own a mobile phone, it is as well to ensure that:

■ he knows how to use it properly and in a way that minimises health risks
■ he knows when and where to switch it on, and when and where to switch it off
■ he knows it is a phone not a fashion accessory
■ he knows how to keep it and its information safe
■ he knows the financial implications of mobile phone use.

THE CULTURE OF CRUELTY

It is no wonder that some boys get depressed when so many of them have to endure what Kindlon and Thompson call a 'culture of cruelty'.[18] This culture is at its most obvious when a boy is coming of age and approaching puberty. The siren call to transfer allegiance from the mother to the father and from the parents to peers is heard. Autonomy beckons and the boy forsakes the security and unconditional love of the home for the allure of conditional acceptance outside of the home.

The trouble is that the conditions set for acceptance can be hard, resulting in a number of boys foundering on the rocks. The boy who is most likely to be wrecked can often be the academically able boy, the reflective boy, the aesthetic, the non-sporting boy who finds it difficult to fit the strict conformity demanded of him by 'the group'.

In describing the characteristics of 15-year-old Eric Wilson, who took his own life in 1997, Spurr writes that Eric was a quiet youngster who served as an altar boy, who loved the romantic language of French and playing Mozart on the piano. Unfortunately, the predominant male culture was such that it would not cope with Eric, and the signals were given that he was a nerd, a 'Nigel'. The intelligent, aesthetic, reflective male was not allowed to exist. Eric heard these messages loud and clear and obliged by eradicating himself. A profound tragedy not just for Eric and his family, but for the contemporary male culture of Australia.[19]

A number of boys just cannot cope with the psychological warfare, the humiliation that comes with their inability to be 'cool'. The definition of 'cool' is established by the boy most in a hurry to grow up, and rules are set. Some of these rules can be really easy to follow — what TV shows to watch, what music to listen to, what clothes to wear. The desperation comes from being given rules it is impossible to conform to — be tall, be muscled, have body hair and a large penis, be Caucasian, be in the footy team and don't wear glasses.

Those boys who fail to conform to peer expectations are often aware that they are also failing to conform to parental expectations, particularly of fathers. Spurr described some fathers as being men who have:

> never developed intellectually, spiritually or emotionally beyond that period of conformist puerility and ... pass on its priorities to their sons. It is Bob Ellis's world of 'blokes and football jocks and hard-drinking he-men's men with brains like burnt rissoles dipped in Foster's'.[20]

The jocular world of mateship is not experienced by all boys. Some are 'frozen out' and are left to freeze without the warmth of friendship to keep them alive. Kindlon and Thompson write that a culture of cruelty exists and is allowed to flourish in most western cultures.

> Despite collegial appearances, all boys live with fear in this culture of cruelty. They also adhere to the code and they are loyal to its tenets even though they may not feel as if they fit it, because they view it as an inevitable test of their manliness. It is with this kind of power that the culture of cruelty corrupts friendships, dictates alliances, and depending on the moment, casts boys in the roles of perpetrator, potential victim, or uneasy silent witness.
>
> With every lesson in dominance, fear, and betrayal, a boy is tutored away from trust, empathy and relationships. This is what boys lose to the culture of cruelty. What they learn instead is emotional guardedness, the wariness with which so many men approach relationships for the rest of their lives.[21]

Small wonder that with this existence of a culture of cruelty there will be casualties; there will be depression and anxiety.

DEALING WITH DEPRESSION

Whether depression has reached clinical diagnosis or not, expert medical assistance should be sought as soon as possible. This assistance may well involve pharmacotherapy, which is a frightening term meaning the use of medicines. Then there is a range of other therapies including family therapies, interpersonal therapies, relaxation therapies and supportive management therapies. Perhaps the most common form of therapy is

Table 8.2 A Year 8 survey about factors associated with emotional well-being

In 1997 a survey was undertaken by 'The Gatehouse Project'[22] run by the Centre for Adolescent Health in Melbourne. The survey involved 26 schools and 2678 students. The following findings about factors associated with the emotional well-being of young people were discovered:

Reported problem	Girls	Boys
Recent victimisation	51%	53%
Victimisation 'most days'	16%	18%
No one to talk to if angry or upset	13%	25%
Having no one to trust	15%	28%

Source: Patton, G, Glover, S, Bowes, G and Coffey, C (1997) *The Gatehouse Project: Report to schools on first survey, Year 8*, Centre for Adolescent Health, Melbourne.

Cognitive Behavioural Therapy (CBT) which has shown itself to be particularly effective with severe depression when used in conjunction with appropriate medication.

The capacity to deal effectively with depression will be reduced if an attitude of hopelessness is engendered, and where the depression is chronic. Parental depression will also hinder recovery in the child as will parent-child disharmony. A broad approach is often needed when dealing with depression, with CBT proving effective in many cases, but there is also a need to solve family conflict, parental depression and demoralisation.[23]

Within the family, a number of things can be done to help inoculate boys against depression, including:

- not embroiling children in parental conflict. Parents who love and care for each other produce children who are less likely to suffer depression;
- if a parent suffers depression, expert medical help should be sought, not just for the parent but also for the children, especially if they should show any signs of being adversely affected;
- parents being neither permissive nor authoritarian;
- families being empathetic and having good listening skills; developing a culture that allows the free sharing of feelings without criticism;
- parents giving praise and encouragement;
- teaching relaxation techniques to children;
- encouraging children to reflect on their positive qualities, and parents fuelling those qualities with praise and encouragement;
- actively dissuading children from the use of drugs;
- choreographing opportunities for leadership and service which can serve to both distract children from their problems and provide a reason for praise and affirmation;
- avoiding negative talk and demeaning criticism within the home, maintaining a positive and cheerful atmosphere within the home. Putting a ban on Automatic Negative Thoughts (ANTS);[24]
- developing a sense of personal pride in children by showing them respect and love and giving them encouragement;
- when disciplining children, learning to show firmness and compassion, remembering to hate the sin rather than the sinner;
- monitoring morale daily both indirectly and directly by getting children to state how positive they are feeling on a scale of 1 to 10;
- working in close cooperation with teachers and relevant doctors;
- encouraging a healthy diet and a good exercise regime;
- paying close attention to the spiritual climate in the home. The concept of a loving God can be a great comfort particularly to those who might suffer from depression;

■ teaching coping skills related to bullying, time management and stress control;

■ encouraging children to be involved in the community by participating in activities which are either enjoyable or which might bring some measure of success;

■ obtaining expert medical advice as soon as a bad mood lingers longer than a few weeks;

■ talking to children about the 'culture of cruelty' among children and teenagers, and the positive things that can be done about it;

■ encouraging psychological hardiness by developing conflict resolution skills and problem solving techniques;[25]

■ avoiding over-protection;

■ reducing the reliance on material rewards and increasing the use of interpersonal rewards such as time and affection.[26]

How schools can help

One of Australia's leading authorities on youth depression and suicide, Associate Professor Michael Carr-Gregg, suggests that schools can help combat depression by:

■ conducting a depression awareness program which helps students to understand that depression is not a normal state of mind;

■ helping students not to feel guilty or inadequate if they should have depression;

■ showing students how to recognise the difference between depression and sadness;

■ encouraging students to develop emotional competencies and mental fitness;

■ promoting connectedness to the family, school and wider community;

■ creating a safe, supporting environment with effective pastoral care programs with adult, as well as student, mentors for each student;

■ developing psychosocial competencies such as problem solving, assertiveness training and anger management;

■ creating a pro-social environment where thoughts and feelings can be expressed in a non-judgmental way;

■ assisting parents in their parenting duties by encouraging and informing them of policies and practices within the home that can help minimise the onset of depression in their children.[27]

The Gatehouse Project

The Centre for Adolescent Health in Melbourne runs a project called The Gatehouse Project, which is designed to help schools reduce the incidence of depression in students. As well as researching the issue, The Gatehouse team visits schools to help students develop strategies to cope with adversity. A further service provided by The Gatehouse Project personnel is to do an audit of the school environment and recommend intervention strategies at three levels:

1. the classroom level
2. the school level
3. the community level.

1. The classroom level

Examples of the advice offered to teachers to help improve student morale included:

- encouraging more collaborative student work
- revising seating plans to promote discussion
- devising agreed rules for behaviour with an emphasis on respect and responsibility
- displaying student work
- exercising multiple intelligences
- providing varying ways by which a student might experience success
- giving leadership opportunities
- increasing the amount of positive feedback.

2. The school level

Examples of the advice given to school principals to help improve student morale included:

- instituting a more effective transition program from primary school to secondary school which might involve establishing a middle school
- revitalising the induction program of new students
- putting in place an anti-bullying policy
- introducing:
  - peer mediation
  - peer support programs
  - mentoring programs
  - student representative councils
- upgrading staff professional development
- improving supervision.

3. The community level

Examples of the advice given to parents and friends of the school to help improve student morale included:

- increasing parental understanding of the problem and equipping them to deal with student depression through:
  - education programs
  - support groups
- improving communication between parents and schools through bulletins, meetings and e-mail links
- working towards establishing a more friendly school so that the school models care and compassion to the community.

Those schools that have instituted The Gatehouse recommendations have noted measurable improvements not only in student self-esteem but also in such areas as reduction in the number of students smoking.[28]

CONCLUSION

Perhaps the key to helping boys deal appropriately with issues such as drugs and depression is for parents and teachers to remain approachable, compassionate and positive. A heavy judgmental approach or a predilection to shaming a boy in order to get him to change rarely works. However it is as well to remember that compassion is one thing, condoning is another. It may also be worth emphasising that if boys remain in frequent touch with that which is beautiful in the world, then they may be less inclined to seek to escape it and if boys are reminded frequently of their positive virtues, then they may be less inclined to be consumed by their negative qualities.

ADDITIONAL INFORMATION

For those wishing to have further details on some of the points raised in this chapter, the following references may be helpful. Each number in the text of the chapter relates to a reference number below which will give further information related to the topic.

1	Dent, J (2000)	'Drugs and depression: Grim trend for young Australians'	Sydney Morning Herald, 25/1/00, p 2.
2	Dent, J	(op cit)	
3	Scott, T and Grice, T (1997)	The Great Brain Robbery	Allen and Unwin, Sydney, p 14.
4	Scott, T and Grice, T	(op cit)	p 15.
5	Scott, T and Grice, T	(op cit)	p 94.
6	Scott, T and Grice, T	(op cit)	p 05.

7	Carr-Gregg, M (2000)		Address given on adolescent health problems to The Association of Heads of Independent Schools of Australia, Pastoral Care Conference, Westminster School, Adelaide, July 2000.
8	Scott, T and Grice, T	(op cit)	p 37.
9	Carr-Gregg, M	(op cit)	
10	Weisser, H (1996)	'Marijuana and mental illness'	*Quandrant*, June 1996, p 29.
11	Commonwealth Department of Health and Family Services (1997)	*It's time to talk straight about drugs*	p 20.
12	Knox, M (2000)	'Live fast, live young'	*Sydney Morning Herald, Spectrum*, p 1.
13	Carr-Gregg, M (2000)	'Feeling connected'	*EQ Australia*, Spring 2000, p 35.
14	Mullins, A (2000)	*Youth at Risk*	Information leaflet produced by Redfield College, Sydney, from information by Associate Professor Michael Carr-Gregg, the Australian Medical Association, and Martin Seligman's book *The Optimistic Child*.
15	Brent, D A (2000)		This information was recorded by Andrew Mullins, Headmaster of Redfield College, from a lecture given by David A Brent MD, of the University of Pittsburgh, 30 March 2000.
16	Brent, D A	(op cit)	
17	Pollack, W (1998)	*Real Boys*	Owl Books, Henry Holt and Co., New York, p 321.
18	Kindlon, D and Thompson, M (1999)	*Raising Cain*	Penguin Books, London.
19	Spurr, B (2000)	'Boys in trouble'	*Sydney's Child*, August 2000, p 20.
20	Spurr, B (2000)	(op cit)	
21	Kindlon, D and Thompson, M	(op cit)	p 77.
22	Glover, S (2000)	*The Gatehouse Project*	Address given to The Association of Heads of Independent Schools of New South Wales, MacDonald College, 6 November 2000.
23	Brent, D A	(op cit)	
24	Barrett, P (2000)	*Alleviating Anxiety in Younger Children*	Address given to the Association of Heads of Independent Schools of Australia, Pastoral Care Conference, Westminster School, Adelaide, July 2000.
25	Barrett, P	(op cit)	
26	Barrett, P	(op cit)	
27	Carr-Gregg, M	(op cit)	p 35.
28	Glover, S	(op cit)	

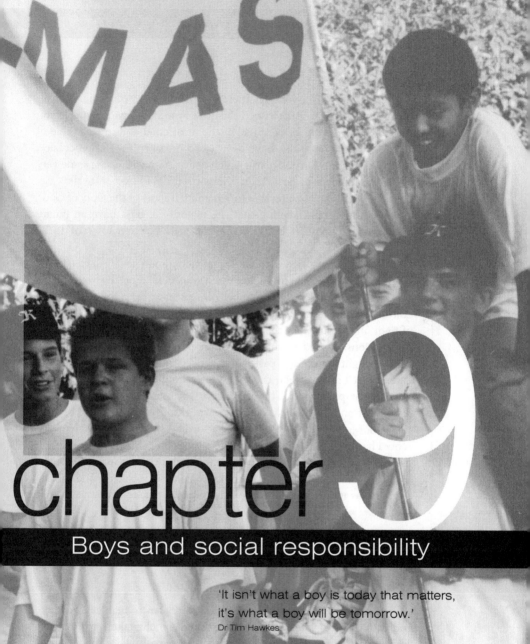

chapter 9

Boys and social responsibility

'It isn't what a boy is today that matters,
it's what a boy will be tomorrow.'
Dr Tim Hawkes

INTRODUCTION

A backward boy is a yob and there are many who would suggest that many boys can best be described this way. Anecdotal evidence is legion that boys can be the perpetrators of the most cruel and irresponsible of acts. Adult conversations have been laced on more than one occasion with the exasperation and alarm which comes from witnessing some very ordinary behaviour by boys. Yet it is important not to over-state the case. Boys are not alone in being able to 'sin and fall short of the glory of God', and it is worth remembering that the majority of boys have an innate sense of what is right and most have a predisposition to want to be responsible.

Although there needs to be some moderation to the accusations levelled at boys, it has to be confessed that defending the young male client is not always easy. A number of boys have been influenced by a culture so characterised by situational ethics and a flexible interpretation of right and wrong, that there is a genuine confusion about behavioural expectations. Added to this is a contemporary youth culture that has been brought up on the pastime of renegotiating punishments to the extent that links between cause and effect and crime and punishment, are now completely lost. This is probably why some boys stare in stunned disbelief if an adult should actually carry through on a threat. Perhaps this is not a boy problem but rather a societal problem. More than one school has been put on trial in the press for taking a stand on issues such as drug abuse, which has led to student expulsions. It is as much for the wonder of an institution to have the courage to set standards and to stick to them, as it is to the severity of the punishment, that engages public interest.

> Train a child in the way he should go and when he is old he will not turn from it.
> Proverbs 22:6

It is a sign of the times that when it is said a boy is 'high calibre' there is confusion as to whether this is a comment on character or fire power. Reviewing the antics of the young is a favourite pastime for those outside this category. This often leads to tuts and mutters about national service, corporal punishment and reminiscences that invariably start with 'When I was a child'. There are other rather more constructive conversations which adults might engage in if they wish to have an influence on developing pro-social skills in boys. One such conversation might profitably put 'the boy problem' in its proper social context.

HONESTY

Let's face it. We are all dishonest, it's just that some are more dishonest than others. We tell tales of the Easter Bunny to explain the eggs, blame Santa for the presents, and the Tooth Fairy is suggested as a major carrier of loose change.

We smile when we want to cry. We say, 'Fine, thank you', when we're not; 'Good to see you', when it isn't.

Some of our models of honesty have disgraced themselves. Politicians have been shown to rort, televangelists to sin, parents to abuse, and our boys and girls in blue have ignited inquiries into police corruption in many of our states.

Lest we grope to remove the speck in our neighbour's eyes when there is a log in our own, it might be as well to remind ourselves that most at some time have fiddled, falsified, fabricated, fibbed, forged, faked or feigned and that's just using the letter 'f'. We could go on . . . Let's try 'd' . . . doctored, distorted, deceived, duped . . . The very existence of thesaurian lists to describe our fallen condition under almost any letter of the alphabet bears testimony to the pervasive nature of dishonesty in our culture.

For example, how many of us have won the 'right to throw the first stone' after considering the following? Who among us has never done one or more of the following:

- fabricated an excuse to avoid an obligation?
- cried crocodile tears over the plight of another?
- borrowed something and never given it back?
- argued a false ruling on a line call?
- taken something which does not belong to us?

Are you the sort of person who would always:

- return money to the police if it were found on the pavement?
- pay the parking fee if it worked on an honesty system?
- ensure your tax return is entirely honest?
- never betray a relationship in order to experience another?

The endemic nature of dishonesty in society threatens to create a new set of laws; laws that are dangerous and not worthy of us. These new laws suggest it is:

- reasonable to be dishonest, as everyone else is
- OK to take someone else's if yours is missing
- fine to lie, providing you're not found out
- not necessary to hand something in if found
- permissible to steal if you are young and going through a difficult stage.

While recognising all of us fall a trifle short of perfection I need to say that we reduce our standards at our peril. We need to fight against the normalisation of dishonesty in our schools and in our society.

▶

We must challenge ourselves to generate, not degenerate; to have the courage to call any form of dishonesty for what it is, rather than seek to accept it. There is little that excuses falsehood and much that condemns it as a practice which is harmful to any society that wishes to call itself civilised.

Therefore, I make no excuse for reminding the school community that any student who steals or uses without asking; or whose verbal testimony is untruthful, threatens to put their place at school at risk. This is because all students must recognise they are members of a community; a vulnerable community; a community which relies upon the honesty and integrity of its members for its well-being and happiness.

Source: Hawkes, T F, Newslink, St Leonard's College, Melbourne, 27 February 1997.

RESPONSIBILITY AND FREEDOM

Many boys are rather impressive and are not totally devoid of morality and purpose, as some would have it believed. It is also worth remembering that the capacity of the young to cause alarm is not a new phenomenon. A casual stroll through Biblical history and/or the social commentaries on ancient Greece and Rome will confirm this.

Curious though it might sound, there is reason to suggest that the growing sense of independence in many youth, together with their increased sense of freedom, might well be creating a number of psycho-social disorders. Without wanting to mandate a repressive right wing reaction, society may need to look rather more closely at the thesis that 'liberty must be limited in order to be possessed'. It is interesting that increased personal freedom has often led to the weakening of a sense of societal responsibility. Society protects its freedom to not work and to go on strike, even if that society is harmed, and society protects its freedom to have guns even if it leads to increased homicide. Drawing lines to limit individual freedom is not popular. Accusations of infringement of individual rights are hurled quickly, and the political mileage thoroughly exploited if one should suggest any curtailment of individual freedom, even if it seems to be in the best interests of society.

In homes and in schools society might need to give boys liberty by limiting their freedom. If a boy wishes the liberty to play and enjoy a musical instrument, many hours of freedom will need to be sacrificed in order to acquire the necessary skills. If a boy wishes to have the liberty of choosing a career, many hours of freedom will have to be given up in order to pass the necessary exams at the appropriate level. If a boy wishes to have the liberty of walking safely in cities, then the freedom of the more anti-social elements of urban society may need to be limited. Parents and educators should not be frightened to advocate the limiting of freedom in certain circumstances, for it is in the limiting of these freedoms that boys can enjoy greater security and achievement.

LAISSEZ-FAIRE DISCIPLINE

Some of the tragedies that have been attributed to boys are probably not due to malignant maleness but to diluted discipline. This has been said of the Columbine School massacre in 1999 where the boys who perpetrated the deed had been allowed to practise anti-social sentiments for some time, presumably in the name of freedom and individual rights. Christina Sommers, in writing on this topic, suggests that many schools have entirely given up on character education and, with this 'laissez-faire' attitude, a great number of children are emerging who are devoid of pro-social skills. Sommers argues that this dereliction of educational duty is like letting children loose in a chemistry laboratory stacked with highly dangerous substances and inviting them to have fun and play.[1] The mortality rate on both building and children is likely to be high, just as the mortality rate on both property and people is unacceptably high because schools are not including character education in the curriculum.

The contemporary age is an age that deplores the concept of accountability. The 'It wasn't my fault . . . I was dropped on my head as a baby' society revels in being able to choose personal standards, but bitterly resents not being able to choose the consequences of those standards. God's gift of free will is exalted, divine judgment is expunged. When asked to excuse the behaviour of a particularly difficult young boy because 'the boy is tired', adults may need to say, 'No, I will not excuse the child's behaviour, but I do now *understand* the child's behaviour'. A brittle response, but perhaps a necessary one, lest the boy begins to realise that bad behaviour is permitted when tired. It is not. Nothing excuses bad behaviour, although explanations can help understand it.

PASSIVITY AND CONTROL

One should mourn the difficult lot given to some boys, but there can also be rejoicing at just how mature and balanced some boys remain despite difficult personal situations. It is important to accept that boys are not passive beings predestined by the vagaries of unknown controls. Most boys have the ability to choose to allow a circumstance to influence their life and no longer allow themselves to drift according to the currents of circumstance. These boys have decided their own direction and, in so doing, determine their own future. Boys need to know they can change the situation. Boys need to know they have the power to determine outcomes. Boys need to be able to hope.

PUNISHMENTS

At times sanctions will need to be applied to boys. Sanctions are best applied in order to:

- ■ deter
- ■ educate
- ■ encourage restitution.

The use of violence as a deterrent should be avoided. Little is gained from demeaning a boy by flogging him physically or verbally. The only eventual outcome is to create violence and anger in the boy and to destroy any relationship that might exist. Boys respond best to sanctions when they know the sanctions are fair and when they know they have transgressed.

Some care is needed as some boys are not above using emotional blackmail to escape a punishment. 'You don't love me anymore' is an accusation commonly levelled by some boys. A boy may need to be shown quite clearly that love is permanent, but what is under discussion are appropriate behaviours which do not appear to be as permanent. Some might call this 'tough love'. Others call it the courage to parent properly.

In relation to traditional battlegrounds such as the amount of TV to be watched, use of the car, bed times and so on, the drawing up of a mutually agreed contract can be useful. It is also useful to draw up mutually agreed sanctions to implement if the contract is broken. Agreements might be reached such as 'I may watch x hours of midweek TV if I can show I can cope with it, that is, maintain sound grades at school, complete homework on time, and fulfil such other responsibilities as are required around the house. Otherwise I may only watch the news and will have to record my favourite programs and watch them on the weekends.'

BEHAVIOUR AND BOREDOM

There is evidence to suggest that the saying 'the devil makes use of idle hands' is true. Boredom in boys cannot be tolerated for long. Boys are bred for action and they will create action, any action, to avoid boredom. This may explain a lot of misbehaviour at school.

One of the most prevalent diseases in schools today is boredom. Dull-eyed students, satiated with wearisome lessons of academia, can be driven to create their own entertainment in a desperate attempt to enliven drab lessons by propelling projectiles, carving on desks and engaging in other subversive behaviours. Incarcerated by law, and instructed by bores, a boy can be forgiven for wondering who took the 'fizz' out of physics — and every other subject for that matter.

Having a dull teacher and suffering dull curriculum is a recipe for behavioural mayhem. 'I'm bored' is a warning statement that some form of misbehaviour is imminent in a boy. Compelling boys into a busy schedule with limited 'time out' is important. Having noted this it is as well to recognise that a boy can be simultaneously busy and bored. Consideration needs to be given to the nature of the task. Busy, repetitive tasks are just as likely to elicit rebellious behaviour. It is a testimony to the dedication and skill of most teachers that inappropriate behaviours are minimalised with most boys. This is no small achievement given the nature of the curriculum that many teachers are required to follow.

THE IMPORTANCE OF EXAMPLE
In the teaching of pro-social skills, little is more effective than positive example, particularly parental example. It is no good giving a sermon to a boy on honesty when earlier in the day that boy watched that parent failing to pay a $2 parking fee which relied on an honour system. Before negative judgments are made, it is as well to look at the behavioural influences in the boy's life. It can be found that parents and teachers may have contributed to the problem through the setting of inappropriate examples or through a lack of clarity or consistency on a matter.

THE PEER INFLUENCE
Before the angry broadside of reprimand is fired in the general direction of an errant boy, consideration may need to be given to a boy's peers. To expect a boy to be able to run counter to a prevailing peer culture is to stake out the moon for a chance glimpse of a jumping cow. The peer influence is immense, and grows in strength significantly during the adolescent years. For this reason one should see boys' behaviour in the peer context. The Australian educators Browne and Fletcher express concern that the treatment of unacceptable behaviour by punishing boys has the effect of making boys responsible for their own behaviours but can sometimes fail to recognise the extraordinary societal and peer pressures that encouraged the infractions.[2] Pathologising a boy is of little use if there is a plague throughout the nation.

Does this mean that parents of adolescents are totally disenfranchised in terms of influencing the behaviour of their sons because their sons are the innocent victims of a national problem? The answer is 'No'. Individuals must recognise that they must still assume ownership of their actions. The awful truth that many boys must learn is that with increasing independence comes increasing accountability. It is also worth acknowledging that the bonds forged in the formative years are such that most parents, irrespective of a boy's growing age, do retain some leverage.

It is still possible for a parent to neutralise some of the less attractive peer values influencing a son, although it must be admitted this is easier when boys are younger.

A little 'social engineering' is possible by parents to ensure that boys are mixing with the 'right' group, and experiencing a culture whose values are such that they are acceptable to the parents. Having noted this, there comes a stage when parental influence is weakened by time and the better tactic might be for parents to resign themselves to accepting their son's peer group rather than risking alienation. Accepting a peer group is one thing, capitulation to their values is another. Parents have every right to expect certain values, attitudes and behaviours to be supported within the family. Yet some sensitivity to the counter values that might emanate from the peer group can be useful. What might also be useful is not turning every contravention of the family rules into a showdown. There is wisdom in choosing the main battles that need winning and in the process being prepared to lose the odd little skirmish.

THE POPULARITY OF GOOD VALUES

Good values are selling well, which is one factor promoting the healthy growth in Christian community and Christian parent-controlled schools in Australia. The Catholic Education Office in Australia found that one of the main reasons parents chose to move their children out of government schools into Catholic schools was the search for better values.[3]

Of course, not everyone can afford private education, and private education cannot always be relied upon to deliver the values expected by parents for their sons. However, the point remains that whether it is through giving support to certain friends, schools, clubs, churches, sports and other recreational activities, most parents to a certain extent can control the cultural 'norms' experienced by their sons. Wisdom comes from choosing the appropriate influence, and even greater wisdom comes from being able to sell these influences to a suspicious and independently minded boy.

Parents and teachers have an obligation to pass on to boys those lessons in history that are helpful to their survival and well-being. Adults can teach that fire can both cremate and create. The trick is to know when to light the match and when to blow it out. In this and other matters, the past can be the tutor. This is worth remembering, for parents can sometimes feel they have little knowledge or experience they can pass on to an adolescent son. The reality is very different and parents should not underestimate the worth of passing on values to their sons. Commonsense is not as common as some might think.

SOCIAL ENGINEERING

Insisting on the demonstration of social responsibility in homes and schools can elicit some emotive reaction. Some might talk of Orwellian values and warn darkly of Nazi social engineering initiatives. Others may argue that in an age of logical positivism, personalism, and pluralism, it is not possible to determine what character should be taught anyway. While wallowing in this moral indecision, boys are being hurt and thus no apology should be made for suggesting that parents and teachers are in the business of social engineering and both should be quite unrepentant about teaching social responsibilities.

Having noted the above, it is well to remember that teaching is one thing, coercion is another. Boys know when they are being coerced and will generally demonstrate this fact by erupting in defiance and anger, or switching off with ears deaf to anything except the call to dinner. Other tactics used by boys include making encouraging noises of agreement before roaring off in total ignorance of what was being said, let alone agreed to.

If coercion is not the preferred approach, then teaching is, and parents and teachers need to be encouraged that the boy is not the toxic force of all evil. There is no question that the curse of testosterone is such that boys have to deal with more aggressive tendencies. It is also true that many boys are trapped in a social convention that requires them to be tough and unfeeling. Yet it should be remembered that the decent young male is still to be found. History books give evidence that the courage and daring of young men has facilitated great achievement.[4] There is nothing to indicate that future books will not be full of similar tales.

When seeking to influence the behaviour of boys, adults may find it effective to:

- Affirm boys in their maleness — 'Being a male is OK'.
- Seek to understand boys before asking boys to understand them.
- Find where boys are at and use where they are at as a base from which to connect and to teach. Common interests, such as sport, and humour can help.
- Hate the sin not the sinner. Leave boys with a sense that there is in them something which is good, something which can give hope.
- Win boys' respect through fairness and consistency.
- Avoid over-familiarity but be approachable.
- Demonstrate a care for boys, not just with words but through action.
- Model the behaviour wanted in boys.
- Seek excuses to praise and encourage.[5]

When a boy does something wrong, he is likely to suffer some fairly blunt expressions of disapproval and advice on the need to change his ways. Many of these arguments will not work because they fail to connect with the boy's understanding of why he should change. The retort 'Why?' is sometimes used as a statement of rebellion, but it can also signal that the reasons for changing a behaviour are not clearly understood by a boy. Teachers and parents might profit from clearly stating the reasons for change, for this can often appeal to the logic in some boys. Examples of the sort of reasons which can sometimes appeal include:

- If you do this, it will help you to get what you want.
- If you do this, it will make you more successful in this area.
- This is what people are looking for in you.
- Doing this will stop you hurting yourself and your friends.

Other responses that can help might include:

- This will take courage but I think you can do it.
- How would you advise your son on this matter?
- How do you think you will feel about this later?

CHARACTER TRAINING

A few schools have reported success with schemes that seek to reward boys for being good. The character education movement has introduced a number of initiatives designed to reward students who are being good. This philosophy is anchored in a behaviourist approach to teaching and is characterised by the frequent use of sticks and carrots.

The great danger of this sort of approach is that a boy can learn that the value of being good is to get rewards, rather than the value of being good being of some intrinsic value in its own right. For this reason, strategies which help boys to internalise pro-social attitudes should be preferred. The occasional reward should not be discounted, providing the reward is not given frequently enough to be relied upon. Not all rewards need be tangible, a word of encouragement or a reassuring gesture may be all the reinforcement necessary.

Teaching social responsibility to boys involves character training. Lickona, in his book *The Return of Character Education*, suggests that character development involves knowing and understanding. This means boys need to:

- be aware of the moral dimensions of a situation
- know moral values
- see things from differing perspectives
- be able to engage in moral reasoning and thoughtful decision making
- have moral self-knowledge.

The second stage is to encourage boys to desire socially responsible behaviour. Boys need to commit to certain values and this generally requires the use of boys' emotions and conscience.

The final stage is the translation of this motivation into moral action, which involves boys acquiring certain competencies such as the ability to listen, communication skills, and willingness to cooperate. Boys need to be given opportunities to mobilise their judgment and develop an inner disposition which sees them responding to situations in a morally good way.

Lickona summarises these three stages as:

1. knowing the good
2. desiring the good
3. doing the good.[6]

USING THE SCHOOL TO HELP BOYS KNOW THE GOOD

Schools may be getting it wrong. When dealing with the matter of morality, some experts are saying that teachers should adopt a 'decision making, moral reasoning, values clarification' approach. The more traditional style of character education, of telling boys what is expected of them, is no longer acceptable because it is judged as being too indoctrinative. Classrooms have been transformed into bull sessions where opinions are shared and teachers transformed into Jerry Springers and Oprah Winfreys, as issues are discussed and non-judgmental therapy is practised. Much of this is commendable, but there is a need to augment the exchanging of opinions and the exploring of feelings with the actual provision of moral guidance, and help with the forming of character.

The modern style is to give information, lots of it, with quite adult data being shared with boys at ever younger ages. However, there is not so much a problem with society being uninformed, but rather with society being immoral.

There is also a danger of desensitisation when discussing matters in a values neutral manner. It is important not to lose the capacity for moral outrage. Even more worrying are clear indications that the very raising of issues with boys can lead to an upsurge in the activity that is being discouraged. This has certainly been shown to be true with some courses in sex education, drug abuse and suicide.

The shopping trolley approach to values acquisition by boys in some schools which sees them picking up the chocolates and sweets and walking smartly by the vegetable stands may need to be questioned. There is a real danger that boys can be encouraged to make judgments with inadequate knowledge of what is appropriate to fostering healthy growth. A valueless syllabus is displayed with sales labels boasting tolerance and children's rights. What society is really saying is that it is lost and unable to affirm that some beliefs are wrong and some are right. Boys need clear guidance in their initial forays into the supermarket of life, at least until they are able to understand the nature of the merchandise on display.

It is not always easy for a school to set standards, particularly as teachers try to thread their way through the minefield of rampant litigation and political correctness. However, schools should proclaim their values on a number of issues in order to give moral direction to the school. The exercise of working through what these values should be can be stimulating and affirming, as well as useful in giving teachers security and direction when seeking to impart these same values to boys.

To teach social responsibility in schools will require the support of students. The school that can attract the allegiance of its boys to its values by methods that are acceptable to the boys, will win for itself the enviable title of 'community'. This accolade is not easily given, particularly in places populated by boys. In a study of over 8000 students in England in Years 5 and 10, Ainsley found that girls valued relationships, community mindedness and obedience to rules and societal conventions more than boys.[7]

The challenge to test conventional boundaries does appear to be stronger in boys. Perhaps it is because boys are less willing to accept constraints and guidelines without first testing them. Once tested, the social conventions are often accepted by boys, but they may not be accepted if they remain unconvinced of either the resolution of society to maintain a standard or the logic of supporting a standard. In short, the fences will be tested, especially by the young bulls.

Parents and teachers can play an important role in helping boys to accept the presence of fences in their life. Schools are a key influence in the guiding of boys towards appropriate behaviours and attitudes. This sounds an obvious statement but the tragedy is that there are some within the educational world who limit their role to imparting knowledge, and who never seek to touch the soul of a boy or to influence his character. The charter of educators is such that it extends beyond the preparation of a boy for an exam. The charter for educators is to prepare boys for life.

School administrators might also need to be reminded that when a teacher becomes disillusioned or burnt out, the most vulnerable aspect of his or her role that can be neglected is the influencing of students' characters. The wounded teacher may retreat to a minimalist expression of the job, which will be interpreted as the dissemination of facts. Helping children with their character can be hugely demanding and can exact an emotional toll which a teacher is not always able to give. For this reason school executives must invest in members of their common rooms to the extent that morale and confidence is such that teachers have the emotional capital necessary to spend on their students.

USING THE FAMILY TO HELP BOYS KNOW THE GOOD

The teaching in schools of social responsibility is best done in conjunction with the home. If there is no accord between the values at home and the values at school, confusion will result. For schools it means that they might have to remove the demilitarised zone at the front gate and invite parents and friends into the school. For parents it means they should, if at all possible, choose a school that is congenial to the values supported in the home. As much communication as possible should occur between the home and the school, for the task of education is best done in partnership. For this reason joint learning adventures might be considered, such as shared student-parent research tasks. Parents cannot only be enlisted and trained to help support a school's maths or English program, they can be enlisted and trained to support the school's social values.

Given the crucial role of the family, there should be concern at parents only spending a few minutes each week in serious discussion with their children.

Then there are the 'Tomagochi children'. These are the sons and daughters born to teenagers who wanted something to play with; who wanted to prove their capacity to procreate. Often born out of lust rather than love, the children of teen parents can, like the electronic Tomagochi babies that were once a craze, have parents who get bored and frustrated with their responsibilities to keep the baby alive and pass that responsibility to others. Unfortunately the Tomagochi children learn that they are not wanted, and the anger and hurt of this realisation can lead to bitterness and anti-social behaviours. These behaviours and attitudes are then passed on to the next generation and they in turn pass them on to their children.

Research has indicated that boys, in particular, have suffered from a lack of parental input from fathers. Steve Biddulph argues that the Industrial Revolution meant that for the first time in history fathers worked away from their sons, and this led to generations of boys growing up without being fathered. The post-industrial society has not seen much of a change in this situation for the busyness of life, together with its growing complexity and materialism, still produces generations of under-fathered boys.[8]

There is no absolute consensus as to the characteristics of the type of adult who is more likely to develop socially responsible children. Even within the same family there can be siblings who were nurtured in much the same way who turn out very differently from each other. One child can be the sort of boy every mother hopes her daughter will marry, while the other can be causing the fathers of those same daughters to invest in double-barrelled shotguns. Nonetheless, there is evidence to suggest that the following characteristics in parents can increase the likelihood of a boy being more socially responsible:

■ The parents who consciously and unconsciously model socially responsible behaviour.

■ The parents who have a genuine concern for the welfare of their son, a concern expressed both in words and actions which leaves the boy in no doubt that his well-being is important to them.

■ The parents who provide security for their son, a security which is physical, emotional and social. This security needs to be provided directly such as protecting the boy from hunger and hurt, and provided indirectly such as a husband loving his wife so that she has the emotional energy to spend looking after the needs of the son.

■ The parents who are not weak in the upholding of values and standards and who have firm views as to what constitutes appropriate behaviour. This should not be interpreted as constant nagging or endless criticism of a boy, and neither should it be interpreted as promoting a restrictive, authoritarian regime within a home. It can be interpreted as parents who have thought through what they stand for and who value these standards enough to want them supported by their children.

■ The parents who can explain their views, who are able to articulate a reasoned argument to support a pro-social attitude can be more effective in passing these standards onto a boy. 'Because we told you so' does not constitute a good example of this practice.

■ The parents who create a stimulating environment that prevents a boy being bored.

■ The parents who encourage a gradual move from an extrinsic motivation for a boy to abide by a code of behaviours to an intrinsic motivation. The development of an 'ownership' of one's own standards is necessary for any boy who wishes to be considered mature.

Divorce and emotional trauma

One hesitates to comment on the effect of divorce on the effectiveness of being able to transmit appropriate values and behaviours to children. The prevalence of divorce is such that it is only the politically naive who venture into these dangerous waters. Having noted this, to fail to recognise that family break-up can lead to grief, anger, disorientation and anti-social behaviour in children, is irresponsible. Also irresponsible is the thought that divorce must necessarily result in sociopathic children.

Some children are better off with their parents apart than together, and many single parents do a wonderful job in parenting their children. A number of parents with their marriages intact are doing an awful job with parenting. After noting these and other caveats, it must also be said that some children, after experiencing the trauma of a family break-up, become disturbed, rebellious and express this anger in anti-social behaviours.

Family disharmony can drive a boy away from the family to the safer and more reliable world of his peers. It is here that some boys, who have been bruised emotionally and physically, will feel accepted and safe in a way that may not always be evident in their home. If this group that they retreat to is an anti-establishment group, then so much the better, for the establishment into which they were born is one that has harmed them too much for them to want to care for it. So they will damage it, colour it in with spray cans, and defy the rules set by that establishment.

The collateral damage in terms of emotional trauma experienced by children when families become dysfunctional must be admitted by society. This is not to pile guilt on the parents, many of whom may be innocents themselves. It is to awaken authorities to the reality of a very real problem which must be admitted, and which must be addressed. Children from broken and dysfunctional homes will sometimes need extra help, extra care and extra assurances of love and self-worth. If these messages are not sent to such children frequently enough, then they may express their hurt by damaging the society that has hurt them.

USING THE MEDIA TO HELP BOYS KNOW THE GOOD

Increasingly it is the media and particularly TV which is defining the social mores of today. The media can propel children into adult life in a way that deprives them of their childhood. As boys' senses become numbed, so the strength of the 'fix' of violence, sex and horror must be increased by the traffickers of shock, and boys in particular like a good shock.

Given that many boys spend more time with the TV than with their fathers, the model of masculinity promoted by the media needs to be critically reviewed. Such a review may well suggest that all too often the male role model is portrayed as having the mental wit of Homer Simpson, the verbal wit of Sylvester Stallone and the social wit of Kramer. All too often the male portrayed in the media is the inadequate male. This may add much to the humour but it adds little to a boy's understanding of maleness.

To be fair, some researchers are not worried by the influence of TV on children and make the point that it is not TV which is the problem but rather the lack of parental supervision of what is watched and how it is watched. In the same vein, the catatonic couch potato sitting passively in front of the TV is not always a fair description of the TV viewer. Some research has shown that TV watching can stimulate a child's imagination.[9]

Perhaps one of the most important points to make on the issue of TV and values is that the influence TV has in teaching a boy about masculinity, values and behaviours will depend on whether there is a congruency with what is seen on TV and what is witnessed in the home. A supportive home with a good culture of behaviour and fine role models will enable a boy to see that some of the role models viewed on TV are untrue and can safely be despatched to the realm of fantasy. Where the home fails to provide that positive modelling then the TV is promoted to the role of teacher and this can be high-risk mentoring.

Music also may need to be monitored. There is music that is inspirational, enjoyable and uplifting. There is music that is destructive and violent; music which advocates the immediate gratification of desires without responsibilities; music that takes adolescent frustration and heats it to irresponsible levels. Some heavy metal bands have described their sound as 'music to kill your parents by'. There are CD covers which depict sexual mutilation, and song lyrics that are destructive and demeaning.

There may be a need to monitor both music and TV and not allow boys to become passive receptors turned on by black wires dribbling from their ears and 24-inch screens in the corner of living rooms. Perhaps one of the main challenges of parents and educators is to help train boys to be selective and critical, to analyse the media and be active rather than passive viewers and listeners, otherwise the media will enslave their minds and, as Aristotle warns, 'the worst thing about slavery is that the slaves eventually get to like it'.

Boys and 'media disability'

'Media disability' was a term coined by Dr Alan Storkey, a lecturer at the Oak Hill Church of England Theological College.[10] It refers to an impairment of emotional, social and intellectual functioning brought about by children having inappropriate exposure to the media. British children spend 45 minutes a day on average playing computer games and Britons are spending over one-fifth of their waking lives watching TV.[11]

The brain is unable to cope with this constant amount of short sequence stimuli so it goes into 'time out' mode. Continual sensory bombardment cannot be mentally digested so the viewer lets it all wash over him in an addictive daze. If the viewer should be stirred from his viewing reverie and asked what is being watched, the response 'nothing much' is probably accurate.[12] Unfortunately, the brain can be conditioned to working in this manner so that even with the TV off, a boy will let life 'wash over him' so that events happen that fail to elicit intelligent analysis and things occur which leave a boy emotionally numb. Because he has been so stupified with stimuli, he now finds it quite difficult to get excited by anything.

The very act of putting on the TV can be very much a 'stop the world, I want to get off' initiative. The TV provides an escape, a diversion from the pressures and responsibilities of real life. Unfortunately, the escapism, whether it be by drugs or the media, can become addictive. A boy can find it increasingly difficult to distinguish between reality and virtual reality; between truth and fiction. Social skills may atrophy, with talking, reading, writing and playing becoming at risk of drying out through a lack of use. Intellectual skills may also wither, such as the ability to concentrate, and even the ability to think.

The greatest users of video games are boys aged eight to 15 years of age. A boy's brain at this age is still developing and requires the engagement in tasks that exercise problem solving, analysis and creativity.[13] The development of these skills may be hindered not so much by physical passivity associated with TV, although this does not help, but by the over-stimulation of the brain to the extent that its mental functioning in areas such as synthesis and evaluation becomes impaired.

Some positive steps that can be taken by parents in relation to controlling TV and video game use by boys:

- remove the TV from the boy's bedroom[14]
- restrict video game use to one hour a day and to four hours over the weekend
- do not allow the watching of TV before school
- switch the TV off during meal times and turn this time into a talking time rather than a watching time
- try to encourage critical, evaluative comments by the family when viewing TV
- be guided by the government viewing codes and do not be bullied by sons to ignore them
- install 'V' chips and such other technology that is necessary to block out unsuitable viewing material
- monitor Internet use and be particularly careful of 'chat lines'.

As can be seen from the above, most of the recommendations are negative and this is likely to cause some angst among boys who have been used to unfettered freedom in this area. Restricting and controlling use is likely to fail unless it is replaced with something else. For this reason, parents must choreograph other activities for their sons to engage in. 'I don't know, go and read a book or something' is not a response which is going to work more than a few times. Story telling, discussions, hobbies, sport, all need to be used to fill the time and entertainment vacuum of limiting TV use.

USING EMOTIONS TO HELP BOYS DESIRE THE GOOD

The apple core in the Garden of Eden reminds society that knowing the good is not enough. One must also desire the good. In this microchip society when people can 'surf the net' to find the mean summer temperature in Wulumuchi in Western Mongolia, knowing things is not a problem. In the same way, knowing what is good is not the problem. This information is readily available to boys in countless different ways. However, the translation of knowing what is right to wanting to do what is right is somewhat more problematic. St Paul acknowledged this even before the advent of the World Wide Web.

> The good that I want to do I don't . . . the
> evil that I don't want to do that is what I do.
> Romans 7:19

One powerful tool available for use by parents and teachers in helping to motivate boys to engage in socially responsible behaviours is the use of boys' emotions. It is strange that teachers can become so hesitant about engaging students' emotions and so abstract when looking at ethical issues. In giving an example, Kilpatrick argues that rather than engaging in a non-judgmental debate over the 'lifeboat exercise' whereby students have to decide which passenger needs to be thrown out of an overcrowded lifeboat, they would be far more challenged if they saw the film A Night to Remember which details the sinking of the Titanic in 1912.[15] This profoundly moving film recounts acts of heroism, cowardice, stupidity, and bravery. Kilpatrick argues that the film doesn't leave the viewer much room for ethical manoeuvring. It is a definitive rather than an open-ended experience and it has something to teach, something to inspire. The more recent interpretation of the same event as described in the film Titanic could serve a similar purpose.

The engagement with a boy's emotions can also be helped through such initiatives as visiting an aged people's home, shadowing a social worker or helping at a soup kitchen. A greater empathy for those with disabilities might also be elicited if a boy were to be blindfolded for a few hours or required to spend a day in a wheelchair. Visits by people working in the developing countries and participation in The 40 Hour Famine are the types of activities that may be successful in encouraging other person centredness.[16]

The capacity for a boy to put himself in 'another person's shoes' is not always as strong as it might be. Some boys can be enormously compassionate, particularly towards their friends. Others can display indifference and a hardness of heart which is positively frightening. Exercises can be engaged in to erode this lack of compassion such as asking a boy to be a 'mentor' for a junior boy, and getting boys to engage in Socratic debate whereby a point of view is argued, then the opposite point of view is presented with participants swapping roles. Taking up local issues in the press and lobbying on behalf of citizens for a change in facility or policy can also help.

Desiring the good can also be influenced by story telling and heroic role modelling. This might mean that students have an opportunity to focus their attention on people other than self-absorbed sports' stars and angry musicians, and look at those of the quality of Gandhi, Martin Luther King, Fidel Castro, Nelson Mandela and Winston Churchill. It is very difficult to study much of Dickens' work without being challenged by the social issues depicted in his writing. A school's choice of literature becomes important. It is worrying that traditional family values seem to be unsupported by so much contemporary children's literature, with some children's books tending to feature characters who are self-obsessed, contemptuous of authority, narcissistic and morally bankrupt.[17]

ENCOURAGING BOYS TO DO THE GOOD

Knowing what is socially responsible and wanting to be socially responsible is but the prelude to the performance. Parents and teachers may need to choreograph opportunities for boys to demonstrate their pro-social skills. As many boys as possible should be invited to audition for the heroic role. It may be that not all can be accommodated in every act, but there is also reward in being able to watch.

Boys identify with heroes and boys identify with boys. If one combines the two and casts boys as heroes, then teachers can have a compelling influence on a youthful audience. Extravagant productions of social responsibility can become a feature of schools. It might be just acting, but it is significant that actors often find themselves taking on the qualities of their character after the play has finished. A schizoid state appears whereby the character is still played when the greasepaint is removed. The ancient Greeks knew this, which is why their ideals of prudence, justice, temperance, and fortitude were frequently celebrated through acting. The internalising and mimicking of virtues occurring 'front-of-house' can seep through to 'backstage'. It is, therefore, not surprising that Aristotle should claim:

> People become virtuous by performing virtuous acts, they become kind by doing kind acts, they become brave by doing brave acts.

A story exists of unknown origin which tells of a particularly precocious starlet who complained that she did not feel like acting a love scene. She was told rather tartly by the producer to 'fake it'. When boys do not feel like they want to be socially responsible, they too can be told to 'fake it' and thus be compelled, as Alexander Pope put it, to:

> Act well your part: there all honour lies.

Those students who study around the world for the award of an International Baccalaureate Diploma are compelled to engage in a range of social service activities which must be diarised by students and verified by staff. Through involvement in these activities, the students begin to realise the joy there is in giving as well as receiving. Perhaps boys not involved in studying for the International Baccalaureate Diploma might also benefit from being compelled into social service activities.

There is nothing quite like the prospect of a critical review in the press to keep a director and cast well focused; so it is with boys. This is why teachers could profit from adding to their school reports a few more 'subjects' to be assessed, such as, the ancient Greek virtues of:

- prudence
- justice
- temperance
- fortitude

or perhaps the Christian virtues of:

- faith
- hope
- charity.

A more contemporary interpretation might be:

- respect for people:
  - self
  - others

- respect for property:
  - own
  - others
- self-discipline
- empathy
- kindness
- fairness
- honesty
- courage.

The reporting on these topics demonstrates that a school is serious about wanting to promote these skills. The current practice of making these qualities a non-assessed subject may promote the marginalisation of these characteristics in boys.

Part of the compelling into experience might involve giving boys responsibility, for it is only the exercise of these skills that will provide the necessary strength to be responsible in later life. Herein lies the tension. Teachers and parents may want a boy to do something but recognise that the boy may not do it if he is involved in the decision making process. The two are not necessarily irreconcilable. Boys can be given some choice but it might be a restricted choice. The range of options from which to choose can be reduced, the parameters of the choice can be given and the teacher might in some circumstances even be a party to the negotiations.[18]

WHY BOYS DO NOT SEEK LEADERSHIP ROLES IN SCHOOL

It is not necessarily true that boys do not accept leadership roles in school. In many ways, a boy will show leadership and give service to others, particularly his friends for whom he can show great care and concern.

Schools often confuse leadership with 'doing duties' and the duties are usually menial administrative tasks on behalf of the school. Many boys are not interested in rendering such service for they have an ambivalent attitude towards schools. Girls are more biddable in this regard and thus they fill most of the official student leadership positions in school. This does not mean boys are into being leaders, they are merely choosing to exercise their leadership skills in other ways.

AN EXAMPLE OF SOME PRO-SOCIAL PROGRAMS

Australian schools have developed a number of social responsibility schemes. Some time ago an attempt was made to collate some of these best practices by the Australian Guidance and Counselling Association Ltd. The project had its genesis in the report *Sticks and Stones: Report on*

Violence in Australian Schools produced by the House of Representatives Standing Committee on Education, Employment, and Training in 1995.

An example of one particular program was the Hokus Pokus Peer Counselling program run at Mentone Girls' Grammar School in Melbourne whereby students gave social support to their peers after having being trained in basic counselling, mediation, and communication skills. The same principles can be used in a school with boys. The Hokus Pokus program had three strains: a junior school Hokus Pokus which was a lunchtime activity for children who were boarders or who lived away from home. The program was conducted by senior students who were also living away from home, with the result that there was a great deal of sympathy and understanding for the student being helped. The second strain was the Hokus Pokus 'drop in centre'. This was aimed at students from Years 6–10 and was run at lunchtime by Year 11 Hokus Pokus helpers. A variety of activities occurred including games, discussion groups and fundraising. The third strain was the Hokus Pokus Peer Counselling Training program which was specifically designed to help meet the counselling needs of students by providing 35 trained Year 11 counsellors.

The USA has also witnessed the development of many social programs, including the emergence of abstinence-based projects. Although not all would support these programs, initial feedback has been encouraging. The American Institute for Character Education found there was a 77% decline in discipline problems, a 64% decrease in vandalism, and a 68% increase in school attendance after schools in the USA had used their pro-social skills program.

The North Clackamas School District in Oregon devised a four-year program cycle whereby certain pro-social themes were targeted each year. The North Clackamas Social Responsibility Program included:

- **Year 1** — patriotism, integrity, honesty and courtesy.
- **Year 2** — authority, respect for others and property, environment and self-esteem.
- **Year 3** — compassion and self-discipline, responsibility, work ethic, appreciation for education.
- **Year 4** — patience, courage, cooperation.[19]

HABITUATION AND RITUALISATION

In their book *Reclaiming Our Schools*, Edward Wynne and Kevin Ryan argue for 'habituation' whereby planned activities are put into the school curriculum which require students to practise good habits.[20] Sanctions are seen as necessary to back up these behaviours.

Ritualisation is also advocated for it is closely linked to habituation. Pro-social behaviours can benefit from becoming ritualised in schools. Rituals can be such activities as peer support programs; cross-age tutoring; the appointment of class/form captains; the appointment of monitors, prefects and senators; the establishment of year level committees and student representative councils; induction programs for new students together with 'buddy' systems; assemblies; chapels; community days; school songs, banners and mottos; student maintenance duties such as sweeping the classrooms, emptying the bins, tending a patch of garden; cross-age coaching in sport; the running of clubs and societies; involvement in social service activities; and publication of a student magazine.

Profound learning

There is a danger with 'gee whizz' social projects that being responsible is equated with episodic rather than permanent behaviours. Parents and teachers do not want a boy participating in Clean Up Australia Day when the other 364 days of the year see the boy's bedroom as a microcosm of the municipal garbage tip. Pro-social behaviours may need to be generalised and a culture of social responsibility may need to be nurtured. This can be assisted by what Wynne and Ryan describe as 'profound learning'.[21] This is learning which occurs through there being congruency between the school's human and material resources, a congruency between the school's curriculum and pedagogy, and a congruency between the values of the home and school, all of which are aimed at reinforcing socially responsible behaviour. Profound learning requires constant reinforcement in rituals, symbols, song, and motto. It requires codes of behaviour and an application to learning. Profound learning is the saturation of a boy in values that are constantly reinforced.

CONCLUSION

Teaching social responsibility is a high calling and one which will involve adults in helping boys to know the good, desire the good, and do the good. Boys need to know that they can make a positive contribution to society other than saving it from digital monsters on visual display units. Adults also need to know that they can make a positive contribution to society by replicating their values in children. This is a huge responsibility, but if it represents one of the greatest challenges, it also represents one of the greatest privileges.

There needs to be an optimism in this process of teaching pro-social skills which recognises the good in a boy. There needs to be compassion in this process which recognises the difficulties in the journey to manhood. The adolescent life is a preparatory life. There can be a frustration in having to wait which can lead to behavioural problems. Stevens writes:

> The tasks we all face as adolescents are formidable indeed: if one is to leave home, support oneself in the world, attract (and keep) a sexual partner and eventually start a family of one's own, then the bonds to the parents must be loosened, a job prepared for and found, sexual development completed, an appropriate persona acquired and enough confidence and self-esteem achieved to be able to hold one's head up in society.[22]

It is unlikely that these tasks are going to be completed without a few errors in judgment. For this reason some understanding is needed. The hair on the adolescent chin and the uncomfortable knack of many boys to grow to a height that blocks out the sun can invite a heavy judgmental hand. Not all boys are uninsurable monsters devoid of social responsibility. Some boys need special help, most boys are fine, all boys are products of a society that has not always been as faithful as it might have been in the nurture of its sons.

ADDITIONAL INFORMATION

For those wishing to have further details on some of the points raised in this chapter, the following references may be helpful. Each number in the text of the chapter relates to a reference number below which will give further information related to the topic.

1	Sommers, C H (2000)	*The War Against Boys*	Simon and Schuster, New York, p 200.
2	Browne, R and Fletcher, R (1995)	*Boys in Schools*	Finch Publishing, Sydney, p 179.
3	Fray, P (1995)	'In the schoolyards of good and evil'	*Sydney Morning Herald*, 16/6/95.
4	Browne, R and Fletcher, R	(op cit)	p 183.
5	Kohn, A (1998)	*What to Look for in a Classroom*	Jossey-Bass Publishers, San Francisco, p 19.
6	Lickona, T (1996)	'The return of character education'	*Educational Leadership*, November 1996.
7	Ainsley, J (2000)	'Some social objectives of schooling'	Paper presented to the National Council of Independent Schools' Association, Barossa Valley, 14–16 July.

8	Biddulph, S (1994)	*Manhood*	Finch Publishing, Sydney.
9	Kohn, A	(op cit)	p 184.
10	Carey, A (date unknown)	'Our children are addicted to the media'	*The Church of England Newspaper.*
11	Carey, A	(op cit)	
12	Gurian, M (1998)	*A Fine Young Man*	Jeremy P Tarcher/Putman, New York, p 220.
13	Gurian, M	(op cit)	p 222.
14	Gurian, M	(op cit)	p 223.
15	Kilpatrick, W (1992)	*Why Johnny Can't Tell Right From Wrong*	A Touchstone Book, Simon and Schuster, New York.
16	Lemin, M, Potts, H and Westford, P (1984)	*Values: Strategies for Classroom Teachers*	Australian College of Educational Research (ACER), Melbourne, The Council for Christian Education in Schools.
17	Kilpatrick, W	(op cit)	p 108.
18	Kohn, A	(op cit)	p 264.
19	Kilpatrick, W	(op cit)	p 238.
20	Wynne, E and Ryan, K (1992)	*Reclaiming Our Schools*	Merrill Books, Columbus, Ohio.
21	Wynne, E and Ryan, K	(op cit)	
22	Stevens, A (1990)	*On Jung*	Penguin, London, p 117.

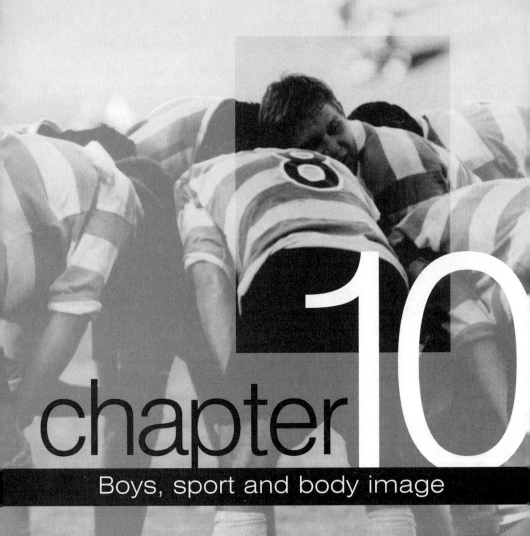

chapter 10

Boys, sport and body image

INTRODUCTION

George Orwell suggested that serious sport had nothing to do with fair play:

> It is bound up with hatred, jealousy, boastfulness, disregard of all rules and sadistic pleasure in witnessing violence; in other words it is war minus the shooting.[1]

It seems that less serious sport can be described otherwise. Stephen Pile, in his book *The Return of Heroic Failures*, tells the delightful tale of the Friendsville Academy Foxes Basketball Team who recorded 128 successive defeats between 1967 and 1973. Examining why this impressive record had come about, it was found the coach had abandoned pep talks as they were apt to make the players nervous. The coach also defended the awarding of MVP (most valuable player) to Phil Patterson, who had not scored a single point, by the response 'You don't think scoring is every-thing do you?' Prominent in the Friendsville gymnasium were signs such as 'character, not victory, is the important thing'. This might have gone some way to explaining their closest score line (2–0) which was achieved by a Friendsville player putting the ball through his own hoop.[2]

THE POSITIVES OF SPORT

Sport can have an extraordinary influence on a boy. Some boys can be addicted to sport and will carry their club's colours as its most faithful disciples. Boys will seek to emulate their sporting heroes in backyard games of cricket and kick-to-kick competitions in parks across the land. These acolytes will watch, will copy and will mimic their sporting icons. This is fine when that which they watch, copy and mimic embraces such behaviours as John Landy stopping to pick up Ron Clarke when he fell in the Australian mile championship in Melbourne in 1956 before going on to win the race in 4 minutes, 4.2 seconds. This is not fine when boys are exposed to cheating, gamesmanship and a 'win at all costs' approach to sport that seems to typify much of the contemporary sporting scene.

Whether playing serious or less serious sport, boys can be captivated by it to the extent they will still want to play despite losing 128 games in a row. However, in the playing of sport there is both risk and reward. The rewards can be:

- physical
- social
- emotional
- academic
- moral/spiritual.

Physical rewards

Sport can improve the cardiovascular system and the efficiency of the human physical frame so that it might allow its owners to do a greater variety of tasks. Healthy pulmonary functions can reduce tiredness and improve the capacity to operate and move effectively. Improved circulation, good muscle definition, resistance to disease and increased vigour can result from the engagement in a responsible level of sport. Through sport, the mind is given a healthier and more efficient body to perform the tasks required of it. The body is described in the Bible as the 'temple of the Holy Spirit' to be honoured and cared for — a directive which can be fulfilled, at least in part, through sport.

Social rewards

Sport can cause a boy to mix with others; to be part of a team; to enlarge his circle of friends and acquaintances. With the growing tendency to recreate in isolation; to engage in virtual sport on visual display screens; the breakdown in connectedness in society has been accelerated. Sport can slow down this fractionating of society and promote interaction with others.

This interaction can occur at many different levels. At the micro level it can be a game of ping-pong with the boy next door. At the meso level it can be playing in or watching a regional football team. At the macro level it can be the celebration of sporting excellence by applauding one's country's effort in the Olympic Games or winning the World Soccer Championship. The pride and pleasure in such an achievement can be incalculable in terms of improved morale and goodwill.

Playing sport gives boys the experience to operate within the rules; to recognise and live within the boundaries of proper and fair play. For some boys who find the very existence of any rule in their life a challenge to remove, the playing of sport within the rules can be an important discipline.

A sport might also bring within the orbit of a boy's life important role models. Not all people accede to the dictum that they are paid to be athletes not role models, and thus their lives can be a real example to a boy.

Emotional rewards

Sport is one of the very few areas within a boy's life wherein he may express emotion; where he might cheer, cry and scream with excitement without arousing the ire and condemnation of others. The rigid male code which prevents the overt display of emotion is relaxed and team mates can hug or put an arm over another's shoulder. Emotional sterility can be rescued in a boy through his involvement with sport. A boy might enjoy a level of intimacy with his team mates which is not otherwise allowed. The uninhibited way in which feelings can be shared with team mates can encourage a connection with others which is not generally permitted in boys.

As one of Howard Gardner's 'multiple intelligences', physical ability provides a boy with an alternative area to succeed in. Not everyone can be gifted academically or in music. Sport can provide another way by which a boy might do well; might succeed; might rescue what might otherwise be very low self-esteem.

At a time when fathers often find they have very little time to interact with their sons, a common enjoyment of sport expressed in rumbles, touch footy games in the driveway, or even watching the cricket together on TV, can help create a bond that might not otherwise exist. The shared interest, the coaching and skill development, the time spent in each other's company can be important, particularly to the young boy who is beginning to move away from his mother in order to discover his male identity.

Academic rewards

A brain tends to function well when the body functions well and thus a healthy body that has been kept fit through engagement in sport is able to assist the brain to function more effectively. The slothful mind can become energised and be more creative if non-excessive amounts of exercise are undertaken. The 'lounge lizard' may become prone to somnolence not just in the lounge but everywhere, including the classroom. The brisk walk to clear the brain bears testimony to the power of exercise in advancing academic performance.

Moral/spiritual rewards

Sport can provide an arena for the battle of good and evil. Participants exercise choice in deciding whether to operate within the rules or not. In this, sport can be a positive and a negative experience. A boy may be taught to be morally moribund and to ignore the rules. On the other hand, with the proper coach, a boy may, perhaps for the first time in his life, be encouraged to obey laws if only because he wants to continue to play sport.

SPORT AND TESTOSTERONE

Engagement in sport can teach a boy something about team work, courage and the ability to moderate an aggressive spirit to acceptable levels. Moir and Jessel remind their readers that testosterone levels in boys soar to 20 times the level in girls. This anabolic steroid helps to beef up the body and assists the body to repair and grow, through the capacity of testosterone to facilitate the storage of phosphorous, calcium and other elements in the body.

The testosterone levels can be influenced by a boy's involvement in sport. Moir and Jessel write:

> Testosterone can be burned off during vigorous physical exercise like combat training ... hence the traditional advice from the school-master to Jones Minor that he should go for a long run to purge himself of profane thoughts ... is well founded in biophysical fact. But a word of caution; the exercise should be specified, because the expenditure of energy in short bursts actually increases the testos-terone level — just as participating in the brief energy bursts of an ice-hockey game increases aggression at the end of the match. Jones Minor should not practise his 100 metre sprints. He needs a long run ... a very long one.[3]

THE NEGATIVES OF SPORT

> If W G Grace were alive today, he would turn in his grave.
> Anonymous

Sport is also able to subvert the morals of a community through the generation of passions which are expressed in unadulterated violence and ethical amnesia. Some boys are being told by their coaches not just to get into the opposition's face, but to crawl down their throats and rip their hearts out. Some boys worship sportsmen like Mike Tyson. However, Tyson does not want to just win, he wants to inflict pain and bite chunks out of the opposition. Some boys lose sight of the talents of the opposition and fail to acknowledge their skill. A few boys can also lose sight of the humanity of the opposition to the extent that they fail to see them as people. The other side are vermin to be exterminated, interlopers who have dared to challenge; who must be chased away lest self-esteem be lost.

The stakes are now much higher in sport. Schools must win or else lose enrolments. Coaches must win or else lose employment. Boys must win or else lose their place in the team. The adult world does nothing other than reinforce the stakes when parents challenge refereeing decisions from the sideline, clap opposition errors and boo opponents. In a game, the self-esteem of not just the boy is at stake, but also that of the parents who must have victory to prove the worth of their genes.

For some boys, their personal sense of worth is inextricably linked to their success in sport. Unfortunately, neither winning nor losing can be very good for a boy. If winning promotes a lack of humility and losing, a lack of self-esteem, then sport is not serving its participants well. Sport can challenge the traditional virtues of truth and loyalty and this is exacerbated by the huge amount of money which is at stake. Cheating takes on a plurality which is positively frightening. Truth needs to be supported not only by neutral referees and video replays but by a recovery of the noble sentiments of sport.[4]

What might well be at risk is the extinction of play.[5] The fun and frolic with bat and ball is being threatened by competition. This is probably why the term 'game' is being heard less and the term 'match' is being heard more. A game evokes a picture of recreation; a match evokes a picture of confrontation.

The taunt 'you are a loser' has developed a currency only because being a loser is so distasteful to boys. There is little interest in how a team plays and more interest in how the scoreboard looks. If a boy should fail to win, the label of 'athlete' is removed and replaced with 'loser'.[6]

For some boys, the male preoccupation with sport has resulted in both anger and frustration. These are boys not of the body weight, temperament and skill to be able to excel in sport. Although relatively innocent in being the cause of limited athletic ability, this has not prevented them being humiliated time and time again both on and off the field of play. The derision of their peers is such that the sporting experience becomes intensely painful, resulting in a withdrawal from physical activity which does little else than compound the problem.

Many boys tend to worship the body more than the brain resulting in the sporting 'jock' being given a status well beyond that of the academic. Schools can reinforce this by devoting the majority of the school magazine space to sport, and the majority of school 'awards' to sport.

HEALTHY SPORT
1. The right amount of sport
Too little physical activity and too much physical activity should to be avoided. Getting the heart rate up to about 70–80% of its maximum for 30 minutes at least three times a week is to be recommended. Too much physical activity will reflect itself in an obsessive preoccupation with sport which leaves a boy tired and unable to fulfil other duties including schoolwork. Unless training at an elite level, more than two hours of sport each of the week days could be excessive. For some boys a lesser amount could still be excessive if they have neither the physique nor the temperament to cope with a significant amount of physical activity.

2. The right type of sport

Not all boys can cope well with physical contact sports. This should not necessarily disqualify a boy from participating in team sports. For example, in rugby union there are positions on the field of play for many different builds. Those with strong upper body strength and who are naturally gladiatorial can play in the front row of the scrum. The small, cheeky one can play half back. His tall mate can play in the second row of the scrum. The all-rounder can play in the back row of the scrum, and the 'fleet of foot' can be in the back line with those least comfortable with physical contact being moved furthest away from the scrum.

Through a boy exploring many sports it should transpire that he chances upon one which matches his interest and abilities be it tennis, cross-country running, rowing, sailing, swimming, cricket, football, handball, volleyball or whatever.

3. The right coach

The coach who excuses bad language and uses bad language because of a passion for the game should be a worry. Also of concern would be the coach who denigrates the opposition and even his or her own players if they should make a mistake. The coach who is adversarial and who advocates violence is best avoided, as is the over-zealous coach who pushes players too far and is insensitive to a boy's pain, both physical and emotional.[7]

A good coach is knowledgeable about boys as well as the game and puts more store on rewarding good play than punishing bad play. Such a coach is able to transform individuals into a team, transform sport training into life training and transform the chore of practice into the joy of learning. What is generally recognised by the good coach is that sport has a technical side involving skill development and physical conditioning, and a moral side dealing with such things as determination, honesty and courage.[8] Good coaches will be demanding but they will also be sequential and measured in helping a boy to realise potential. The good coach will like the players more than the game and will have a sense of humour that puts everything in perspective; even the dropped catch which cost the team the premiership.[9]

4. The right skills

Sport should teach not only the rules of the game but the rules of life, the importance of honesty, commitment, working well with others and the knowledge of one's strengths and weaknesses. Adaptability, quick thinking, strategic thinking, courage, determination and the value of commitment are just a few of the other skills that might also be taught.

Even the rough and tumble of informal games and wrestling matches with the father can be important. Biddulph states:

> It's been found that what boys are learning in 'rough and tumble' is an essential lesson for all males: how to be able to have fun, get noisy, even get angry and at the same time, **know when to stop**. For a male, living with testosterone, this is vital. If you live in a male body, you have to learn how to drive it . . . A dad who knows what he's doing stops the action . . . a little lecture takes place — not yelling, just calmly explaining, 'Your body is precious (pointing at boy) and my body is precious too. We can't play this game if somebody might get hurt so we need a few rules like no elbowing and no kneeing or punching. Do you understand? Can you handle it?'[10]

5. The right attitudes

Sport can be an outstanding way of smuggling into boys a number of pro-social skills and teaching them to share, be honest and to acknowledge excellence in another without jealousy or guile. An example of this was in the Annual Rugby Union Match between St Joseph's College and The King's School in Sydney in 1999. One of the parents of a boy playing in the 1st XV for St Joseph's wrote the following in a letter to The King's School:

> . . . Congratulations on the result. King's were deserving winners of a game played in the spirit and intensity that these two great schools stand for. It was on Sunday when discussing the game that [my son] brought to our attention something I am sure you and the school should be proud of. He said 'That was the best loss I have had'. Wondering where he was coming from, we asked him to explain, and this is what he had to say. 'After the final whistle, there was the initial feeling of disappointment and emptiness, and the thought of a long walk off the field through the opposition stronghold to the dressing shed. It was while leaving the field we received many pats on the back, congratulations and many positive comments (from The King's students) all in appreciation of a good, hard game and the manner it was played in.' [My son] thought the response was fantastic and as parents we feel you should be very proud of your students, players and the school in general for displaying a level of sportsmanship and behaviour that we are all trying to achieve.

In sharing this letter, I added:

> We need to be careful that we do not lose the intrinsic reward in playing a sport, nor forget the joy of participation in our search for a win. We need to be careful we do not peddle the tired clichés of only winners being able to grin, and that winning being the only thing. We need to be careful that in competition we do not negate the humanity of the opponent. They too can be noble, fine young men with a generosity of spirit . . . Let us honour our opponents both on and off the field, and let us leave a game proud not only because we have given our best, but also because we have displayed the qualities of a gentleman. For this reason we should acknowledge good play on both sides, we should respect our opposition and we should play as fair as we do hard . . . and King's men can play very hard indeed!
>
> *Source:* Hawkes T F, *The King's Herald*, The King's School, Parramatta, 27 August 1999.

BOYS AND BODY IMAGE

Most research in the area of teenagers and body image centres on girls and their battle with anorexia or bulimia. However, boys can also suffer body image problems which drive to depression or, for the more proactive, to the gym where they work on their 'six-packs' and the sharp definition of their muscles.

Boys are not immune from anorexia or bulimia with some 10% of cases being male. Neither are boys immune from body image neurosis and an obsessive preoccupation with size, shape and strength. This can become pathological. The terms 'reverse anorexia nervosa' and 'muscle dysmorphia' have been added to contemporary vocabulary with both describing an obsession about body shape. However, the 'Baywatch' body is not easily gained by every boy.

Consideration needs to be given to those boys who are not sportsmen. One initiative that schools can take is to expand the range of sports on offer so that they include options other than physical contact sports, thus allowing a chance for the less bulky, less aggressive boy to succeed. Sports like tennis, table tennis, swimming, volleyball, cross-country and orienteering should be considered as complements to the team games offered by a school. Drummond and West write:

> . . . boys are very anxious about their body image. 'Hey, sir, look at the six-pack I got by working out in the holidays!' This refers to the highly-defined stomach muscles some males develop; the fact that

> boys know the names for so many muscles tell us a great deal about
> their concern for the right body image. Unfortunately boys who see
> themselves as fat or skinny have a poor self-image . . . boys who cause
> trouble at school often feel unconfident about their bodies and have
> bad self-esteem. These boys get sick, or cover their bodies up if they
> have to display them, for this can expose them to ridicule.[11]

In response to these concerns, Drummond and West suggest that schools
should model a more caring masculinity and stress sport as enjoyment
rather than competition. Drummond and West also suggest that championship sporting events which cater for the elite athlete could be
augmented by less intense sporting activities which enable all students to
participate. Weight training and body-building programs can also be
supplemented by aerobics, jazzercise, rap and break dancing.

Boys' love of sport presents unique opportunities to smuggle into
them those values, attitudes and behaviours which society deems to be
worthy. If schools and parents combine to harness that which is good in
sport for the benefit of their sons, the interpersonal skills and intrapersonal skills of boys might well be significantly advanced.

A CHANGE IN THE IMAGE OF MALENESS

The encouraging news for some boys is that the call to be macho, to have
a clearly defined 'six-pack', an appetite for physical contact sports and
V8 engines is beginning to diminish. There is a place for the sensitive,
thinking male who enjoys reading and computers and whose physical
exercise might be limited to an occasional game of chess. The popular
question 'What do you call a nerd in 10 years time?', answer: 'Sir', is a
popular joke proving to be true often enough to cause some boys to re-
evaluate their attitude to 'the wuss'.

The gradual acceptance of the less overtly masculine type of boy by
his peers has been assisted by films such as *Billy Elliott*, *Strictly Ballroom*
and *Romper Stomper*. Books like *A Heartbreaking Work of Staggering Genius*
by Dave Eggers, and the campaigning by individuals such as R Eirik Ott,
an American who described himself as somewhere between 'guy' and
'gay'. The acceptance of Leonardo Di Caprio masculinity is by no means
universal among boys, but there has been a noticeable expansion in some
boy circles of the types of boys who are acceptable.

A number of forces have been at work in the broadening of boys'
minds as to what might be considered masculine. As indicated above,
the media have helped. Another very powerful force has been that of the
feminists who have shown by their own success in winning better

recognition for females that cultural opinion can be changed. Girls are also signalling to boys that the loutish and high-risk behaviours sometimes associated with boys is actually a turn-off. Professor Garry Egger, scientific director of the Gutbuster program has found from his research that men wanted a body which was 13 kilograms more muscular, while women did not desire this change in their men. Most women were very happy for their men to have the Hugh Grant figure and did not really want their men looking like Arnold Schwarzenegger.[12] There is a redefinition of what is attractive to the herd, so the bulls need to listen. The small-bodied, large-brained boy can actually be attractive to a girl and there is nothing like a shift in consumer taste to cause producers to alter their product. For this reason boys can thank feminists for contributing towards a broader definition of maleness.

Another force at work in changing what society sees as attractive in a boy is the incursion of the computer into contemporary society. IT and its place in society is such that it is changing perceptions as to what it means to work. It now has nothing much to do with fleetness of foot and muscle bulk. There is less need to hunt mammoths or even till the soil. The contemporary provider is likely to succeed if he has shown he can communicate well, relate cooperatively with others and can understand the bewildering world of 'techno speak'. The provider today does not bash heads, he taps keys.[13]

ADDITIONAL INFORMATION

For those wishing to have further details on some of the points raised in this chapter, the following references may be helpful. Each number in the text of the chapter relates to a reference number below which will give further information related to the topic

1	Orwell, G quoted in Daintith, J, Fergusson, R, Stibbs, A and Wright (eds) (1998)	*Thematic Dictionary of Quotations*	Bloomsbury Publishing, London, p 399.
2	Pile, S (1989)	*The Return of Heroic Failures*	Penguin Books, London.
3	Moir, A and Jessel, D (1989)	*Brainsex*	Mandarin, London, p 104.
4	Grace, D (1999)	'Preserving the spirit of play: Values and ethics in sport'	*Values*, New College Institute of Values Research, University of New South Wales, Spring 1999.
5	Grace, D	(op cit)	

6	Drummond, W and West, P (1995)	'Getting more boys involved in sport'	Unpublished paper, University of Western Sydney, Faculty of Education.
7	Pollack, W (1998)	*Real Boys*	Owl Books, Henry Holt and Co., New York, p 289.
8	Grace, D	(op cit)	p 2.
9	Pollack, W	(op cit)	p 282.
10	Biddulph, S (1997)	*Raising Boys*	Finch Publishing, Sydney, p 71.
11	Drummond, W and West, P	(op cit)	p 5.
12	*Sunday Telegraph* (2000)	'Men's quest for muscles'	*Sunday Telegraph*, 8/10/00, p 46.
13	French, N (1999)	'It's been tough for boys'	*New Statesman*, Vol 128, Issue 4463, 22/11/99, p 40.

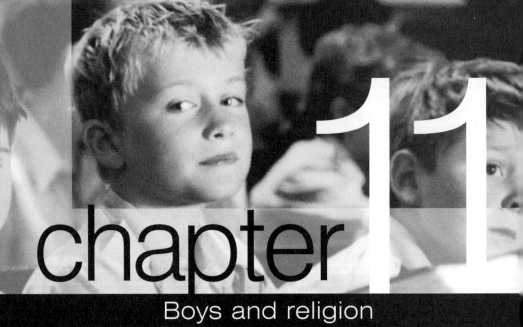

chapter 11

Boys and religion

INTRODUCTION

Boys have learnt from Arnold Schwarzenegger, just as their fathers learnt from John Wayne, that to be male is to be tough, independent and entirely able to cope using courage rather than faith. The idea of religion is not attractive to many boys who are trying to demonstrate to others and to themselves that they are man enough to cope. 'Thank you God, I no longer need you. I may have needed you when I was younger, when at night my dressing gown on the back of the door would turn into Darth Vader, but not now because I am older and at night my dressing gown stays as a dressing gown.'

Despite this denial, many boys are innately spiritual and have a predisposition to put their faith in a God. Religion can still give boys answers to questions, meaning for life and help in trouble.

SECULARISM AND THE NEW AGE

The decline of religion in the lives of many boys is symptomatic of a growing secularisation of society. This decline can leave a void, as secularism fails to provide answers to the great questions, resulting in a vacuum in the lives of many children. Nature abhors a vacuum and so it is filled with the worship of oneself. It can also be filled with new-age superstition, a preoccupation with psychic energies and a range of cults and 'isms'.

RELIGION IS FEMININE

A particular problem for many boys is that religion can be associated with the feminine and the weak. For boys, the two are synonymous. It was mum not dad who said the prayers; it was mum not dad who read the great religious stories; it was mum not dad who went to church and took the children to Sunday school. Dad was elsewhere being a male, and on Sunday males hit a golf ball, fix the car and get the barbecue fired up.

This pattern of behaviours is not found with all religious groups. Some faiths see a dominant spiritual role being played by the adult male. It is hardly surprising that these same faiths have greater success handing on their belief to their sons.

As a boy grows up, dependence on the mother is reduced and a growing association with things masculine becomes a priority. The warm security of a mother's arms becomes less attractive as societal expectations teach a young man not to be 'a mummy's boy'. The male code is practised in playgrounds and parks. The trusting and dependent child becomes the cynical and independent young man and religion is put away and stored in the attic with the stroller. Some boys may chance upon their faith in later life but many do not unless, of course, a personal tragedy makes a visit to the attic a necessity. By then the dust is probably too thick on the remnants of childhood faith to offer any spiritual comfort which is useful. Small wonder Jesus should require His disciples to have the faith of a child, for society has conspired to ensure that faith is not found in the adult.

Many religions have congregations and gatherings that are dominated by women. Men are not well represented in some churches. This may be because some congregations are ageing and women tend to live longer than men. It may be because employment obligations require more men to work during times of worship. Much more likely is the fact that generations of men have copied their father's attitude to church and religion. This attitude suggests that religion is a private thing, like grand-dad's incontinence — 'you don't talk about it'. So no one talks, and nothing of spiritual value is handed from father to son.

Another attitude among males is that of humanistic convenience. 'God is best kept on the fringe of one's life, for one should not become a religious fanatic, and besides you do not have to go to church to be religious.' This sentiment is often linked to tales of religious hypocrisy and the realisation that the favourite TV show clashes with the times of the evening service. Adults practise a defensive rhetoric to justify the marginalisation of their God. Little ears listen and little eyes watch and the excuse is learnt by heart and transferred to another generation.

GOD AS A JUVENILE SENTIMENT

Boys tend to move away from religion at much the same time they move away from their mothers. Religion is often seen by some boys as something which is associated with infancy, something which is associated with femininity and something which is associated with inadequacy. All three associations are significant enough to ensure that, for many boys, the spiritual dimension of their lives remains underdeveloped.

A steady diet of legend and story is fed to infant boys, who accept the existence of Santa and Jesus. The primary school years see the gradual realisation that it is all a story, a nice story, but a story nonetheless and God is dumped along with the Tooth Fairy. Belief in God is met with the same incredulity as belief in the Easter Bunny. These are stories to be associated with Fisher Price toys and 6 o'clock bed times.

Adults conspire to help children shed the trappings of youth. Children are praised for looking so old; for growing so tall; for being advanced a grade in school; for learning to read early; for a myriad of things that suggest to a boy that childhood and all the stories that go with it should be abandoned as soon as possible. Boys can be robbed of their childhood and their faith by a society that continually signals that it wants its sons to grow up and to shed the things of youth: the innocence; the ignorance; the faith; the teddy, it all goes . . . or does it?

RELIGIOUS THOUGHT IN YOUNG BOYS

The concepts of God and religion have baffled adults for thousands of years and have caused war and division throughout the world as answers have been sought. The idea of an all-powerful God is not a concept that is too hard for young boys to grasp. Their world is full of wonder and magic, and they have had to learn to trust and have faith in so many things that the translation of that faith into a spiritual awareness of there being a God is not difficult. Boys have had to learn to trust in others for the provision of food, shelter, love and support. To expand this trust to encompass a God is not difficult for a child.

One of the key variables in the presence of religious thought in a boy is the home. If there is an expression of faith by parents and siblings, the boy is likely to inherit this faith. In his early years a boy might have an 'adopted faith', a faith borrowed from parents and principal carers. In the initial stages of a boy's life, faith is likely to be literal. God is actually a big man in the clouds with power to punish naughty children. The young boy is also relatively compliant and will accept teaching from adults about God without a great deal of questioning. Boys have been used to having things explained to them by adults which have all proved true. Some insects can sting you; having a bath makes you clean; too many sweets can make you ill; God loves you and will reward you when you do good; fire can burn.

While many families support spiritual values, some are somewhat less keen to support the theology that lies behind it. 'I can accept the value of trying to be kind to your neighbours and help them but not the value of trying to convert your neighbours and save them' is the sort of senti-ment that is often voiced. The 'religion is significantly improved if you take God out of it' mentality is strong. Even some mainline churches are marginalising God in favour of social service. Far easier to share the soup than share the gospel. Others would argue that in sharing the soup one is sharing the gospel.

Sometimes the spiritual vacuum in contemporary society is being filled with fringe religions. Some of these fringe religions wear the face of fanatical fundamentalism and this has helped to scare many families away from religion.

All of this can mean that there can be something of a spiritual void in many young boys although it is unlikely that a young boy is going to escape some exposure to religious ceremony: a bar mitzvah; a wedding; a Christmas pageant. These occasions may foster some embryonic faith even in a faithless home. However, if the home expresses no spiritual faith, it is unlikely that the young boy will develop much of an awareness of God or of religion. What faith does develop may well be more of a superstition or even a fear.

RELIGIOUS THOUGHT IN ADOLESCENT BOYS

With growing independence, and an ability to understand abstract concepts, a boy will begin to seek ownership of his own faith during the adolescent years. The influence of the adopted faith from parents is weakened and the boy must now find his own religious belief. If the faith of the parents is a sort of 'agnosticism with a hint of atheism' then this sort of faith, or non-faith, tends to be accepted by adolescents. This might be because it is hard for an adolescent boy to flex his own spiritual muscles if years of neglect have left these muscles undeveloped. As a result, the adolescent boy is even denied the satisfaction of rebelling against the faith of his parents. There is simply nothing to rebel against.

Boys will rarely wake up to their spiritual impoverishment until something happens, such as a death in the family. A grandparent's funeral, the death of a friend can cause confusion in the adolescent boy if he is given no framework with which to make sense of it all. Not many boys have been acquainted with death — their life has been a continual celebration of the glorious inputs into the cosmos — they have rarely had to experience the outputs. Baptisms, bar mitzvahs and weddings have been enjoyed but not funerals. When one is young, no one dies — if you get shot, all you have to do is count to 20 and then you can play again. Then something shocking happens, and there is no resurrection at the count of 20. Such occasions can motivate spiritual enquiry, although the overwhelming sense of anger, shock and deprivation does not always create the ideal climate for the clearest of thinking.

GOD IS DEAD

'Marx is dead, God is dead and I'm feeling unwell myself' is the sort of graffiti that entertains because of truth as well as humour. So where does this leave boys who, as one unknown commentator put it, are having to deal with scientists who offer theories that God doesn't exist; agnostics who say that it's important to keep an open mind on the issue; atheists who say bluntly that there is no God; psychoanalysts who suggest one might have a 'God fixation' and offer treatment at $250 a go; cynics who will mock a boy's belief; and humanists who say that you are the God? And then there are the liberal theologians who will tell you to 'un-God' your God.

Confusion about things spiritual can be exacerbated by the moral and ethical uncertainty of the post-modern era. If there is no God, there are no rules, there is perfect freedom . . . until one realises that one person's freedom is another person's jail. With a divine imperative to keep to certain codes of behaviour comes boundaries; comes a spiritual and social civility; comes a check on godless activity. Without God, humankind is not frolicking in unfettered freedom; without God society is producing sons who are all too often imprisoned by dejection, discouragement and depression. Even more frightening is the overwhelming sense of hopelessness which can be found in the faithless. If there is no God, there is no purpose. If there is no God, there is no power that can intercede. If there is no final judgment, there is no final justice. Taken together it is small wonder that adolescent depression is found less frequently in families with a strong religious faith.

Perhaps it is not fair to say God is dead and more accurate to say God has changed. With the new millennium came the change from the Age of Pisces to the Age of Aquarius; from the Christian symbol of the fish to a new-age symbol of nature; from a Judeo-Christian era to an era of cosmic energy; from the divinity of God to the divinity of nature. The new creed could read:

> I believe in nature the mother of all
> Maker of heaven and earth
> And that cosmic power her holy force is good
> We were conceived by the creative host
> Born of ancient energy
> Suffered under environmental neglect
> Were used, discarded and buried
> We descended into hell
> Until we controlled our emissions and grew new trees unto heaven
> We now sitteth with others to chant
> Our thanks for dolphins and whales
> I believe in the holy place; the holy place of peace
> The communion of saints, the forgiveness of sin
> And the recycling of all things everlasting.

Growing environmental awareness is to be encouraged for it is vital to the health and well-being of this fragile planet. Increasing awareness of the holiness of nature is also to be encouraged for the character of God is revealed within God's creations. Yet, care is needed that the search for meaning is not just limited to the natural world, for there are other worlds that harbour spiritual clues. It is true that the natural world and the spiritual world can be found together. It is also true that the natural world and the spiritual world can be found apart.

RELIGIOUS REMAINS STILL TO BE FOUND IN BOYS

There was a time when eternal damnation could be threatened to induce compliance from boys. An offence against the school was an offence against God. Six strokes and a guilty repentance before God was the penance paid if found dipping Pippa Ruth Hoskins' pigtails in the inkwell. This no longer happens and it is because inkwells, God and the cane, and possibly even Pippa's pigtails, have all gone. However, God is proving remarkably difficult to be shifted entirely from families and the lives of many boys, despite a contemporary culture that is witnessing declining church attendance, cultural diversity, growing secularisation, and moral and ethical confusion.

Perhaps there is some truth that in all boys there remains a 'God-shaped blank', which boys might try to fill with sport, music, friends and sex — but none are completely the right shape to fill the void, and thus, despite the best efforts of humanism and a lot of other 'isms', a latent spirituality remains. Aboriginal people call this *dadirri* — the deep spring within us, that place of listening, of quiet awareness and spiritual contemplation.

There does seem to be an innate spirituality in boys. Richard Dawkins, the Oxford biologist, explains this as being because children become 'infected' with religion when they are young and impressionable. One only has to walk beside the terrifying rows of examination desks in schools to see vestiges of some sort of faith. The array of lucky gonks, charms and bracelets, together with the significant number of crucifixes dangling from around necks, bears testimony, if not to some sort of faith, then certainly, to some sort of superstition.

Although significant numbers of mainline churches have been ineffective in attracting boys, this should not necessarily be confused with a lack of spirituality in boys, but rather a signal that the established places of worship in their antique buildings, quaint vestments and old prayer books, are having some difficulty in convincing adolescents that the message they bring is relevant for today. This has resulted in what one cynic has described as many of the young abandoning church in favor of a relationship with God.

Boys may not want to admit it, but many, even in their adolescent years, find they have spiritual questions which modern day secularism is having difficulty in answering; such questions as 'Who is it that made this world, and what is the mind behind the cosmic system? Is all the order, the beauty, the interconnectedness just an accident?' These questions may not be admitted, but they are still asked by many boys.

Even scientific minds such as that of Paul Davis, wonder at the awesome complexity to be found within creation. Suggestions of a primordial swamp from which it all began are just about as fantastic as tales about a God taking only six days to make it all. It is valid, even for boys, to wonder at these things.

The poet Gerard Manley Hopkins talks of the earth being 'filled with the grandeur of God'. Boys are not generally given to such poetic exclamations but this does not mean the question of God does not pass through their minds, particularly a mind being entertained by the marvels of nature.

SUNDAY WITH MY SON

Not long ago on a Sunday morning, I joined my son for a walk along Sorrento Back Beach in Victoria, having swapped my *Hymns, Ancient and Modern* for *A Visitor's Guide to the Mornington Peninsula*. We found ourselves gazing at the crashing waves on Derby's Rock, fortified by a hot chocolate and marshmallows from the Sorrento Back Beach Restaurant.

The sight was breathtaking, full of foam and fury, with a brisk south-westerly stirring up a significant swell that exploded on the rock shelves, then sucked greedily at the kelp as it gathered itself, white with rage, for yet another frontal attack on the rocks.

The rocks were winning, splintering the waves into shards of spray, but they were wounded, with the strata-ed shelves scarred and scabbed by their constant attrition with the sea.

This, then, was our opening hymn, the base boom of imploding waves giving harmony to the hiss and bubble of the receding waters.

The readings came from the melaleuca and coastal tea tree along Coppins' Track. They spoke to us of adaptation and endurance. The tortured twists of the tea tree told of the agony there can be in growing. Their deformed spines were beyond chiropractic help and yet they not only survived, but bloomed, with their small, white petals imparting a confetti-ed blessing.

Humbled and inspired, we were then baptised, be-goggled and be-snorkelled, in the tranquil kingdom of the rock pools in which there was peace beyond all understanding. 'You are in the world, but not of the world', the stands of Neptune's necklaces reminded us. 'For everything there is a season', said the red sea anemones, opening up with the incoming tide, and a small shoal of translucent fish reminded us of the strength and security there is in fellowship. Enriched beyond measure, we returned to the slightly martyred company of friends who had been to church. 'Skipped church today then . . .' they accused, to which we replied,'No we haven't. Just decided to worship somewhere else today.'

Source: Hawkes, T F (1998) 'Old religion and young people', *Ministry*, Vol 0 No 1, Spring, p 6.

Very few have been able to explain to boys the marvelous complexities of the natural and human world, the patterns, the beauty, the relationships without some reference to a creator God. Many boys have no difficulty in acknowledging the existence of some great architect of the universe. Despite the 'big bang' and various theories of evolution, one of the strongest intellectual justifications boys have in entertaining some form of faith, is in the clear evidence of a 'divine' creator.

Creation is not the only question in the minds of boys. There are other age old questions such as:

- Where do I come from?
- Where am I going to?
- What is the purpose of my life?
- What is the purpose of my death?

In the past, it was suggested that God existed to explain the unexplainable. Thus there developed the 'God of the gaps' syndrome, where, if there was any gap in knowledge, the answer was God. Then as the gaps in knowledge decreased, the need for God decreased. However, there still appear to be enough gaps to fill boys with curiosity, and to cause them to ask 'Why?' and to wonder whether the hand of God is involved.

This theme should not be over-developed or the spiritual appetite of boys made to be more significant than it really is. For a great number of boys, the great questions do not really bother them and neither do the implications of whether God exists or not. Religion is often just an irrelevance, something to be associated with one's younger days and mother's milk. Now that other beverages are being enjoyed and dad's Sunday worship is directed to the car and the local soccer team, a man's place, and a boy's place, is not in the pew.

Nonetheless, absence from the pew should not necessarily be interpreted as an absence of spiritual sensibility. Some boys have a dormant faith and even a real appreciation of religious tradition as seen at baptisms, weddings, confirmations and funerals. It is also seen at different times throughout the religious calendar, such as at Christmas and Ramadan. Although a significant number of boys are sucked into the vortex of commercialism at Christmas where cash-card convenience replaces sacrificial service, and where love is quantified on cash dockets, Christ is still searched for by some among the snowy windowsills, sleighs and stockings. Although the unfashionable Christ has been removed from Christmas and has been replaced by the spiritually anonymous 'X', midnight communion will often witness the presence of some adolescents. Although many adolescents grumble 'Bah, humbug', others are haunted by the 'ghost of Christmas past', and they remember the story of 'The First Christmas' when a baby was born, who grew into a man, who was crucified for the sins of all humankind. Such is the comfort that some boys draw from the familiar cadence of the Christmas carols and readings, and the Easter songs, that it is sometimes difficult to move them on from the love of the ceremony, to a love of the meaning. There is no reason to suggest that other religions may not have similar challenges.

SUGGESTIONS FOR DEALING WITH ADOLESCENT SPIRITUALITY

1. Teach the dominant spiritual stories

Despite being a multicultural society, the western world is still founded on the basis of a Judeo-Christian heritage — a heritage that has permeated the law, the parliamentary system and culture. So western schools should not be too apologetic about introducing their students to the basic tenets of the Christian faith. For other countries this may well involve other stories and other faiths. This is not to say that schools should involve themselves with indoctrination, for this would be an abuse of power. But neither should schools shrink from education. Schools need to seek not so much to cause their students to be religious but rather to understand religion. There is value in teaching the history, the symbols, the stories, the rituals, beliefs and value systems that are associated with a country's cultural heritage.

2. Teach religious tolerance

Although Australian society once enjoyed a Dreamtime 'religion' rich in ancient truths, it was to be largely replaced a little over 200 years ago by the English Anglican and Irish Catholic traditions. These were subsequently enriched by European Catholicism, Jewish migrants and, more recently, Buddhists and Muslims from the Middle East and Asia. More and more, Australia, like many other countries, is adopting the characteristics of a plural society and unless that society wishes to be splintered by cultural schism, it must teach cultural understanding and acceptance in its schools.

An understanding of, and knowledge about, other major world religions and traditional beliefs is important for boys, for not only does it contribute to their own spiritual journey, it can encourage the sort of tolerance that Bertrand Russell advocates.

3. Teach the affective domain of religion

Teaching the affective domain of religion means allowing boys opportunities to consider their own personal faith by introducing them to moments of spiritual wonder and reflection. Most of the great world religions touch not only minds, but hearts, and work not only at the cognitive level, but at the emotional level.

This particular domain is fraught with danger, for it can lend itself to emotional manipulation and proselytising. On the other hand, schools need to acknowledge that wonder and reflection can be encouraged responsibly in schools. For example, a field trip which involves taking students into a cathedral, a mosque and a synagogue might not just educate, it might also be emotionally uplifting and thought-provoking, causing students to reflect upon their own personal faith and relationship with their own God.

4. Provide ethical and moral reference points

With the decline of strong ethical guidelines, there is a real moral confusion in society so that some boys are genuinely confused about what is wrong. Perhaps God is to blame. If She had not allowed herself to be marginalised, society would have a set moral code that defined good and bad. But even God is having Her problems. The church is split on whether to ordain homosexuals, ordain women, or ordain guitars in church. Theologian Barbara Thiering is denying the gospels, bishops are denying the virgin birth and clergy are denying charges of sexual misconduct. In all of this, boys are becoming genuinely confused and, thus, one of the great missions for spiritual educators in schools is to provide boys with a number of firm reference points from which they may take their bearings on their journey of life. Schools need to meet not only the temporal needs of boys, but their eternal needs.

In seeking to provide these reference points, schools might lay themselves open to the charge of social engineering. Any school that takes its charter of education seriously must be involved in the business of social engineering, and of daring to suggest that some behaviours are appropriate, and others are not. It is impossible to divorce religion from character education and the teaching of pro-social skills. Just as faith can be translated into action, action can be translated into faith.

5. Stress the sacredness of the individual

How much are humans worth? Do we have some intrinsic value? There is enough phosphorous in each person for several boxes of matches, fat for a few bars of soap, iron enough for one medium-sized nail which, together with a few assorted salts and a number of buckets of water, means that a person is probably valued at about $10. Is this all a person is worth? Are humans merely a higher order ape; an accident; an evolution from jellied lumps in the sea? Is there anything that sets humans apart? Do we have a soul? Do we bear the image of God? Is there an external element within each person that is sacred, or is this a monstrous presumption, a pathetic grasping for immortality?

If boys are shown that people are not sacred, there need be little respect for each other or themselves. Society can use people as objects and throw them away as mangled foetuses, homeless children, derelict adults or institutionalised elders. The bruised, abused and used society might profit from the discovery of the worth of the individual and convey this to its sons. This is particularly important for adolescent boys, for they are being heavily targetted by advertisers who would want to suggest that unless they have the body of Rambo, the intellect of Einstein, or the wealth of Bill Gates, they have failed. It is one of the important tasks of schools to remind its boys that every one of them is precious, if not to themselves, then to those who love them, and if not to those who love them, then to God.

6. Teach students to care for their soul

Cholesterol and carbohydrate consciousness is now endemic. Health is injected through vaccines and spread using 15+ sunscreen. Although society cossets its physical frame, does it take as much care of its soul?

Soul does not necessarily mean a religious sensibility so much as that seat of consciousness, character, morality and meaning — that place where nature and nurture forge the deep you; a place where imagination and reality meet; a place where consciousness and unconsciousness meet. In the fifteenth century, Marsilio Ficino described the soul as giving coherence, relatedness and substance by bringing together mind and body, dreams and reality, spirit and world. The soul is responsible for making good people glow *goodness*, and bad people, *badness*.

Thomas Moore, in his book *Care of the Soul*,[1] suggests that the great malady of our time is the neglect of the soul. This is revealed in shallowness, loss of meaning and a failure to recognise the sacredness of ordinary things. Society needs to care for the soul with deeds and thoughts that enrich the inner being, and boys should not be excluded from this obligation.

It is significant that many of the Amazon tribes are not so much afraid of the white man's world but they are horrified by its toxicity to their soul. Perhaps the western world should also be horrified, and seek to counter the soullessness within. This is why boys should watch sunsets, practise reflection and feed their minds with those things that edify and enrich. Perhaps boys need to engage in 'soul watch', with frequent checks as to their soul's depth and health.

Thomas Moore reminds us that the parish priest used to be charged with the responsibility known as *cura animarum* — care of the soul. All boys can be curates of their own souls, an idea that implies an inner priesthood. Caring for the soul involves an awareness of a fourth dimension, a fascinating dimension in which can be found health and healing. Schools and parents need to encourage boys to keep their souls healthy by a diet of noble action, moving and aesthetic experiences, love, wisdom and reflection.

7. Protect adolescents from exploitation by damaging cults and 'isms'

There are many who would compete for a boy's spiritual allegiance. Cults and 'isms' abound, as do promises of eternal life. Massacres in Wako, Texas and ritualised death pacts in Jonestown, serve to remind that society must be careful with its young, particularly those who are lonely, gullible or vulnerable. Unfortunately, the modern messiah seems to have developed a penchant for guns, poison and war gas. Religious fanaticism and dangerous egos have seen the modern sermon reinforced by plastic explosives and automatic weapons.

The Age of Aquarius is also bringing with it Shirley MacLaine videos, crystals and star sign necklaces. It is also bringing the questioning of traditional beliefs. Some of this thinking can be helpful, but some of it can also be quite damaging. So society needs to ensure that its sons make informed decisions about their faith and remain in control of their decision making in all matters spiritual.

8. Adopt age-appropriate approaches to teaching religion

Developmental psychologists like Jean Piaget[2] describe a staged development in children towards intellectual maturity moving from a reliance on concrete things to an appreciation of abstract thinking. Another developmental psychologist, Lawrence Kohlberg[3], was more interested in the development of moral thoughts which he saw as moving from an initial dependence on the morality of others to the capacity to decide on ethical matters for oneself. James Fowler[4] built upon Kohlberg's work and suggests the following stages in faith development or 'enfaithment'.

1. **Imitation faith** — in the first few years of life a child will have a faith that imitates that of his or her major carers. It is a compliant faith, an inherited faith and one that is unsophisticated. 'Mummy, John didn't close his eyes for grace.'
2. **Literal faith** — up to about eight years of age a child is able to recount some of the great religious statements and stories. However, these are accepted literally and there is no ability at this stage to cope

with the symbolic or abstract elements of faith. '. . . Then this big snake said to Eve, you like apples don't you . . .'

3. **Conventional faith** — this is a pre-adolescent phase which sees individual faith being influenced by the faith of peers and of the media. 'You don't still believe in Santa, do you?'

4. **Individual faith** — at adolescence a child is usually able to show some individuality in his or her own thinking about faith and may even drift away from the faith inherited from parents. 'I don't believe in it anyway so why should I go to church?'

5. **Consolidated faith** — all of life's experiences to date have led to a gradual consolidation of belief which has been cemented by reflection to the extent where the person feels comfortable defending his or her faith stance. 'Dad, I think you ought to know . . . I've become a Christian.'

6. **Demonstrated faith** — this is where a person's faith is congruent with his or her life. Faith is consistently seen in action as well as in words. 'I'm sorry, I don't feel comfortable doing that, it's against my beliefs.'

Educators should be guided but not constrained by the conclusions of these developmental psychologists. While there is wisdom in building faith in a way which is congenial to a boy's age, it should be remembered that spiritual maturation can vary a great deal in boys. Nonetheless the stages of faith development described above reinforce the importance of encouraging a personal ownership of faith in later years.

9. Develop a 'whole school' approach to developing faith and character

The Christian educator Tim Macnaught suggests that schools should work with the home in adopting a 'whole school' approach to the development of faith and character.[5] Among a number of ideas, Macnaught suggests:

■ Using all subjects as potential areas to discuss matters relating to morality, values, reason and purpose. The sciences provide unique opportunities to study creation and to explore the implications that there might exist a 'grand architect' of the universe. The arts also allow opportunities to comment on the human condition and the positives and negatives of that condition.

■ Encouraging individuals to search for truth and meaning. A cooperative learning environment allows each to tell his or her story. This can enrich others in their search for spiritual reference points in their lives.

- Inspiring students to adopt certain attitudes and interests through the use of real life testimony and also through the use of appropriate literature and films.
- Providing opportunities for students to develop responsible behaviour patterns by giving students duties associated with being a mentor, coach or leader.
- Providing opportunities within the curriculum to exercise moral reasoning, to discuss past and present values and to compare both local and international perspectives of truth and meaning.
- Putting in place age-appropriate camps and retreats to enable students to be less distracted by everyday life and to concentrate on issues of faith, purpose and lifestyle for a while.

10. Consider adopting the 'five-strand approach'

The author Peter Vardy has studied how religious education was transformed in Britain throughout the 1980s and 1990s. An increasing number of students studied religious education in British schools during this time and Vardy suggests that part of this growth was due to a new approach to the teaching of religion in schools. This approach included:

- an appreciation of the Bible and Christian tradition:
  - the main Bible stories
  - a broad understanding of the character of God as shown in the Bible
  - the exploration of the truth and relevance of the Bible stories
  - the role of metaphor, analogy and symbol in Christian teaching
  - the Bible, Catechism and Sacraments
  - the underpinnings of the Judeo-Christian faith.

- values education:
  - exploring ethical issues
  - age-appropriate exploration of values, law and ethics
  - age-appropriate exploration of values rich issues, such as social justice, sexuality and human rights.

- philosophy of religion:
  - arguments for and against the existence of God
  - suffering, evil and judgment
  - love, forgiveness and redemption
  - the character of God.

■ world religions:
   – a basic understanding of the main world religions with particular reference to Judaism, Islam, Hinduism, Buddhism and Aboriginal beliefs.

■ reflection and feeling:
   – the value of silence, stillness, reflection, feeling and emotion.[6]

Vardy also offers advice on how schools can encourage the effective religious education of boys:

■ Allow boys to express their religious ideas without fear or ridicule.
■ Incorporate religion in the values and ethos of the school.
■ Ensure a strong spiritual example is given by the school principal.
■ Employ quality teachers of religious education.
■ Draw up a detailed religious education curriculum with clear educational targets.
■ Encourage a cross-curricular approach to the teaching of values.
■ Make sure religious education programs are sequential and age-appropriate.
■ Encourage open-minded intellectual enquiry among students.
■ Ensure that the religious education curriculum is designed to increase knowledge rather than promote faith. Faith-promoting experiences have their place in a school but should be built within the school's voluntary program. With this approach, charges of indoctrination should be avoided.

CONCLUSION

Boys may exhibit the post-modern traits of being materialistically focused and morally confused. However, in some boys one can still find a genuine interest in matters spiritual. One can also see in boys a demand for justice and a desire for meaning, and some way to make sense of it all. Despite disillusionment with much of what is offered by many churches, there remains a spiritual hunger in some boys. This hunger will not often be admitted for boys often feel obliged to 'spit in the eye of the devil', to take risks both spiritual and physical and to be independent of their parents and their God. Yet, despite the bravado, a spiritual being can still be discovered in a boy. Some boys discover that the nihilism of a godless world might be 'cool' for a time, but it fails to give the sort of reference points they are happy to take their life bearings from.

When encouraging the young to discover something more about their God, Peter Corney advises:

- Don't tell adolescent boys what the 'truth' is, but explore what 'needs' boys have and how some of these needs might be met through the development of a mature faith.
- Don't push it, use several steps when introducing boys to a better understanding of God.
- Don't use words and written texts too much. Use experiential, visual and musical means to help get the message across. Stories and testimonies work well.
- Establish a proper relationship with the boy first. A person will be listened to by a boy if he or she is both known and respected.
- Don't come over as the 'know all'. Show humility, concern and a touch of humour.[7]

Many schools and churches will need to rethink their approach to teaching religion, for boys will not be won by meaningless ritual. Consideration might be given to using modern technology, music and the modern idiom in order to have ancient wisdoms accepted.

What boys demand of their religion is that it be authentic. They are not particularly interested in perpetuating the spiritual schism of existing generations for denominationalism is meaningless to contemporary youth. Neither may it be presumed that boys will accept the cultural norms they were born into, for they have grown up as children of another world and another time.

In dealing with boys on matters of spirituality it should be remembered that the issue of relevance needs to be tackled. Boys may have to be persuaded of the value of the spiritual dimension of their world. Some boys are spiritually thirsty, but the job of adults is to direct boys to the water, rather than forcing them to drink. In being given the privilege of directing boys, it must be recognised that, in the end, the spiritual realm remains a mystery, and thus all must approach spiritual matters with some humility, recognising that in the very lack of certainty, faith is born.

ADDITIONAL INFORMATION

For those wishing to have further details on some of the points raised in this chapter, the following references may be helpful. Each number in the text of the chapter relates to a reference number below which will give further information related to the topic.

1	Moore, T (1992)	*Care of the Soul*	Piatkus, London.
2	Piaget, J (1959)	*The Language and Thought of a Child*	Rutledge and Kegan Paul, London.
3	Kohlberg, L (1963)	'The development of children's orientation toward moral order. 1: Sequence in the development of moral thought'	*Vita Humana*, 6:11–13.
4	Fowler, J (1981)	*Stages of Faith*	Dove, Melbourne.
5	Macnaught, T (1997)	*Towards a whole school approach to developing character in today's young people*	National Anglican Schools' Consultative Committee 6th Annual Conference, Conference Report, p 84.
6	Vardy, P (1997)	'Towards a new approach to religious education'	Paper presented at the Australian Conference on Religions and Values Education, Geelong Grammar, Victoria, September 1997.
7	Corney, P (1995)	'Seeking hope in the ruins of modernity'	*Zadok Perspectives*, No 49, July 1995.

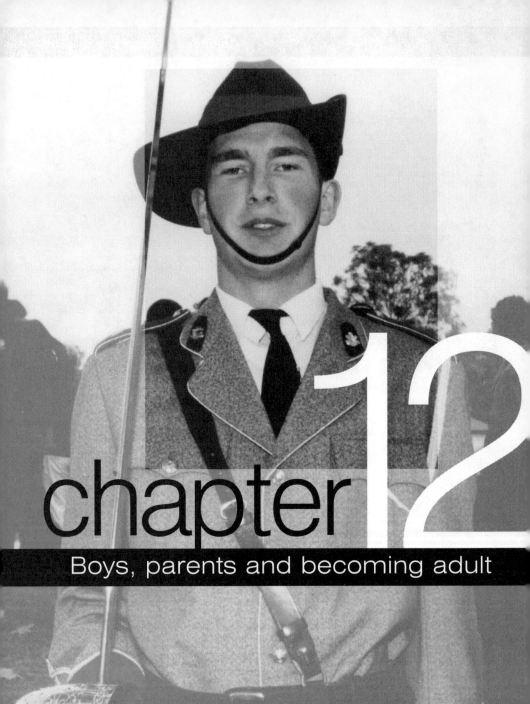

chapter 12

Boys, parents and becoming adult

PARENTING

Parenting has never been more demanding. Three clear bits of evidence support my claim and they are now 17, 15 and six years of age. It was Francis Bacon who suggested that those who have children 'hath given hostages to fortune; for they are impediments to great enterprises' . . . such as McDonald's-free car journeys! Parents engage in a daily battle to meet their children's needs, to finance, fetch and feed. The night brings little respite, with even the simple task of getting children to bed being fraught with potential conflict.

Although Monday's child may be 'fair of face' and Tuesday's child 'filled with grace', it should be remembered that Wednesday's child is 'full of woe' and Thursday's child 'has far to go' . . . usually to a basketball match in Templestowe followed by a music exam in Camberwell and a sleep-over in Frankston.

John Irvine writes in his book *Coping with Kids* that raising children is harder today that it has ever been, suggesting there is no sane parent or grandparent who would disagree. The job carries less prestige or authority than it ever has and yet it is more demanding, more confusing than ever.[1]

Trapped between the children's rights movement on the one hand and the accountability movement on the other (a movement which has started putting parents in jail for offences committed by their children), the job of parenting is becoming somewhat pressured. Intergenerational crossfire is not a new phenomenon. G B Shaw said of his daughter, 'She has lost the art of conversation, but not, unfortunately, the power of speech'. To this must be added single parents, double incomes, increased family isolation and decreased family values, and we have the potential for some angst and a few slammed doors.

Heaping coals upon our head are the painfully accurate accusations of social commentators, such as John Abbott, who wrote:

> Parents on average . . . watch television for 25 hours each week. Very many have no direct involvement in their children's learning and, therefore, miss out on an essential lynch pin of emotional bonding. Parents have grown to see those 25 hours as 'their' time. Children can be bought off with Nintendo or videos. Family meals are replaced by convenience foods, taken whenever appropriate. Family discourse almost disappears. Children can be a bore: relationships are disposable: and one in two marriages it appears will end in divorce. And the schools are left to pick up the pieces.[2]

I don't watch much TV but I am still guilty of dining in communion with the microwave rather than with the family on far too many nights, because of other commitments. We can but try to encourage each other as parents, as we search for ways and means to be more effective in the care of our young.

Source: Hawkes. T F, *Network Magazine*, St Leonard's College, Melbourne, October 1996.

INTRODUCTION

Although some are suggesting that parenting has never been more difficult, there are signs that conflict between children and parents has been going on for some time. Even the ancient spiritual text needed to carry the injunction to, 'Honour your father and mother'. (Exodus 20:12)

Nearly 2000 years ago, St Paul was moved to write: 'Children, obey your parents in everything for this is your acceptable duty in the Lord'. (Colossians 3:20)

Such words should be an encouragement to parents, for there are many other words written which do little else than provide guilt generating prose on what duties should or should not be undertaken by parents. This chapter offers some guidelines and hopefully some encouragement in the task of parenting boys and helping them become inducted into the world of manhood.

WHY FATHERS ARE IMPORTANT

Fathers are important biologically. Even with the advent of sperm banks and wondrous chemicals in petrie dishes, for simple convenience, a man still remains very useful in the act of procreation. However, the importance of a father extends beyond the function of keeping alive the species — the father has duties to perform which are vital subsequent to reproduction. This might come as a shock to a few of the younger 'studs' who seem to be so totally consumed with the act of impregnation that they have little energy or inclination left to fulfil the subsequent and associated duties of fathering.

True, these other duties are not always so attractive, but attraction has never been a reliable guide to value. After helping to produce a child, a father has a duty to help nurture a child. Nurturing responsibilities must necessarily be limited by virtue of a father lacking a number of the biological assets of the mother but this should not prevent the sharing of feeding and nappy changing duties even if it means just being with the mother and giving her emotional support and a good back massage from time to time. A contented and well-supported mother tends to result in a contented and well-supported baby.

There is the temptation to think that in the initial years an infant boy must bond with his mother. Wrong. In the initial years, an infant boy should bond with his parents. It is true that the biological and emotional predisposition of the mother combines with social conventions as to who must leave the nest to collect worms which results in a baby boy spending most of his time with the mother. Yet these conventions must not be allowed to marginalise the father in a baby's life. Even in the formative years, a baby must hear the baritone voice, must feel the love and the strength of the father so that the infant learns that strength need not be disassociated from gentleness; that men need not be disassociated from emotion; that males need not be disassociated from empathy and care.

As the child becomes a toddler, the father's role continues to be important. When breast feeding ceases, the father is able to be even more actively involved in the nurture of a child. Unfortunately, societal habits are such that learning to share in the nurturing duties does not always come easily to a father.

THE SOOTHING VOICE

Picture the scene . . . a young father is wheeling a stroller in which his infant son, freshly fed, washed and changed, and without any apparent motive, is screaming his head off. 'There, there William, there is nothing to worry about,' soothes the father. The baby greets these words with a fresh fury of rage to which the father responds calmly 'There, there, William'. A woman watching our hero's predicament, and touched by his new-age gentleness as a father, leaned into the stroller and mewed 'There, there William, now what is bothering you?' 'Excuse me,' said the father, 'I'm William, the child is called Geoffrey.'

Much has been written about the importance of the father being on hand when the young boy begins his search for his own male identity. This advice is flawed. A boy searches for his own identity the day he is born and fathers should in no way be encouraged to withhold their involvement in representing the male world to the child until the infant years have passed. The modelling of maleness by the father needs to begin the day a child lies wet and messy in his arms in the delivery ward.

The early teens can often witness the demise of the heroic father and the birth of the adversarial father. The process of change typically begins with puberty when a boy begins to realise that his father's feet are made of clay. This results in the boy beginning to project himself into the dominant role and search for greater power. The transfer of this power is not always smooth.

MODELLING INTIMACY AND FEELING

Something must be done to break the cycle. The sins of the fathers are being visited upon the sons and this must now stop, for the sons don't want these sins. In particular, they do not want the emotional barrenness inherited from their fathers. The standard criticism of many sons of their fathers has been the father's relative absence in their lives, the aloofness when present and the incapacity or unwillingness of many fathers to school their sons in the important things in life.

The disappointing father has led to generations of new fathers vowing to do a better job of fathering. Tragically, this does not always happen, for nature and nurture can conspire to ensure a repeat performance. For this reason a conscious and concerted effort needs to be made to break the cycle. In particular, fathers need to give more encouragement to sons and express feelings of warmth and intimacy towards them.

Society has been bruised enough by the man without feelings. Contemporary partners want to see more emotional transparency in their men. Contemporary employers want to see the ability of a man to work closely and effectively with others. Contemporary sons want to see approachability and understanding in their dads.

A son must not only find the sportsman in his father but also the aesthetic, the reflective thinker, the compassionate father. If not, Spurr suggests, the fathers will forever hand on to the sons the legacy of being a:

> fat, lazy and puerile brain-dead moron, permanently trapped in puberty. Novelist Tim Winton has said that the 'costume' of males which Australian men are forced to wear is 'killing them; ruining their families; terrifying their wives and children; making beasts of them.'[3]

Fathers need to ask themselves when was the last time there was a genuine expression of warmth and appreciation by them towards their son? This should occur daily and not just be saved up until the eighteenth birthday party speech. Sadly, some fathers even miss this opportunity. Boys can probably survive with fewer presents from a father but not with less presence from a father.

For those fathers who do not feel as comfortable as they might in the overt display of feelings and emotions there is some encouragement, for such feelings can best be shown, not so much by words, but by actions. Kindlon and Thompson write:

> Between men the talk may be centred around action instead of reflection. A physical expression of affection may come in sharing a space — sitting side by side to assemble a model or standing at opposite ends of the field for a game of catch; the arc of the ball tracing the bond of affection that is clearly there.[4]

REMAINING RELEVANT

It can be a struggle for fathers to remain relevant in the lives of their sons. When a son is an infant, the mother can be the omnipresent figure. When the son is older, the peer group is the pervasive influence with peer interaction consuming nearly three-quarters of the teenager's waking hours. In between there is not much room for a father and thus it is a challenge for a father to remain relevant at every stage of a son's life.

Efforts to remain relevant must be more than tokenistic. It is no good going on a father-son school camp and spending half the time behind a newspaper and the other half restoring body fluid levels with other fathers in between taking calls on the mobile phone.[5] Neither is a son going to be greatly persuaded as to a father's relevance if this strange man suddenly becomes 'sharing and caring' for 14 hours when for the last 14 years this same man has been distant and unknown. By all means choreograph such time together but let it never be a substitute for the interest and involvement of a father in a son's everyday life. It should not always need a tent and campfire to stimulate meaningful discourse between father and son.

The trouble is, fathers can be trying so hard to be someone outside of the family, that they forget to be somebody within it. They get so pathologically consumed by collecting twigs for the nest that they rarely find time to sit in it. Steve Biddulph, in his book *Manhood,* suggests that sons in particular suffer from a lack of paternal influence. Biddulph argues that the Industrial Revolution meant that for the first time in history fathers worked away from their sons and this led to generations of boys growing up without being fathered. Before the Industrial Revolution, fathers and sons lived and worked in close proximity and, by doing so, they were taught the craft of being a man.

> What children get from a career father is not his happiness, nor his teaching, nor his substance, but only his mood and at 7.00 pm, that mood is mostly irritation and fatigue. Men show their love by working hard and long. They do not get appreciated for it — since it is their presence, not their bounty that is hungered for by their children.[6]

It would seem that even the contemporary father is not content with producing 2.3 children and must also produce 2.3 cars and 2.3 houses and this can lead to him being marginalised in his own home. Just when the father struggles to find significance in his children's lives after having collected his quota of sticks, the chicks are ready to fly. The father becomes an embarrassment or, even worse, irrelevant, having to resign himself to the role of financial teller and emergency driver.

INVOLVEMENT OF FATHERS IN THEIR SONS' EDUCATION

Education can be both formal and informal. As one unknown wit has quipped, 'One should never allow the classroom to interfere with education'. This hints at the huge amount of informal learning which can directly involve a father outside of school. Pollack calls for a father to be 'generative', to interact with his son in everyday life so that a son is stimulated to learn and to grow in understanding.

Much has been said in earlier chapters on how fathers can help their sons learn by modelling good learning behaviours themselves. A father who rarely reads, who rarely displays higher order thinking skills and who is reluctant to view learning as a lifelong experience is likely to produce a son who rarely reads, who rarely displays higher order thinking and who is reluctant to learn. This is particularly true of a boy in the pre-adolescent years who is looking to adopt the masculine traits of his father.

A crucial area where a father can help his son is in the area of literacy. A father who reads and, even better, a father who reads to his son, can do much to counter the lack of literacy skills in boys. That same father might also write e-mails and letters to his son, compose prose and poetry with his son and choose books for his son to read. (See Chapter 5 for further detail.)

Literacy skills are influenced by articulacy skills. The language used by a father can reflect the written skills of a father and both can bear upon the literacy skills of the son. It is extraordinary how long it takes a son to remember the words a father uses to compliment someone and how quickly it takes a son to remember the words a father uses to curse someone.

The language a father uses towards his son's mother is particularly important for the words used betray attitudes and values. If a son hears words of warmth and appreciation, he is likely to use these same words in relation to women in his own life. For this reason, the father who is divorced, separated, or at odds with a boy's mother needs to be particularly careful. The venting of his own hurt in the hearing of a son can sow the seeds of misogyny.

Educational and social programs should be designed which involve fathers. Some fathers may need to arrange priorities so they can interact with their son's teachers rather more. As a little test as to how effective fathers are in this regard, the following questions can be attempted:

A TEST FOR DADS WITH A SON AT SCHOOL

- What are the names of your son's teachers?
- Have you attended your son's past three parent-teacher evenings?
- Do you regularly read the school's newsletter?
- What were the three major recommendations for improved learning made in your son's last school report?
- What book is your son currently reading?

Any score less than five may indicate the need for a father to connect rather more with a son's formal education.

TEACHING THE RULES

Fathers can be particularly effective in teaching a son the rules of life. These rules are better modelled than lectured. A father who berates a son for intemperate behaviour at school and then enters into a high-decibel confrontation with his wife which is concluded by a slammed door, stomping feet and several hours of injured isolation, is sending very mixed messages.

Dealing with hurt, disappointment, anger, stress, boredom, love, affection, lust, surprise, embarrassment and responsibilities can all be taught a son by a father. Some fathers wear the teacher's tag with some reluctance but, whether acknowledged or not, fathers are the teachers of their sons. Whether they are good teachers is another matter.

Steve Biddulph stresses the importance of rough and tumble play with dads for it teaches a son to have fun while keeping to emotional and physical rules.[7] Pollack calls this kamikaze play between father and son 'enthralment'. This type of play may put the paint work at risk but it can teach a son to regulate behaviour and to explore the limits of acceptable force; of acceptable action; of acceptable competition. Pollack writes:

> Fathers show a unique capacity to draw out the infants' emotional expression along a wider scale of intensity and so help the infants to learn how to tolerate a wide range of people and social situations. When their sons become toddlers, fathers boost the stimulation ante, revving up the emotional systems of their sons by playing games such as tag or wrestling.[8]

In persuading sons to keep to the rules, fathers may have to use sanctions. Punishments that demean a boy, or indeed the father, should be avoided. The dignity of the father evaporates if the air thickens and turns blue. The dignity of the son evaporates if he is given a punishment that degrades. As far as possible, punishments need to be creative, restorative and positive. This should not be interpreted as giving weak or ineffectual punishment, for the deterrent value of a punishment should not be underestimated.

It is also important that with the sanction applied, the son experiences a reassurance of two things:

1. love
2. forgiveness

Parents must bring the act of disciplining a child to closure by dealing with these two matters or else there may be unnecessary insecurity in the boy and a weakening of respect for the parents and a weakening of communication between both.[9]

Garrison Keillor reminds his readers that the punishment spectrum used by a father needs to be consistent, even among children of different sexes, and writes:

> A father turns a stony face to his sons, berates them, shakes his antlers, paws the ground, snorts, runs them off into the underbrush, but when his daughter puts her arm over his shoulder and says 'daddy, I need to ask you something', he is a pat of butter in a hot frying pan.[10]

THE WELL-FATHERED BOY
A badly fathered boy is more likely to be:

- overly male in his orientation, with a derogatory view of any who are different such as women, homosexuals and people from other cultures
- consumed with male 'toys' such as cars, guns and pool tables
- obsessed by male looks — muscle tone, hair
- emotionally immature with difficulty in controlling and expressing emotions
- subject to periods of depression and low self-esteem
- a behavioural risk in terms of delinquency and violence
- academically weak and linguistically limited
- gang-oriented rather than family-oriented.[11]

A well-fathered boy is more likely to:

- be close to his father and see him as a companion as well as a dad
- be loving and respectful towards his mother
- want to be like his father
- find it easy to share and show feelings
- be emotionally stable
- be morally strong
- be spiritually mature
- be socially adept
- be academically well supported.

The well-fathered boy is also unlikely to experience 'paternal hunger' and may be better able to cope with change in his life.

Hearing accounts of fathering can involve tales of neglect, abuse of power and disappointment. There can be a sense of bereavement and a profound sadness borne of a lack of real connection at anything other than the superficial level. Society needs manly fathers who love their sons not by controlling or criticising them but by being a provider, friend and positive example of what it means to be a well-balanced man at peace with himself and his God.

WHY MOTHERS ARE IMPORTANT

Ambrose Bierce, with his usual acerbic humour, describes a mother as 'an animal usually living in the vicinity of a man and having a rudimentary susceptibility to domestication'.[12] This definition is hardly adequate as indeed are most definitions of a mother for it is difficult to give adequate enough credence to the importance and value of motherhood. A mother represents more than the womb of life, she represents the nurture of life. Thomas Jefferson saw the mother as 'the keystone of the arch of matrimonial happiness'.[13] However, the edifice supported by mothers is somewhat bigger — it is society itself.

The vital role played by a mother is what is usually described at this stage in a text on parenting. This can be a mistake, for mothers need to be acknowledged not just for what they do but for who they are. Mothers vary greatly in personality and type but general consensus would have it that mothers have been provisioned with a warmth and acceptance, a tolerance and forgiveness, an empathy and compassion which has saved this world from more wars than they have started.

Mention 'father' and one might see in eyes a sense of respect mixed with a little sadness. Mention 'mother' and those same eyes will invariably soften with the countless memories of undeserved favours.

Not all mothers perform their maternal duties well, but most typically display a devotion which is constant, and a dedication which is humbling, particularly as the task of being a mother is complicated significantly by having to look after fathers. The orbit of a mother's love also encircles the children, the relatives, the friends and the sponsored child in Nigeria whose picture lies behind the ladybird fridge magnet. Mothers need to be celebrated and thanked for who they are as well as for what they do.

It is perhaps significant that mothers are not mentioned by St Paul in his advice to the Colossians: 'Fathers, do not provoke your children, or they may lose heart'. (Colossians 3:21) Evidently, the warning then, as now, is seldom needed for mothers as there is a natural predisposition towards pacification rather than provocation.

THE MOTHER'S HANDS

It is easy to get sentimental and maudlin about such topics and to wax lyrical on the wonders of a mother's healing touch. Yet behind the verbiage is a scientific fact that the caress given by a mother to a child can act as an analgesic.[14] The tactile comfort given works on the brain to release a morphine-like chemical which, quite literally dulls the pain. Given the frequency with which little boys skin knees, this healing touch becomes important in a boy's life and all the more so when it comes with the promise of security and a doughnut for afternoon tea.

The cosseting, cooing and cuddling by a mother of her son is invaluable. Pollack writes:

> How we respond to our baby boys and younger sons — the manner in which we cuddle, kiss and reassure, teach, comfort and love — not only determines a young boy's capacity for a healthy emotional start in life, but deeply affects a boy's characteristic style of behaviour and development of his brain. A behaviour fundamentally, and at times, irrevocably, alters a boy's neural connections, brain chemistry and biological functioning. The capacity to use language, to tolerate distress, to show and name feelings and to be timid or eager to explore, are all dramatically affected by the emotional environment created for a boy during early childhood.[15]

For this reason, boys who have suffered from maternal deprivation can become emotionally inert, psychologically damaged, socially inept and morally bankrupt.

The nurture given by a mother for a son is also vital to the son's sense of self-worth. By doing absolutely nothing other than gurgling, sleeping, crying and soiling nappies, a baby becomes the object of his mother's pride and pleasure. From a very early age, a baby boy will learn there is nothing that has to be done to earn his mother's love. Freud writes:

> If a man has been his mother's undisputed darling, he retains throughout life the triumphant feeling, the confidence in his success which not seldom brings actual success with it.[16]

THE FREEDOM TO GO

The mother can give a security to a boy from which he might eventually draw courage to venture away. This, in many ways, is the tragic role of a mother — to prepare her son to leave. There will be several leavings. The first will generally occur about the age of eight or nine years when a boy increasingly wants to align himself with his father rather than his mother. The second occurs in the pre- or early teens when a boy increasingly wants to align himself with his peers rather than his parents. The third occurs in late teens or adulthood when a boy increasingly wants to align himself with his partner. A mother has a crucial role in preparing a boy for all three departures.

It is a curious truth that the greater the emotional support given to a son, the less dependent a boy is of it. A mother's love can provide the social and emotional strength necessary for a boy to leave and to explore. The safe haven of the mother remains a constant in a boy's changing world, but it is a haven from which a boy will venture on many voyages.

TOLERANCE AND UNDERSTANDING

Another crucial role a mother performs for a son is to model femininity. Quite what expression this femininity takes will vary from mother to mother, but nonetheless a boy is exposed to another gender and another perspective. This can have the effect of preparing a son for a multi-gender world and for a world in which there are great differences between people. The result of this instruction can be a young man with a greater tolerance and a better understanding of the complexities of the human condition.

With the emergence in boys of the desire for sexual and affectional relationships, adolescent boys need the approval and understanding of their mothers and, indeed, hints and instructions as to what works well in such a relationship. It can be difficult for a mother to share her son's affection with another, especially if the 'another' is an alarming young lady with dyed hair, a 14DD bra and a nose ring. Mothers may have to be reminded that boys will need to go out with all types of partners in order to build up for themselves an understanding of the type of values that are important to them in a lifelong commitment.

MALE-MAKING MOTHERS

There is evidence to suggest that unwittingly and unconsciously, many mothers may begin the process of emotionally hardening their sons. Some researchers are suggesting that even at birth mothers encourage a greater self-reliance in boys. Subliminal messages are sent to the infant boy to curb emotions, to not cry because its something that big boys don't do.[17] No suggestion is made that this parenting is in any way callous or uncaring. In fact, it is born out of love to have a boy adjusted to the cultural imperative that they should be strong and 'copeable'.

Unfortunately, this style of nurturing combines with other influences from peers to create a need for a boy to mask his feelings and to cope privately with any emotions. This can result in loneliness and depression. It can also result in the wearing of a 'macho mask' so frequently that a boy forgets what he really looks like. Others can also forget, which is a shame, for the face behind the mask is generally far more attractive.[18] Sometimes the 'macho mask' is removed but only in the presence of someone the boy really trusts and perhaps when he is drunk, which is one of the reasons why girl friends and drink can be so popular with older boys.

Mothers may need to be encouraged to help their sons not to be 'masked crusaders' by allowing and even encouraging the transparency of emotion in their sons. Female writers such as Babette Smith are now saying that the psychological clichés which are stunting sons need to be abandoned in favour of an expression of masculinity which does not leave boys emotionally dumb and socially clumsy.[19]

FATHER HATING AND RE-MATING

The emotional fall out from a marriage break-up can be considerable with relative innocents, like children, becoming casualties. The collateral damage done to children has often been concealed because the frequency of marriage break-up is such that it can be politically expedient not to dwell on this fact. As soon as one should dare question the injury to children, anecdotal evidence is given of happy children with single parents and unhappy children with both parents still married to each other. Some of these tales are true but what is even truer are the many instances of children being psychologically damaged by marriages that should break up and by marriages that do break up.

Another reason why damage to children is seldom proclaimed is that the parents themselves are experiencing quite enough pain, anger and guilt without the accusing finger being pointed at them. A fractionating family needs reassurance and understanding, not accusation and blame.

When a marriage is disintegrating the mother needs to cope with the growing sense of despair and disillusionment and, at the same time, have the emotional capital left to meet the needs of the children. This is not easy. What is also not easy is maintaining a positive attitude towards males and a son who is the spitting image of that unconscionable heel that is now the 'ex'. The capacity to love such a child is even further reduced if the boy should react with sullen suspicion to the new male suitor who appears on the horizon. Difficult though it may be, warring parents should declare a full and unconditional cease-fire in the presence of their children. Mothers and fathers should be allowed to be loved by the son even if one should hate the other. Family celebrations should continue to be observed, a boy's grief for the absent parent should continue to be respected and the right of access, if granted, should continue to be maintained.

SHARING NOT SNARING

In their exasperation, mothers can assume parenting duties that should never be theirs. Some mothers have no alternative for they may be single parents or their partner may have work commitments which make it difficult for them to play the father role. Sometimes the nurturing side of a mother has invaded a father's responsibility. This can be due to the absence of a father or the absence in a father of the emotional and physical energy to be a father.

If this scenario is one that a mother can identify with then a rather honest discussion is needed about the importance of sharing the parenting duties. This sharing is not just for the benefit of the mother, but also the benefit of the boy who needs to spend quality time with the father.

The 'servant mother' is also not good for a boy if it means his mother becomes a domestic slave trapped into service by her love for a son. As it has been said a mother who does household chores for $200 a day is doing domestic science. A mother who does household chores for nothing is married. Some esteem needs to be given to mothers; esteem expressed by the male folk in her life rendering assistance. This should translate into a son doing a number of chores such as keeping his room clean, taking his laundry to the proper place, making his bed and helping with the washing up. On top of this there should be other duties which are part of his education program such as cooking a meal, shopping for groceries, and washing, ironing and cleaning. A son may need to be compelled into a number of these experiences but they should nonetheless be engaged in lest a boy become egocentric and possessed of minimal life skills and a poor sense of social responsibility.

Also needing to be shared is the task of having fun with a son and disciplining a son. Boys have an uncanny knack of being able to divide and conquer parents, particularly when they are in their teens. Common standards need to be agreed on and a determination shown to support the other partner when they undertake the less pleasant tasks of disciplining their son.

MOTHERING — A JOB WORTH DOING

Moir and Jessel warn mothers against accepting the current societal doctrine that sees mothering as the sabotaging of a woman's capacity to do real work.[20] It is pointed out that the modern mother tends to spend about 25% of her time in close physical contact with a child, whereas in more primitive cultures the figure is closer to 70%.[21] Moir and Jessel write:

> . . . just at the moment when women are freest to enjoy and exploit their natural, superior skills in motherhood, a stern sisterhood tells them that this is an unnecessary low-value, and socially regressive role.[22]

Society must recognise the importance of mothering and mothers must be encouraged that the job they are doing is vital. Mothering is a task women should be proud of, honoured for and supported in. The nurture of children is not only a fulfillment of personal design and purpose, it determines the character and well-being of society in general. In a very real sense, the hand that rocks the cradle rules the world.

INVESTING IN SONS

The most significant influence on a boy is usually the parent. There are other significant influences but the parental influence is generally the greatest. Of course, boys will probably deny this, particularly in their teens. Mark Twain wrote:

> When I was a boy of 14 my father was so ignorant I could hardly stand to have the old man around. But when I got to 21, I was astonished at how much he had learned in seven years.[23]

The uncomfortable implication is that if something is not quite going right in the life of a boy, that one variable that needs to be looked at by parents is themselves. The help of external observers both professional and lay can assist this task of self-examination.

The imperative of getting it right as a parent is even stronger when it is realised parents are not only investing in a son, they are investing in grandchildren and great-grandchildren. The strengths and weaknesses of parents will be felt by several generations. Hugh Mackay, in his book *Generations*, states:

> The most powerful influences on most young people is the example of their parents. The biggest difference between your generation and your children's generation is not likely to have been the advent of the computer and the threat of AIDS, nor the level of unemployment, it is more likely to be the fact that for better or worse, you had your parents for children and your children had you.[24]

BOYS BECOMING ADULT

Two of the strongest impulses in a boy are to belong to the tribe and to grow up. Both of these impulses can be satisfied, at least in part, by a boy going through an initiation ceremony. Throughout time and across many cultures, boys have undergone initiation, a period of ritual and celebration as a boy is embraced as belonging and as being a man.

In some countries, the initiation can be a test — an endurance of pain. This is often accompanied by a physical transformation such as scarring, removal of teeth, tattooing and circumcision. In the more developed cultures there are also tests. These are usually done in a car with 'L' plates. This transformation may be less physical but just as significant with the boy now able to drive; able to vote; able to marry without parental consent.

There are other differences between the initiation experienced in more developed countries and that experienced in tribal cultures. One difference is that tribal cultures often seem to celebrate initiation rather more formally and significantly. The eighteenth birthday bash, the confirmation or bar mitzvah pale beside some of the initiation ceremonies found elsewhere in the world.

Whatever else may be said of some of the more painful initiations which involve endurance, separation and training, it can be argued that experiencing such trials can cause a boy to know with some certainty that he has journeyed from boyhood to manhood. In undertaking this journey, the boy can spend time with men who teach him. The boy then experiences the affirmation of belonging which comes from being accepted back into the tribe. There is also a sense of accomplishment at enduring the pain, separation and trial.

While not all will rate these characteristics as important or desirable, it might be said that rites such as these can tell a boy in an unambiguous manner that he has made it, that he has 'arrived'. Ceremonies such as these might do something to counteract something of the neurosis among adolescent boys in the western world as to whether they are really men.

It is probably no surprise that the men's movement has been characterised by a return to tribal rituals and all-male gatherings in secluded settings. However, this need not be the only option. There are ceremonies that can be devised that leave out drums and campfires. This is not to say that a father and son spending a number of days camping together is not an excellent initiative. It is. There may also be virtue in rather more public proclamations of the arrival at the state of manhood for a boy which involve the sharing of the experience with a community. A Christian example of a simple initiation service is that found at Athelstone Uniting Church in Adelaide whose minister, Nick Hawkes, uses the following service outline:

INITIATION TO MANHOOD

Welcome.

A brief talk on the important features of maleness and the threats facing males in contemporary society.

An apology by the men present for any failures they have had in not modelling true manhood.

A declaration of the 10 marks of manhood which are:

1. to have integrity
2. to work well:
   - in mind
   - in body
3. to be responsible
4. to be generous
5. to have the ability to endure pain (At this point, molten wax is poured into the palm of the father who then presses it onto the palm of their son)
6. to honour and protect the weak
7. to seek wisdom
8. to learn how to be a good husband, good father, a good example
9. to care for the environment
10. to be spiritually mature.

A challenge is given to the boys to build the 10 marks of manhood into their own lives.

These words are said: 'The men of this community charge you, our sons, to live these marks of manhood. Do not shrink from passing on the baton of faith, character and wisdom to the next generation. Improve on them and hand them on.'

Prayers are said for the sons that they will have the strength, courage and wisdom to know and adopt the marks of manhood.

An affirmation is given for each son of his gifts and abilities, together with the public declaration of each father's love for his son:

■ A meaningful gift is given to every boy. This wrapped gift is usually given by the father and is not necessarily large or expensive and is opened at home to avoid comparisons.

■ A list of the boy's forefathers is given to each boy. If the forefathers are not known, appropriate men in the church are listed as members of the boy's spiritual family.

The declaration is given that the son is now an adult.

A blessing is given to the son by the father/father figure with the son kneeling before his father and the father placing a hand on his head and praying the blessing.

Each son who is admitted into the adult fellowship of the church is then given a certificate of manhood (see Figure 12.1).

Figure 12.1 Certification of initiation into manhood

CERTIFICATION OF
INITIATION INTO MANHOOD

On this _____ day of _____ Year _____
At Athelstone Uniting Church

_____
was formally invited to take his place
as an adult in the Athelstone Uniting Church Community

As a man, you stand in the following line of men in your family or in your church:

Great-great-grandfathers _____   _____

_____   _____

_____   _____

_____   _____

Great-grandfathers   _____   _____

_____   _____

Grandfathers   _____   _____

Father   _____

The message that your father or father figure has for you is:

_____

_____

The gifts and abilities seen in you are:

1. _____

2. _____

3. _____

Today we declare our love for you and congratulate you on becoming a man.

Signed: _____
(Father's or father figure's signature)

Formal initiations into manhood are not necessarily advocated as always being desirable or even appropriate. It is entirely possible that the ceremonies that currently exist, when linked to a loving family, are more than sufficient to affirm a boy in his growing maturity. Having noted this, there may be virtue in having clear signposts in a boy's life which remind him of his maturity and acceptance by the 'tribe'. Birthday parties might serve, but other signposts can also be added. The most valued signposts are probably the ones which are not expected, and which are initiated by the adult members of the community to celebrate the son's growing maturation.

Not all signposts need to be formal. An informal time spent on holiday, a camping trip, a visit to relatives can all be used as times to pass on the collective wisdom about being male from one generation to another. This need not always express itself as 'secret men's business' for the transmission of knowledge can be all the more effective if adult females, as well as males, are involved.

Quite what form the celebrations take will need to be determined by each family but some form of recognition of a boy's transition into the state of manhood can be important to a boy. The affirmation and encouragement given can be such that a boy is released from the burden of having to prove continually that he is a man.

ADDITIONAL INFORMATION

For those wishing to have further details on some of the points raised in this chapter, the following references may be helpful. Each number in the text of the chapter relates to a reference number below which will give further information related to the topic.

1	Irvine, J (1994)	*Coping with Kids*	Horwitz Grahame, Sydney.
2	Abbott, J (1993)	'Preparing hearts and minds for the 21st century'	Paper presented to the Association of Heads of Independent Schools of Australia, Biennial Conference, St Peter's College, Adelaide, 7 October 1993, p 31.
3	Spurr, B (2000)	'Boys in trouble'	*Sydney's Child*, August 2000, p 20.
4	Kindlon, D and Thompson, M (2000)	*Raising Cain*	Penguin Books, London, p 118.
5	Legge, K (1995)	'Some mothers do have 'em'	*Australian Magazine*, 11/3/95, p 26.
6	Biddulph, S (1994)	*Manhood*	Finch Publishing, Sydney.
7	Biddulph, S (1997)	*Raising Boys*	Finch Publishing, Sydney, p 71.

8	Pollack, W (1998)	*Real Boys*	Owl Books, Henry Holt and Co., New York, p 114.
9	Dowrick, S (1991)	*Intimacy and Solitude*	Mandarin, Melbourne, p 90.
10	Keillor, G quoted in West, P (1996)	*Fathers, Sons and Lovers*	Finch Publishing, Sydney, p 87.
11	Biddulph, S (1997)	(op cit)	p 140.
12	Bierce, A quoted in Brussell, E (ed) (1970)	*Webster's New World Dictionary of Quotable Definitions*	Prentice Hall, New Jersey, p 608.
13	Jefferson, T quoted in Brussell, E (ed)	(op cit)	p 378.
14	Kindlon, D and Thompson, M	(op cit)	p 194.
15	Pollack, W	(op cit)	p 57.
16	Freud, S quoted in Pollack, W	(op cit)	p 111.
17	Pollack, W	(op cit)	
18	Pollack, W	(op cit)	
19	Smith, B quoted in Legge, K	(op cit)	p 22.
20	Moir, A and Jessel, D (1989)	*Brainsex*	Mandarin, London, p 165.
21	Moir, A and Jessel, D	(op cit)	p 149.
22	Moir, A and Jessel, D	(op cit)	p 147.
23	Twain, M	Quoted in the *Concise Dictionary of Quotations*	Pocket Reference Library, William Collins and Sons, London, p 325.
24	McKay, H (1997)	*Generations*	Pan Macmillan, Sydney, p 2.

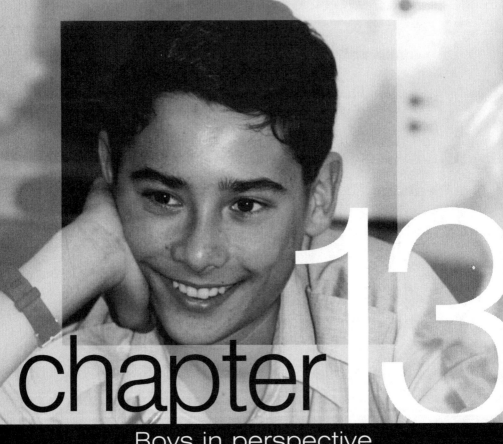

chapter 13

Boys in perspective

'The boy stood on the burning deck
Whence all but he had fled;
The flame that lit the battle's wreck
Shone round him o'er the dead.'

Felicia Hemans, Casabianca

INTRODUCTION

The heroic individualism in boys can be more imagined than real. In fact there can be a compliant sameness about a boy which is disturbing. Perhaps one of the greatest societal challenges is to cultivate a climate that will allow a boy to be different without having him standing on a burning deck surrounded by carnage.

Somehow or other boys need to be persuaded that searching for their own identity does not mean a total subjection to a perceived definition of what it means to be a young male. The irony is that in the search for personal identity, boys conform to the cultural anonymity of their peers. In searching for intergenerational difference boys adopt intragenerational sameness. A uniform is worn, attitudes adopted, speech patterns rehearsed in order to belong. In defiance of conformity, boys conform.

Is there a way a boy can celebrate 'unity in diversity', whereby the cultural rules can be relaxed to accommodate a greater diversity in 'boyness' which still recognises that a boy has value even if he is different from most others? Can the stifling requirement to conform be relaxed a little or are social insecurities such that strict group discipline and tribal obedience must be maintained?

There is some ground for hope in this regard. Despite the world being 'Microsoftened' and corporatised, there are counter-cultures at work — cultures that appeal because they are different, because they are unique. Stereotypes are being questioned as much as they are being conformed to. There is a market for the non-customised product; you can now buy cars that are not black.

Something of this growing individualism is being seen in the classrooms. Phrases such as 'differentiated learning' are now being heard; de Bono is allowing many differently coloured hats to be worn. Teachers are recognising the existence of 'multiple intelligences' in their students and are talking about left and right brain activities. Moral guides are urging to take 'the road less travelled' and gender stereotypes are now being questioned.

The repressive societal grip on boys is beginning to relax a little and open its hand to allow greater freedoms in the expression of how to be male. The sensitive boy can be found in films; the computer nerd can be a hero; the hairless boy still gets the girl and the modern Romeo can weep at the death of his friend, Horatio.

Whether boys themselves have relaxed their grip is another matter, although there are signs that this might be happening. There are the beginnings of a cultural shift in what boys perceive to be 'cool'. The growing influence of IT in contemporary society is helping to redefine what is considered clever. There are opportunities here for boys to grasp in helping to promote a wider definition of what it means to be acceptable as a male.

Further hope for a societal shift in a broader definition of the acceptable male comes from the strengthening female voice. Many women have judged the current male product to be deficient. They will no longer tolerate the oafish bore devoid of feeling and social responsibility. Women are leaving such men in droves with most divorces in the western world being initiated by women. To this can be added the increasingly strident feminist voice — it may not be subtle, but it is certainly effective in reminding the male world of its deficiencies.

Perhaps the greatest hope is the steady ticking of the clock. Each successive generation of fathers seems to want to do a better job of raising its sons. Some fathers are beginning to break the cycle of perpetuating the emotionally barren son given to coercion and conquest. Although it is slow and although it is patchy, fathering is probably improving.

BELOW THE SURFACE

Another area of 'sameness' in a boy that needs to be challenged is the sameness which makes a lie of the statement, 'Deep down he is really different . . . deep down he is a real softie . . . underneath he is pure gold'. Whereas this may well be true in some cases, it is not true in all. Deep down in some boys can be found the very same attitudes and inclinations as there are at the surface. The promise of gold deep down is not always a reality and even if it was, is it fair to expect others to prospect at such a depth? After days of counselling, weeks of therapy, years of teaching, will the shovel be decorated by anything other than dirt? Even if gold be discovered, it might need to be checked that it is not 'fool's gold' where:

- ■ lust masquerades as love
- ■ greed masquerades as investment
- ■ cruelty masquerades as toughness
- ■ cynicism masquerades as wisdom
- ■ prejudice masquerades as loyalty
- ■ self-centredness masquerades as altruism.

Are the geophysical conditions such that real gold can reasonably be expected in a boy? Are boys 'deep' people, or is shallowness a common feature in the boy terrain?

Shallowness and frivolity have their place in barbecue banter but there needs to be the promise of depth in a boy, a deep down value which has not been corroded by a culture committed to the instant fix, the minimal effort, the maximum pleasure. Somewhere there needs to be found the spiritual faith, the personal dream, the moral inheritance.

Shallow thinking and thoughtless action may be understood from time to time, for all are prone to behaviours that do not always edify or enrich. The trick is to know that they are shallow and thoughtless. There is nothing much wrong in being a total 'airhead' from time to time providing one realises one is being a total 'airhead' and that one has the capacity to cease being an 'airhead'.

It is when a boy does not have the knowledge of what he could be and what he should be, that he is in trouble. If there is no place deep within that is different, that harbours the noble sentiment, then the youth of today is in strife. Fortunately, most boys know intuitively, deep down, what sort of people they should be. A worrying few do not but they are generally a minority. This should be an encouragement to any who are working with boys. There is little need in most cases to teach goodness or to argue for kindness. On the surface a few boys may reject these values; deep down most appreciate them.

How might society ensure that its sons and young men have depth and value? Michael Gurian, in his book *A Fine Young Man*, suggested that there are 10 'integrities' which should be encouraged in a boy.[1] In a similar manner, the following six virtues are suggested as being important in a boy:

1. social virtues
2. emotional virtues
3. physical virtues
4. intellectual virtues
5. spiritual virtues
6. moral virtues.

1. Social virtues

Social virtues include those social graces within a son that enable him to mix freely and at ease with those he knows and with those he does not know. Not everyone will have a temperament that is naturally gregarious but every boy should have the skills to:

- be helpful
- be polite
- be inclusive
- be kind
- be forgiving
- be compassionate
- say hello and goodbye
- say thank you
- say sorry.

All too often these skills are seen as optional 'extras' in a boy. They should not be. A baseline in social competence needs to be established or else humankind will become less human and less kind.

Of particular importance is teaching a boy how to deal with those who are different:

- in age
- in sex
- in ethnicity
- in ability.

2. Emotional virtues

Having emotional virtues requires the capacity to show emotions and the capacity to not show emotions, and having the wisdom to know which of these options is best at any particular time. It can call for a certain emotional resilience so that a boy is not crushed by disappointment. It can also mean that a boy learns not to become an emotional puppet whose strings are manipulated by others. Surrendering the control of one's emotions to others is losing personal control to the vagaries of fate. A boy should be taught to own his emotions. Care is needed not to confuse controlling emotions with no emotions. The Biblical injunction to 'weep with those who weep' incorporates a timeless truth that empathy and compassion are the characteristics of the strong. It is the weak who will have a personal insecurity that prevents them from exhibiting emotion. It is important for a boy to know how to cry and when to cry, and how to laugh and when to laugh.

3. Physical virtues

Many boys are physically strong and very fit. Running around like mad things does tend to build up a certain anaerobic and aerobic fitness. However, a growing number of boys are compromising the male reputation for fitness through changing from active to passive recreation habits. Changing diet and a reduction in exercise is producing a large number of 'jelly bellies'. When a national identity centres on the meat pie and cold stubby, lectures on the nutritional worth of fruit and vegetables tend to be subverted. 'You are what you eat' and, in the case of the boy, a growing proportion of his limbs are made up of Big Macs and chips. The erosion of the immune system through inappropriate diet is frightening with some 35–40% of Australian children being overweight.[2]

An Australian survey found that 55% of children aged between five and 16 engaged in exercise for less than 100 minutes each week. Fewer than half of children in public primary schools are participating in interschool sport.[3] For overall well-being, about 180 minutes of exercise a week is needed for boys with about half that time arranged so that the heart rate is working to about 60–80% of the maximum. As a general rule of thumb, the maximum heart rate should be a commonly accepted formula of 220 minus one's age in years. However, professional opinion should be sought on a case-by-case basis when planning an exercise regime for a boy.

4. Intellectual virtues

Developing the intellectual virtue of boys will require the complicity of the boys themselves. In the seventeenth century Duc de la Rochefoucauld stated that 'the height of cleverness was to be able to conceal it'. Either the Duke was wrong or the world has a vast number of boys who are very clever indeed for there is much concealment. A new dictum needs to be advanced that 'the height of cleverness is being able to show it'. Boys need to be taught that short-term popularity with peers is no price to pay for long-term unpopularity with employers. More importantly, the failure to fulfil design expectations is a waste of God-given gifts which will be adversely felt by society in general and by the boy in particular. Unfortunately, this realisation of waste tends not to occur until adulthood and long after a man is able to atone for the sins of his youth.

Society needs to be careful not to be complicit in the academic underperformance of boys by so feminising the schooling experience that it provides little to capture a boy's interest or to keep it. Not only is the academic agenda in schools in danger of being feminised, the social agenda in schools is also under threat. Christina Sommers writes:

> Socially divisive activists, many of whom take a dim view of men and boys, have been allowed to wield unwarranted influence in schools. They write anti-harassment guides, gather in workshops to determine how to change boys' 'gender scheme' and barely disguise their anger and disapproval.[4]

A renaissance in learning is required of boys supported by a culture that recognises individual differences in preferred learning styles in schools. The temptation to 'dumb down' learning needs is to be resisted. The compulsion to 'crank up' learning standards needs to be accepted.

5. Spiritual virtues

For there to be a spiritual richness in a boy, there need not necessarily be a regular commitment to formal worship, although this would probably help. For there to be a spiritual richness, a boy needs to explore his place in the scheme of things and to contemplate the purpose for his existence. A boy needs to communicate, if not with his God, then with himself. A boy needs to ask the question 'Why?' and to wonder at the beginning and end of his life.

In God's great cathedral there are 100 000 million lights in one section alone. It is called The Milky Way. There are at least 100 million other sections of the cathedral. The sense of awe at figures such as this should be encouraged in a boy, together with a wondering. 'Am I the product of the random mix of some amino acids or is there a mind behind the system? If there is a mind, then can I connect with that mind?'

Evidence of God's presence around us can lead to the reality of God's presence within. A sense of being part of some great purpose can launch a boy on a pilgrim quest which can give both direction and hope. Removing oneself at the epicentre of one's life and replacing the void with God can help remove the self-orientation that can be so crippling to society. A person focused on God is a person focused on man in that a relationship with God tends to translate to service to others.

Most boys believe in God. There is an innate spirituality in boys which the world sets about removing through diversion, distraction and derision. To encourage spiritual virtue, a boy will need experiences that interrupt him. A boy will need to experience places where he can rest from concentrating on the immediate in order to concentrate on the eternal. Sometimes this might be a camp in a wilderness setting; sometimes it might be a life interrupted by crisis; sometimes it might be serendipitous words of wisdom from an elder.

Parents and teachers need to plan on how they might encourage the growth of the spiritual dimension in a boy, for relating well to one's God brings pleasure both to the divine and to the mortal.

6. Moral virtues

Some may be tempted to think that there is not much moral virtue in a boy. The Columbine High School killers have been allowed to become the metaphors for young males — violent, dangerous and destructive. However, all boys are not the pathological beings that some would believe.[5] Much that is good and proper in the world can be found in boys. Their daring and energy has served society well. Some 99% of all inventions patented are by males and much of this creativity has been learnt in their youth.[6]

Boys need to develop a moral richness and society needs to develop the courage to put in place behavioural boundaries for its boys. Society must also model the morals it wishes its sons to learn. The guaranteeing of individual freedoms has reached a point where community freedoms are now at risk. Increasing secularism and the removal of moral absolutes has also contributed to the problem of moral aridity in some boys.

A moral environment is required whereby everyone, not just boys, see themselves as connected to others and as having obligations towards others. These obligations include living by a code that enriches rather than despoils the society within which a boy lives. Morality must not just be linked to people but should encompass the physical environment as well.

DO NOT ROB BOYS OF THEIR YOUTH

VALUING OUR TIME

When young, time can be seen as a hostile barrier between you and adulthood, so we hurry through childhood despising its limitations. Society is involved in a conspiracy to rob our young of their youth: 'Don't be so childish . . . now I want you to be grown up about this'. We boast at how young our baby walks, at how mature our son looks, at our boy being advanced a year in school. It is hardly surprising that those cursed with youth become impatient to advance beyond this state. Time is killed to speed up the clock. We skip and run through graveyards, subtracting birthdays from deathdays, but go very still when we reach our own headstone. Gordon Bailey, in his poem Playing Out Time, writes:

At birth they wheel you into life's great slot machine arcade;
At death your epitaph describes the kind of game you've played.
But gravestones hide not just a corpse, they cover countless sins,
And lie about achievements in a game where no one wins.
A man sits in the 'change' kiosk — the kind of change he pays
Is months for years, or weeks for months, or moments for our days.
Some games cost just a moment, others cost a day per try;
The younger punters act as though each year was worth a dime,
and fail to see death waiting for the fools who play with time.

Source: Plastic World, Send the Light Trust, 1971. Gordon is the author of several books including Mix and Match.

I would encourage our young men to savour their youth and not rush through it. Heaven does not lie in a 2.00 am bedtime, increased access to social drugs and a semi-reliable car! I would encourage our young men to luxuriate in the gift of life, to enjoy the present, to roll and splash and shriek and play in the shallows. There will be time enough to swim in deeper waters for we are all eventually borne to the deep by the tide of time, with only the ripples of celebration around each birthday beacon to mark our ageing. Some panic when the tide gets swift and try to swim against the flow, but the 'youth creams' and 'stay young' chemicals eventually fail, and leave us exhausted and curiously fatalistic as the land of our youth shrinks on the horizon and we progress to our inevitable burial at sea.

Time is precious and cannot be held, for it trickles through our fingers. The more we grasp it, the less we can hold it. So we must drink of it while we may and allow it to give us life. We must make the most of our alloted years and even endeavour to make some sense of it all.

Source: Hawkes, T F, The King's Herald, The King's School, Parramatta, 27 August 1998.

Boys musts have time to grow, time to mature, time to prepare themselves for the future, yet they are being rushed through their childhood.

Having noted how it is important not to rush boys through their childhood, care needs to be taken not to keep boys in a perpetual juvenile state with stunted brains and a blundering liability when let loose in society. Boys will be boys, but they should not remain boys, perpetual Peter Pans wanting to fight with swords and lead their gangs against other gangs. Boys should not be excused from the obligation of growing up.

DO NOT ROB BOYS OF THEIR MASCULINITY

The answer to the problems being faced by boys is not to feminise them, it is to masculinise them within a broader context of what it means to be male. Strength and power present only part of the picture of maleness. The complete male is also the provider and the protector. What society is in danger of doing is allowing a definition of males to exist which does not capture those qualities of maleness which have always existed. Where are the qualities shown by the great male artists, inventors and theologians, by the great philosophers and academics whose work has changed the world? The answer is not to emasculate boys — it is to encourage them to accept a more complete and accurate picture of maleness.

Society may need to develop a definition of what it means to be a male. This can involve recognising that a boy can have some characteristics which are traditionally seen as female without entirely losing his masculinity. The psychologists call this 'androgyny'. It does not necessarily mean that gender swapping is either advocated or advanced as acceptable boy behaviour. It does mean that boys may still be considered male even if they do not fit the 'blokey' macho image. A broader definition of acceptable maleness is proposed, not a denial of maleness.

There are innate differences in the male and the female brain and in the male and female body. These differences can be described clinically and even humorously, but the differences are real and to pretend that they do not exist is a nonsense. The time has come to acknowledge the differences between the sexes and to celebrate these differences as the 'Yin' and 'Yang' of God's glorious creation.

CONCLUSION

One should neither triviliase nor sensationalise the problems being faced by boys. To triviliase is to be irresponsibly dismissive of very real problems that need to be owned by society. To sensationalise is to have out of perspective the great number of thoroughly decent boys and the capacity of those who are somewhat less decent to become decent through firm but compassionate instruction.

Care must be taken not to punish boys for being male, or to punish boys for attributes they can do little about. What society in general and schools in particular need to do is to allow maleness in its many manifestations to have a place, and to celebrate its positive virtues such as its strength, athleticism, energy, daring and mateship. There are elements of maleness which, if not trained, can run wild. This can be to the detriment of society which has the right to suggest and enforce civilised behaviours. This is best done by training, not constraining. It is best done by making an example of best practice, not worst practice. It is best done from the premise that maleness is a valued attribute in our society; rather than something that should be feared.

ADDITIONAL INFORMATION

For those wishing to have further details on some of the points raised in this chapter, the following references may be helpful. Each number in the text of the chapter relates to a reference number below which will give further information related to the topic.

1	Gurian, M (1998)	*A Fine Young Man*	Tarcher/Putnam, New York, p 256.
2	*Sunday Telegraph*	'Schools fail the exercise test'	*Sunday Telegraph*, 21/5/00, p 44.
3	*Sunday Telegraph*	(op cit)	
4	Sommers, C (2000)	'The gender project'	*Sunday Telegraph Sunday Magazine*, 9/7/00, p 8.
5	Sommers, C	(op cit)	p 10.
6	Moir, A and Jessel, D (1989)	*Brainsex*	Mandarin, London, p 186.

Index

Page numbers in *italics* refer to figures.